Fitness Culture

Consumption and Public Life

Series Editors: Frank Trentmann and Richard Wilk

Titles include:

Mark Bevir and Frank Trentmann (*editors*)
GOVERNANCE, CITIZENS AND CONSUMERS
Agency and Resistance in Contemporary Politics

Magnus Boström and Mikael Klintman
ECO-STANDARDS, PRODUCT LABELLING AND GREEN CONSUMERISM

Jacqueline Botterill
CONSUMER CULTURE AND PERSONAL FINANCE
Money Goes to Market

Daniel Thomas Cook (*editor*)
LIVED EXPERIENCES OF PUBLIC CONSUMPTION
Encounters with Value in Marketplaces on Five Continents

Nick Couldry, Sonia Livingstone and Tim Markham
MEDIA CONSUMPTION AND PUBLIC ENGAGEMENT
Beyond the Presumption of Attention

Anne Cronin
ADVERTISING, COMMERCIAL SPACES AND THE URBAN

Amy E. Randall
THE SOVIET DREAM WORLD OF RETAIL TRADE AND CONSUMPTION IN THE 1930s

Roberta Sassatelli
FITNESS CULTURE
Gyms and the Commercialisation of Discipline and Fun

Kate Soper, Martin Ryle and Lyn Thomas (*editors*)
THE POLITICS AND PLEASURES OF SHOPPING DIFFERENTLY
Better than Shopping

Kate Soper and Frank Trentmann (*editors*)
CITIZENSHIP AND CONSUMPTION

Harold Wilhite
CONSUMPTION AND THE TRANSFORMATION OF EVERYDAY LIFE
A View from South India

Consumption and Public Life
Series Standing Order ISBN 978–1–4039–9983–2 Hardback
978–1–4039–9984–9 Paperback
(*outside North America only*)

You can receive future titles in this series as they are published by placing a standing order. Please contact your bookseller or, in case of difficulty, write to us at the address below with your name and address, the title of the series and the ISBN quoted above.

Customer Services Department, Macmillan Distribution Ltd, Houndmills, Basingstoke, Hampshire RG21 6XS, England

---

Fitness Culture

Gyms and the Commercialisation of Discipline and Fun

Roberta Sassatelli

University of Milan, Italy

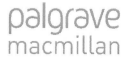

palgrave
macmillan

First published 2010 by
PALGRAVE MACMILLAN

Palgrave Macmillan in the UK is an imprint of Macmillan Publishers Limited, registered in England, company number 785998, of Houndmills, Basingstoke, Hampshire RG21 6XS.

Palgrave Macmillan in the US is a division of St Martin's Press LLC, 175 Fifth Avenue, New York, NY 10010.

Palgrave Macmillan is the global academic imprint of the above companies and has companies and representatives throughout the world.

Palgrave® and Macmillan® are registered trademarks in the United States, the United Kingdom, Europe and other countries.

ISBN-13: 978-0-230-50749-4 hardback

This book is printed on paper suitable for recycling and made from fully managed and sustained forest sources. Logging, pulping and manufacturing processes are expected to conform to the environmental regulations of the country of origin.

A catalogue record for this book is available from the British Library.

A catalog record for this book is available from the Library of Congress.

Printed and bound in Great Britain by
CPI Antony Rowe, Chippenham and Eastbourne

Contents

Acknowledgements

This book took several years to mature. It comes out of a long and laborious process of research, writing and analysis which was initiated in the early 1990s and has spanned, with very varying degrees of intensity, over 15 years. Fitness culture has been a fantastically portable research topic, travelling with me from Italy to Britain and back numerous times. The book has effectively grown with the global expansion and institutional consolidation of fitness gym culture and the broad fitness phenomenon. I have tried to reflect such complex ongoing development in my writing. Fitness can surely be approached from a variety of angles. The way I did it was mainly through the sociology of consumption, being interested in how the "need" to keep fit was stimulated or otherwise by fitness culture as experienced through interaction in the gym.

As befitting a long-lasting research interest, this project has accompanied the ups and downs of my personal and intellectual life, some friends and colleagues were important at the beginning of it, some have continued to contribute to my intellectual growth and others have become very important in more recent times. While my gratitude extends to all, I now limit myself to acknowledge those who have directly contributed to the development of this book. I have been fortunate enough to meet and discuss my work with a giant of twentieth-century sociology, Harold Garfinkel; his comments on some of the chapters have encouraged me to keep writing when I would have easily done otherwise. Gary Alan Fine and Paul Willis have read draft chapters and have provided precious suggestions: I mention them in gratitude with the obvious disclaimer that, if my writing is no better, it obviously is my sole responsibility. I am also thankful to Tim Dant for his helpful general comments on the final draft as well as Kate Nash and Alan Scott for their careful suggestions on many aspects of my writing, including style, and for their unfailing friendship and support. I am grateful to Stefania De Petris, Paolo Magaudda, Chiara Pulici and Daniele Tricarico who variously helped me in collecting some of the empirical material. I feel obliged to Elizabeth Beck for her valuable editing of part of the manuscript, to Joel Jones for editing in the final stages of production, and to Philippa Grand at Palgrave for her editorial assistance. Thank you indeed to the editors of the book series Frank Trentmann and Rick Wilk for their stimulating interest in my research. A unique, sincere thank you goes to my husband and fellow sociologist Marco Santoro, not only for his companionship but also for his poignant criticisms in my pursuit of an adequate rendering of the micro-macro link. I also thank my son Riccardo, for he has been a major source of both happiness and fitness while writing this book. I also feel obliged to his London babysitter Sonia "Grande" Scavuzzo for having been a great company to the whole family, allowing me some time for fieldwork. Last, but not least, I owe a resounding thank you to all the people whom I have encountered in the fitness world during my exploration of gyms and the gathering of interviews and documents on fitness participation and expertise. This book could not have been written without their help and collaboration.

I had the opportunity to present my work in progress on fitness at a number of stimulating occasions: for helpful feedback I am grateful to audiences at the bi-annual meeting of the European Sociological Associations in Berlin and Amsterdam; at the conference "Time and Value", University of Lancaster; the TCS conference "Body Modification", University of Nottingham; the conference "Women's Bodies, Women's Minds", University of East Anglia, Norwich; the Norwegian University of Sport and Physical Education, Oslo and finally to the Department of Anthropology at UCL, London. Many of the papers presented have subsequently been published as articles in journals and books. While I have not reused previously published material as such, my earlier work on the Italian fitness scene has had an impact on my thoughts and research strategy for this further endeavour. My Italian ethnography was published as *Anatomia della Palestra*, il Mulino, Bologna (2000) and aspects of it were discussed in "Interaction Order and Beyond. A Field Analysis of Body Culture within Fitness Gyms", *Body and Society*, 5, 2–3, pp. 227–48 (1999); "Fitness Gyms and the Local Organization of Experience", *Sociological Research Online*, 4, p. 3, www.socresonline.org.uk/ (1999); "The Commercialization of Discipline. Fitness and its Values", *Journal of Italian Studies, Special Issue on Sport*, 9, 4, pp. 332–49 (2000); and "Bridging Health and Beauty. A Critical Perspective on Keep-fit Culture", in G. Boswell and F. Poland (eds), *Women's Bodies*, MacMillan, London (2003).

The book is dedicated to the four most important women in my life, so different, so close: my grandmothers, Vittoria and Ines, my mother Angela and my sister Monica.

Introduction: Bodies, Consumers and the Ethnography of Commercial Gyms

> You say "I" and you are proud of this word. But greater than this... is your body and its great intelligence, which does not say "I" but performs "I".
>
> Nietzsche, Ecce Homo

In most cultures throughout history a variety of body decoration practices – in the form of clothing and adornment, or even tattooing and piercing – are fundamental to mark social identity. In Western modernity the human body has been invested with instrumental rationality, being disciplined as an instrument for work and labour, a utility, a function, while continuing to operate as the paramount symbol for the subject to demonstrate his or her being self-possessed, civilised or otherwise valuable. Ever more sophisticated bodily markers indicate both "diffuse social statuses" and individual "character", that is, the actor's "conception of himself", his or her "normality" or "abnormality" (Goffman, 1963a). The process of individualisation largely means that the sacred is translated at the level of the embodied self: a particular "civilised" bodily conduct based on the internalisation of social controls has become widespread as the norm (Elias, 1939) and a sort of "air bubble" around the body in ordinary life helps people project a sacred, deep self (Goffman, 1963a; 1967). In contemporary Western societies, the fit body has in many ways replaced body decoration as a potent symbol of status and character, both for men and women. As clothes are ever more revealing, what is fashionable is the actual sculpting of the body itself. The fit body appears to reconcile both instrumental and ceremonial values, ready to be dressed up or shown, it displays vitality and control, power and utility.

The lithe and energetic body, tight and slim, with its firm and toned-up contours is a powerful icon of contemporary Western culture, especially as proposed by advertising and commercial culture. Not only has the toned, fit body become a commercial image, but also fitness gyms and health centres have become highly visible as the sites where such a body is produced. While fitness culture is broader than the gym (comprising informal practices

1

such as urban jogging, sports carried out for keep-fit purposes such as swimming, and being practised at home with the help of videos or, increasingly, simulational devices such as Wii Fit) fitness gyms are at the core of such culture. A number of indicators support this claim: the professionalisation of trainers has happened around the development of the fitness gym, fitness magazines repeatedly offer advice on how to choose a gym or how to get the best out of it, training equipment has been developed around the gym, and even keep-fit manuals which are written for DIY fitness mention the gym. Gym scenes are themselves increasingly glamorised beyond fitness culture. Advertisements portraying the gym as a fashionable environment, full of interesting people and stimulating activities, have multiplied: the fitness gym is evidently so much part of our shared experience that it can easily act as a backdrop for the most diverse types of products, from cheese to sanitary towels, toothpaste to chocolate.

Given its powerful iconic status, there is the temptation to understand what happens in the fitness gym as the direct result of a vaguely defined "consumer culture". Contemporary fitness gyms thereby appear as the by-products of, or the reaction to, commercially led normative injunctions which have been described as inviting individuals to joyfully take responsibility for their bodies and to invest in body maintenance in order to perform culturally appropriate self-presentation (Amir, 1987; Baudrillard, 1998; Bordo, 1993; Le Breton, 1990). A similar reading does not account for the specificity of gym practices with respect to other forms of body transformation, with fitness being grouped together with arguably quite different techniques such as plastic surgery. Detailed examination is often replaced by reference to broad cultural critiques of late-modern individualisation – as different and distant from fitness such as "narcissism" (Lasch, 1979) or, more recently, the "corrosion of character" (Sennett, 1998). Such readings have accompanied the broad reception of fitness in the quality press and high-culture circles. For example, *Perfect* – one of the early movies to exploit the world of fitness to tell a story about love and success featuring John Travolta – was reviewed in *The New York Times* by influential film critic Vincent Canby suggesting that "body-fitness" had been presented "as a form of self-promotion and the kind of narcissism that, in our society, produces journalists who are more important – more celebrated – than the stories they cover" (Canby, June 7 1985). Highlighting the corrosion of character in an era of obsessive self-presentation, this view contrasts markedly with fitness discourse according to which fitness demonstrates character. Fitness discourse is indeed closer to another set of grand theories which have been drawn upon to understand the fitness boom. These theories offer a more positive view of individualisation and revolve on the notion of "body projects": the idea that in late-modernity the self becomes a reflexive and secular project which works on an ever refined level of body presentation (Giddens, 1991). These views may be further sociologically qualified, and made more critical, by relating reflexive body projects to the particular self-presentation needs of the new middle classes that compete in job and relationship markets where high levels of "physical capital" are required (Bourdieu, 1977; 1978; 1984; Featherstone, 1982; see also Chapter 1).

These theoretical insights are in many ways intriguing, as intriguing is the game that social theory and cultural criticism seem to play on the fit body. We may gain perspective from such a game and delve more deeply into what fitness culture actually means by providing for a longer historical scope. Contemporary fitness culture occurs on the historical background of an increased power/knowledge investment in the body via the use of expansive, positive disciplinary techniques (Foucault, 1977; 1983; 1991), but inserts discipline at the heart of largely commercial institutions such as the fitness and health centre. We may thus recall that the subjectivity effects of discipline are both active and passive: providing the subject with new capacities and subjugating it to new forms of power. Such dual subjectification is ever present in the culture of consumption, as people are asked to be both creative and committed, desiring and reliable, self-oriented and accommodating. To capture such dual process, however, we must also get into the lived culture of the fitness gym; a lived culture which, despite the theoretical paraphernalia deployed to refer to it, remains largely unexplored. Grand theories indeed do not describe the world of the gym, their interaction mechanisms, the situated body practices of fitness training and the meanings that these practices have for those who decide to participate, drop out or continue to train assiduously.

The two main English books available on fitness culture in the West treat it as either a demand-side phenomenon of body transformation (Glassner, 1992) or as a supply-side phenomenon of commercialisation (Smith Maguire, 2007).[1] As a result fitness is either traced back to the late-modern subject and its new middle-class incarnations, or is conceived as a leisure industry, the mirror of mounting commoditisation with the ensuing individualisation of social problems such as obesity. This book takes a different perspective. With the objective to move beyond over-generalised, production-led views of fitness, it looks at keep-fit culture neither as a series of commercial images (in fitness magazines, fitness manuals or more broadly in market-driven cultural values) nor as a leisure business driven by a promotional outlook. On the contrary, it looks at gyms as places of consumption, where producers and users contribute to the fitness culture development as an ongoing dialectic achievement.

This book also avoids tracing fitness to a modern, post-modern or late-modern subjectivity with its body projects, or to the distinction requirements of a particular class such as the (new) middle class. Sure, as compared with characteristically working-class institutions such as body-building gyms studied ethnographically by Alan Klein in his *Little Big Men* (1993) or boxing gyms vividly rendered by Loïc Wacquant in his *Body and Soul* (2003), fitness

gyms may be said to be "middle class". But this characterisation may objec-
tify fitness: not only do we know how complex it is, in reality, to pin down
the middle class (see Sassatelli et al., 2008), but also, and more fundamentally, we risk failing to account for fitness as *lived culture*. Just like Klein or
indeed Wacquant, this book aims to provide a "carnal" approach, one which
deploys ethnography to account for the lived experiences – of fun and frustration – of fitness gyms' participants. Inevitably these experiences negotiate
with images of social classification, such as class and gender. But my emphasis is on the *negotiation* of distinction rather than on *objectified distinctions*. I
have thus worked on the assumption that motives for joining and for going
to a gym are to be understood in their own right in their translation into
practices and accounts and on the basis of actual empirical observation of
interaction. Finally, this book aims to qualify the notion of body discipline,
looking not only nor primarily at fitness discourse, but at lived bodily experiences of gym participants, and the often creative ways through which they
appropriate fitness and are transformed in the process.

1. Fitness gyms and fitness culture

If you wander around urban spaces, in Europe as well as the USA, Australia
and Japan you can easily come across the entrance to a fitness gym. Whether
tiny and half-hidden between a shop and a cafe, or imposing and brightly
lit, fitness gyms have become part of late-modern cities. The contemporary
world of gyms is an extremely complex and varied reality, yet, as I will show
in more detail in the next chapter, since the late 1970s there has been a
considerable growth in commercial recreational centres which have presented themselves in a new way: gyms have been tightly associated with
the notion of "fitness", and old labels have been replaced in professional
texts by neologisms such as "fitness centres" and "fitness clubs", and more
recently as "health centres" or "wellness clubs". These neologisms have a
more luxurious feel attached to them, as well as diverting attention from
the competitive, harsh and often very masculine world which was originally
associated with the term "gymnasium" (see Craig and Liberti, 2007). Still,
most fitness participants I have come across refer to their clubs using the
word "gym", something which reflects the fact that, even in large fitness
centres, the core training space is indicated as such.

Fitness gyms are a special breed of leisure institutions (Rojek, 2000). Gyms
are different from social clubs – both working class and upper class – in that
a set of specific tasks are to be carried out, with sociability being either a by-
product or a facilitator of those tasks. In some ways, going to a fitness gym
is a form of "serious leisure" (Stebbins, 2009) which allows the development
of a project and to a degree a "career" within one's own free time. In others,
it is a form of "therapeutic leisure" (Caldwell, 2005) which is believed to prevent negative life events, can help us in coping with them and can generally

have healing functions. In many ways, different from casinos and theme parks (see Bryman, 1999; Gottdiener, 1997), which aim to provide for emotional release and chance playing, fitness gyms are best understood under the banner of "rational recreation". A notion of Victorian heritage according to Foucault (1977), rational recreation stresses that recreational activities should be morally uplifting for the participant and have positive benefits for the wider society. At a difference with more informal, spontaneous forms of leisure, or with sub-cultures of commodity appropriation (see Willis, 1979) they appear, at least at first glance, functional to social order and dominant classifications, rather than "anti-structural" or "subversive".

Considered in this light, fitness gyms are a special breed of gyms as well. Of course, gyms which concentrate solely on one competitive physical activity, such as boxing, martial arts or on muscle development and body-building, do still exist, but they represent niche phenomena as compared to the often much bigger premises which offer a variety of exercise possibilities collected under the banner of an ever-shifting notion of fitness. Body-building gyms, and even more so, boxing gyms, are often strongly connoted in terms of sex, class and ethnicity, and provide for the consolidation of veritable sub-cultural environments, quite markedly cut out of mainstream cultural formations (see Klein, 1993; Lowe, 1998; Wacquant, 2003). For the most part, fitness gyms present themselves as unisex and appeal to an as wide as possible public of consumers. The fitness phenomenon is commercial at its core. And fitness gyms are generally modelled as spaces to be consumed, used and appropriated via some sort of commercial relation (see Urry, 1995).

To be sure, different countries across the Western world have different traditions of physical recreation provision. Nordic countries rely more on public provision in the context of a strong voluntary sports sectors and strong links between sports, non-profit idealism and volunteerism (Steen-Johnsen, 2004), the USA relies more on market relations (Smith Maguire 2007), and countries such as Britain and Italy rely on a fair mixture of private health clubs and fitness schemes in public facilities (Crossley, 2006; Sassatelli, 2000c). Still, fitness gyms as such are heavily imbued with *promotional culture* (Wernick, 1991), and the idea that leisure products have to be targeted to clients or consumers (see Chapter 1). Taking a look at the international expansion of fitness, there seems to be a trend in many Western countries for commercially owned fitness centres to take over other, community-based, forms of fitness provision and in fact dominate the market; there also seems to be a correlation between the presence of large sections of the population with the financial means to pay for commercial fitness services and the rise of fitness training in general (IHRSA, 2006).[2] As I shall show later, this partly reflects the official objective of fitness training, namely the improvement or maintenance of individual body qualities and well-being. Emphasis on individuality, the duties and pleasure of "taking care of oneself", is paramount in fitness culture, which also speaks in the seemingly universalistic voice of a fight against the ills of urban living and its desk-bound patterns.

Fitness gyms are non-competitive environments aimed at providing recreational exercise to boost physical form and well-being. As such, they are at the *core* of a much broader fitness culture. All in all, fitness culture is a constellation of hybrid, shifting and rather diverse phenomena which are growing across the world. It comprises a variety of commodities: news-stands are full of magazines on physical exercise, health and beauty, which promote an increasingly nuanced vision of the fit body and offer advice about exercises and diet that may help to get it; bookshops have an increasingly large and varied collection of exercise manuals; fitness festivals are increasingly getting media coverage and contribute to the professionalisation of trainers. Besides this, there has been a remarkable diffusion of fitness training aids – from aerobics videos to home-fitness equipment – for individual use at home. Urban jogging is still popular and traditional sports may be practised for fitness purposes rather than competition or play. Accurate figures of the amount of people involved in fitness training across the population are not readily available, as workout routines may be exercised alone in front of the television set, at the workplace, on an urban sidewalk, in a class set up by a community leisure centre or indeed in a commercial fitness gym. Furthermore, fitness culture can be said to be much broader than the people who actually and regularly train, as the growing market for sportswear clearly witnesses; indeed fitness outfits are not only increasingly sold to the fitness fan, they are also bought by casual consumers and have long influenced other types of clothes. Even more broadly, as hinted before, keep-fit activities in the gym and the fit body have become commercial icons in themselves, signs used in the patchwork images surrounding commodities.

Reflecting the increasing diversity of fitness culture, keep-fit exercise is increasingly hegemonic within contemporary physical recreation activities, attracting in its orbit a number of different, even rather established, forms of recreational physical practices such as boxing, martial arts or Nordic walking. Today, a number of activities are coded as "fitness", including established sports such as swimming which are increasingly practised for fitness purposes rather than competition; oriental techniques such as yoga which have been both incorporated within fitness exercise in the gym and are available in more "pure" forms in specific institutions; leisure activities such as orienteering, walking, gardening and dancing whose fitness benefits are increasingly underlined both within and without the fitness world narrowly defined; physical activities such as jogging whose birth is indeed co-extensive with the emergence of contemporary fitness culture; and, as suggested, fitness exercise at home. As is apparent, these activities are diverse and varied: some are highly institutionalised and commercialised, some are not; some are more clearly geared to body maintenance, others refer to sociability, recreation and spirituality. It was not possible within the scope of a single volume to offer an in-depth study of each of these activities, nor would it be advisable. Rather than try and zoom in on the whole spectrum of places and activities which can be coded as fitness, I have focused on gym practices as the more iconic, if not significant, aspect of the wider family of keep-fit exercise.

Typically organised via market relations, fitness gyms are central to the fitness market. On a global level, the USA stands out as having a significantly stronger commercial fitness sector than any other country. In 2005, in the USA there were 29,000 health clubs with a clientele of about 14 per cent of the population. In comparison, the EU states taken together had 33,400 fitness clubs with a mean penetration rate of 8.1 per cent (IHRSA, 2006). The gym obviously occupies a crucial symbolic space in fitness culture. Gyms are firmly present in fitness discourse on exercise as the main site where the fit body is both produced and consumed, they are specific institutions where trainers translate their expertise for the public to meet the expectations, illusions and delusions of consumers, and they provide a dedicated space where the meanings and objectives of fitness training are continuously negotiated alongside participants' identities. The negotiation of meanings and practices which takes place within fitness gyms between clients and trainers is crucial to the dynamic of the fitness world at large. Recreational physical activities are indeed being continuously monitored and selectively exploited by the fitness industry which is firmly grounded on fitness gyms. Fitness gyms draw on emergent, grassroots or parallel phenomena to continuously define the content and meaning of fitness, broadening their scope to include fun, sociability and psychic fulfilment. While increasingly complemented and challenged by a host of less institutionalised or emergent phenomena, commercial fitness gyms are hegemonic formations within fitness culture. All in all, they do offer a vantage point to consider the family of activities branded as fitness.

2. Keep-fit training and its accounts

Fitness gyms are the primary empirical research setting of this book. This reflects a specific research strategy, namely to address the ever-changing and rather ill-defined reality of fitness culture capturing its commercial thrust and considering its core, culturally hegemonic and clearly institutionalised instance, that is, fitness training within the gym. My objective is to offer a perspective on fitness culture by entering the gym world and sharing clients' embodied experiences – from frustration to joy to fatigue to embarrassment. So people's experience as fitness consumers is the primary focus of the research. As suggested, commercial fitness paraphernalia is often surrounded by commercial images emphasising body ideals and spectacular exercise results, yet the gym world is made up of routine physical exercise, of the ongoing emotional work performed by trainers in order to help clients sustain their routines, and of the ceaseless negotiation of meanings which clients accomplish in their gym practices. To understand how and why training in the gym is becoming important for an ever-increasing number of people while others find it neither attractive nor compelling, I needed to get inside the gym world and consider how space, time, relationships and bodies are organised in order to offer meaningful experiences to the participants. As I shall show, the fitness gym is experienced not simply as an ingredient in the search for a perfect body, but as a well-organised place where a vast array of meanings and identities are negotiated. Wider cultural values, the ideals of the fit, toned and slender body, coded as both a conspicuous sign of personal worth and a matter of individual choice, are indeed mediated and reinterpreted in locally prescribed ways.

This book will thus look at fitness culture starting from the microphysics of its main institution, the fitness gym. This demands a meticulous analysis of *how* the gym realises its ascribed cultural goals by focusing on the interaction arrangements which are locally sustained without reifying the discontinuity of the gym from everyday reality. I have thus, initially, studied gyms as ecological systems whose internal shifting equilibrium is relatively autonomous from the outside world, or at least responds in a selective manner to the context of general cultural values. Such a naturalistic and pragmatic approach attempts to understand the mechanisms of social life from the bottom-up, starting from the local organisation of experience and practice.

Erving Goffman's lesson on face-to-face interaction and the interaction order has been crucial to my endeavour (Goffman, 1971, 1982). Interaction can be defined as a face-to-face sphere of action maintained primarily by implicit rules about how to proceed, express one's desires and emotions, present oneself and behave with others.[3] These are tacit ceremonial rules which give form to the experience of participants, maintaining their ability to feel involved while performing the exercises and promoting specific definitions of what is taking place and the various resources which are brought into play. Some of these rules, such as role-distance or deference, operate in many domains of action and symbolic worlds. Yet the fitness gym defines its boundaries as a symbolic world by putting these general interaction mechanisms to work in specific ways, which, we shall see, work on the negotiation of a specific motivational logic, a certain gym etiquette, a vision of the body and its relation to the self. The observation of participants' experiences in the local reality of the gym thus provides privileged access to the meanings of fitness. Clients' experiences in particular appear as the outcome of a negotiation between the modalities of interaction which participants are encouraged to adopt in the gym, and the cultural values associated with fitness. This, as I shall expand in the next chapter, is "loosely coupled", to borrow Goffman's (1982) term, with the social structure: gender, class and other external identity specifications being translated and re-worked within the gym in specific ways which reveal its commercial and yet disciplinary character (see especially Chapter 4). In this light, the gym is a *living world in the making*, recognisable in its continuous negotiation of its specificity based on the participants' performance of fitness training. This active and creative participation of subjects is both a threat to the stability of the meanings of fitness and a fundamental ingredient in the success of the gym. Gym culture thus helps address the issue of agency, but it also obliges us to move away from textual models and embrace action as embodied practice. It is by engaging with clients sense of selves through their five senses – through the particular visuality of the gym, its aural culture combining loud music, client's strain grunts in the machine areas and trainers' screams during classes as well as a vast array of touch, smell and taste details – that the gym constitutes itself as a meaningful world.

With these problems in mind, I have conducted a multi-site ethnography in several gyms in two European countries, Italy and Britain. I started my research conducting an extended ethnographic project in Florence, Italy, in the mid 1990s (see Sassatelli, 1999a, 1999b, 2000). This ethnographic fieldwork considered in particular the spatiality and temporality of the gym world, the management of interaction during the exercise and gym etiquette among clients and instructors, the tone of social relationships in the gym and the negotiation of body ideals by fitness fans and more detached gym participants. Two Italian gyms representing the extreme opposed poles of the commercial fitness provision in the same middle-class neighbourhood were studied for a nine-month period. This has been fundamental to get into the world of fitness, grasp the main local patterns of interaction, appreciate the relational dynamics inside gym environments, explore the motivational accounts of a variety of gym-goers as they join the gym and progress through their gym careers, and consider the motivational role of trainers and the way gym-going helps clients to negotiate the broad discourse on fitness. The initial ethnography has been complemented later by two shorter periods of ethnographic observation in Norwich, Britain at the turn of the millennium conducted in a commercial local club close to the city centre and in a newly constructed university sports centre. A further reprise of ethnographic observation finally took place in the winter of 2007 in Britain, and in the spring of 2007 in Italy. As the purpose of these final observations was not to compare countries, but to widen and diversify the empirical basis, checking findings and hypotheses developed earlier and monitoring the development of fitness practices and culture in a variety of Clubs, I visited and attended the activities of about 20 gyms in three rather different urban realities such as London, Bologna and Milan. In a couple of cases I enrolled for three months, but more often I just spent a day or two in each gym, chatting with clients and trainers, and of course with managers. I was particularly interested in monitoring gym chains and in moving up-market, getting into more exclusive clubs, something which proved rather complicated on a free-trial basis. My observations were conducted at all times of the day, for several days a week, and took place in the changing-rooms, in the different studios available in the gyms I went to – ranging from aerobics and step-aerobics, to stretching and Pilates, to spinning and aquagym – in the relaxation areas, including saunas, in the bars, corridors and lobbies of the gyms.[4] While each of the gyms I visited deserve a thorough description, the book works in a typological fashion, concentrating in particular on the management of the training scene. In what follows I will try to offer rich, structured descriptions of the many gym interactions I witnessed, while using pseudonyms for all personal and company names.

As a result of my fieldwork I have come to spend a remarkable number of hours in gym environments. Yet, this has been initially unintentional: I have started this project out of intellectual curiosity rather than fandom or personal experience, and during fieldwork I have initially been a reluctant participant myself in many settings, having only quite slowly developed something of a "liking" for fitness training, as my body and mind gradually learned to respond to the training scene. Recalcitrant as I might have been at the beginning, I have learned much from my apprentice as a fitness client in the initial extended ethnography of two Florentine gyms. And among the things I have learned is that inside the fitness gym there is nothing comparable to what in sports activities are the ritual events which help in formalising internal hierarchies and clearly structured practitioners' career paths. In his ethnography of the boxing gym, Wacquant (2003) progresses to the centre of the art – the ring, the fight night – and indeed devotes quite a substantial part of his precious book to these dramatic events. The fight night is "the focal point of the boxing field, and quite necessary to sustaining the excitement and *illusio* which generates it" (Crossley, 2001, 109). *Illusio*, in Pierrre Bourdieu's (1998) terminology, is a "belief in the game" or "enchantment" with it – something that is required from participants in every social field if it is to function as such. Not that the *illusio* is absent in fitness though. Indeed, like all regular participants I have come across, I managed to get involved, to work in accordance with the basic stakes of keep-fit workout, and even got to the stage that for me the game was very much "worth the candle". But stakes in fitness are different. Fitness is all training: the fitness gym never gets frenetic with the anticipation of contest as in body-building and boxing gyms, or of public performances as in the ballet studio. Fans may become trainers, they may become familiar with the techniques, but by and large they just remain more or less keen trainees. As I have become acquainted with fitness and its discourses, as my body progressed through training, I have been able to experience more clearly the *illusio* of fitness, the difficulties and pleasure of the trainee. This did not mean that I was totally submerged in the activity. As Robert Perinbanayagam (2006) has shown, strategic agency is compatible with involvement in the game. And I have learned, so to speak, to exploit the spaces offered by the fitness gym: in this individualistic, universalistic environment patterns of participation may range from strict to quite loose – something which incidentally has allowed me to complement the initial extended ethnography with shorter observational studies. Reflecting back on my gym experiences, I must now recognise that attendance at fitness gyms has ended up accompanying a significant portion of my adult life. But just as for many other gym-goers, I was allowed a rather fluctuating participation, being institutionally encouraged to adapt training to the different needs of my body and my work or family requirements across the life course. And the constant renovation of techniques together with the familiarisation with rather urbane but intensely cheerful local patterns of relations were very much helpful in keeping me going. Presently, I am more of a swimmer than a gym-goer, and I largely rely on fieldnotes to explicate embodied experiences which are not central to my current body disposition. But I doubt that I could have managed to write about fitness culture as a practical accomplishment without direct, sustained embodied participation. Ethnography pushes the participant observer to experience, with her own embodied self, the spatial, temporal and social environment of the gym, and it allowed me to collect a wealth of irreplaceable data. It proved to be the best research option in order to shift attention from the psychological or demographic characteristics of gym-goers to the ways in which physical activity is performed, and from the aims of training to the social mechanisms which account for participants' experiences of involvement.

Fieldwork has provided me with the chance not only to gather participants' impressions on the spot, but also to collect formal interviews taking into account a variety of participation profiles and social backgrounds. In particular, in the course of 15 years, I have collected a rich archive of long and rich stories from clients and trainers. The book relies on 67 long interviews: 49 with clients and 18 with trainers and gym staff, conducted in Italy and in Britain.[5] In-depth interviews have helped chart peoples' conscious experiences in a more systematic way, eliciting self-reflexive accounts about reasons for joining, continuing or leaving the gym which have greatly helped to situate the local organisation of experience into a wider picture. Together with participant observation they helped me to come to terms with the main acknowledged frustrations of clients and the main professional preoccupations of trainers. Although fitness activity takes place in a very orderly manner, not all clients are satisfied, and alongside the many enthusiasts, there are a great number of irregular clients, and an array of people who quickly get disaffected and drop out. Interviews with clients and trainers helped in figuring out how self-narratives are marshalled to account for the give and take of gym-going.

Fitness fans have described the fitness gym as an environment which offered them "a space for themselves", where everyone can and must "withdraw from the outside world". On the contrary, the comments made by irregular clients or by gym-dropouts have shown how difficult it can be to enter the world of physical activity and concentrate on its specific local demands. Although they were prepared to say that gym training could be "a rational solution" to get fit, leavers were unable to "enter" the spirit of the exercise, in the gym they felt "bored" and "uninvolved", "alone" and at the same time "tense" and exposed as if they were "in a shop window". Interviews with clients and trainers have offered very vivid descriptions of the emotional codes which are to be managed by participants to continue training (see Chapter 5). In particular, the interviews with trainers provide a spotlight on the kind of work which trainers do in order to boost participation. Trainers work as body and exercise experts as well as emotional workers, mediating between the precise promotional needs of the fitness industry and the often vague body aspirations of the clients.[6] Like theme park animators, fitness trainers have to get consumers to partake in a meaningful experience, inducing them to experience things in a particular way, furnishing them with a series of cognitive and emotive instruments to read and enjoy the scene which they are entering. They are key resources to qualify as free, self-gratifying, personalised, amusing, and creative a place like the gym which could otherwise be felt as too instrumental, rationalised and standardised (see Chapter 3).

3. Fitness discourse and lived bodies

The organisation of keep-fit practices is predicated on the ongoing negotiation of the notion of the fit body (Sassatelli, 2003). Such a notion, promoted by fitness discourse, is negotiated during interaction within the gym, but this happens in a rather tangential fashion. Fitness participants' accounts of their gym biographies were crucial for this, and trainers' stories about their professional passion helped provide a rounder picture of the meanings associated with fitness. Yet, from the early days of my research, I felt the need to collect other qualitative sources, textual and visual sources in particular. Sure, I had been collecting the many different pieces of written and visual texts produced by the gyms I was visiting in Italy and Britain (brochures, timetables, websites and so on), which provided hints and props for my formal and informal interviews with clients and trainers. But, more importantly, and as a further angle to the research, I have analysed expert discourse on fitness. By this I mean that part of fitness discourse which is produced by fitness experts and fitness cultural intermediaries. As such fitness expert discourse is at the core of a broad set of discourses on fitness which is produced across different fields including body care, sport, health, fashion and popular culture. In particular, I have concentrated on expert discourse as it is fixed in exercise manuals and health and fitness magazines (Sassatelli, 2001). I have carried out a systematic discourse analysis of the specialised press on fitness, health and beauty in Italy, Britain and the USA. Initially the analysis was conducted on all the fitness magazines published in Italy between 1994 and 1996, and on a wide range of fitness and gym manuals on sale in Italy during the same period. This analysis has been extended via an analysis of the most important fitness magazines in Italy, Britain and the USA for the period January–June 2007.[7] In the course of the years I have also collected a vast array of fitness and exercise manuals published in Italy, Britain and the USA starting from the early 1970s when fitness culture begun to consolidate until the early 2000s when it has reached maturity. This collection comprises over 60 manuals, and includes world classics such as Jane Fonda's *Workout Book* (1981) and Callan Pinkney's *Callanetics* (1992).[8] I have used such analysis whenever helpful throughout the book, with the aim to triangulate the magmatic richness of ethnographic materials with the crystalline horizon of expert and commercial discourse.

The clarity, precision and systematic nature of specialist publications helped in gaining a better understanding of the organisational principles which support the efforts made by clients, and which are rarely expressed so explicitly during training. Nothing can substitute lived experience, but lived experience is fuzzy, mixed, ambivalent and paradoxical. Bearing in mind its normative, typically reconciliatory character, expert discourse has helped in offering a more systematic overview of the repertoires of justification and the vocabularies of motives which people draw upon in giving shape to their experiences and motivations. My research here owes much to the different, classic works of Charles Wright Mills (1940) and Harold Garfinkel (1967) on vocabularies of motives and accountability. I have tried to look at people's accounts as motivational narratives and practices of justification which people use both to motivate themselves and to be accountable. Through their accounts, gym-goers perform motivation and desire, modify motivation and account for it to others (see Sassatelli, 1999a and 2000c). Their accounting practices are built upon, and build up, a vocabulary of motives and justifications for fitness. The legitimating vocabulary or rhetoric of fitness is thus the result of many accounting practices carried out from different positions in the lived culture of the gym: to render the multivocal nature of the vocabulary of fitness, I have tried to adequately distinguish between official discourse which is objectified in fitness manuals, lived expert discourse as spoken by trainers and gym instructors, and experiential discourse as spoken by gym-goers. As we move from official to experiential narratives, accounts become, so it seems, more fragmentary, more contradictory but also potentially richer. It is especially fitness fans who seem to master a particularly rich and articulated vocabulary to help them stick to training. And they insist not only on the relevance of external incentives such as body projects or ideals, but also on internal rewards such as involvement, enjoyment and even relaxation. The experiential moment is clearly important in fitness culture, and ethnography coupled with such a performative emphasis on vocabularies of motives has helped to explore how and why this is so.

As I shall show, expert discourse on fitness is clearly characterised by a universalistic and individualistic rhetoric: its growth proceeded by a *differentiating pluralism*, which is largely structured according to subject categories that fix stereotypical images of social divisions (women, men, the elderly, stay-home mums, pregnant women, ex-athletes and so on); to exercise techniques (body-building, aerobics, stretching, yoga, step, spinning and so on); and to body targets (slimming, toning, getting healthier, feeling better and so on) or body parts (legs, shoulders, stomach and so on). As clients and trainers typically translate and transform themes which are widely present in expert discourse, careful attention to such publications has helped provide a richer picture of the meanings attributed to fitness. In clients' accounts as well as in expert discourse, ideas of health and beauty are juxtaposed with the notion of the "fit body" which thereby consolidates as a third, irreducible and partly superior, body ideal alternative to both (see Chapters 6 and 7).

The exploration of the complex, contested and shifting notion of the fit body is crucial to an understanding of fitness culture as a commercially mediated world of practices. As I shall show, the fit body is a relatively abstract ideal which relates to an instrumental vision of the body's underlying features such as resistance and muscle tone compatible with different body shapes. Ostensibly about the body, fitness is primarily a way to negotiate the body-self relation. Fitness training is broadly considered a means to change one's own body – image, capacities, perceptions – and hence one's own self. Changing is not easy, it is embarrassing. Yet must be sought after, deserved and justified. Fitness culture provides a repertoire of legitimating and motivating discourses which revolve around a number of binaries – such as nature and artificial, authenticity and falsity, control and surrender, pleasure and duty, sociability and self-centredness. All in all, fitness culture as being developed in fitness gyms and health clubs works on the notion that, through a careful mixture of fun and self-discipline, our relation with our body can at the same time be more instrumental and more authentic. Significantly, this is in line with the received view of modern subjectivity: the self is a body-owner who chooses to discipline the body in order to obtain happiness, freedom, dignity or more simply to realise subjectivity. Such construction contains a number of paradoxes and contradictions which fitness, as a practice and as a discourse, both brings out and strives to solve. Ultimately, fitness revolves around the notion of individual choice. This study has indeed shown that gym-going is modelled on the notion of individual, autonomous consumer choice, and that choice is often invoked as a normative ideal – a claim which helps clients to account for their practices and a normative frame for self-understanding and self-presentation. Yet, the ideal of choice is not realised in practice: fitness becomes a need and it is actually consumed not because of an abstract, self-contained choice, but because of a situated, contingent learning process, which is nonetheless far from arbitrary or casual. What is more, at least in the case of keep-fit activities, choice requires further normative framings which, as it were, contain its indeterminacy: fitness is good not just because people choose, but also because they choose to realise themselves as authentic subjects through an activity which is constructed as natural and moral.

As is apparent, this book has tried to offer a multi-layered perspective on fitness culture as a culture of consumption. Consumption is surely a matter of taste, but tastes are not the only thing that counts in understanding our desires: institutions and places of consumption are social structures in relation to which tastes become translated into practice (Sassatelli, 2007). To this end, this study has pursued a bottom-up approach to consumption grounded in ethnography. Fitness gyms, and in particular commercial premises, were the main settings. This of course has meant that both informal keep-fit practices, such as jogging in a park or home-fitness, as well as the pursuit of a sport practice for mainly fitness reasons, such as regular swimming, have been largely left out of the picture. However, a focus on the fitness gym as the key institutional context of today's fitness culture has allowed me to consider how needs may be locally created and reproduced as well as addressing the relevance of interaction and its coupling with wider cultural ideals. The choice of fitness culture has certainly been instrumental to pursue my theoretical interest for the study of consumption as an ongoing situated practice. Still, very much in the tradition of classical ethnography, I have endeavoured to provide what has recently been called "peopled ethnography" (Fine, 2003): a rich description of people, practices and meanings coupled with sustained theoretical reflection. The relationship between fitness culture as lived culture in the gym and the broad sociocultural structure is thus often addressed, even though this is done from the perspective of ethnographic experience. Being on the scene is crucial for an ethnographer. I found a place, the fitness gym, where by speaking of small fragments of reality it has been possible to speak of big cultural borders – and of cultural dualities such as consumption and work, discipline and fun, nature and culture, self and body. To accomplish this task properly it was crucial to take fitness culture and its participants very seriously.

4. Summary of the book

With the help of a variety of qualitative data – ranging from ethnographic fieldwork to formal and informal interviews with clients, trainers and managers to expert discourse on fitness in the specialist press and exercise manuals – this book aims to offer access to keep-fit culture as developed in commercial fitness gyms. By actually getting into the world of training in the gym, it firstly deals with the local organisation of experience and then considers more closely the body ideals which are negotiated by fitness participants and fitness experts. The book thus aims to start from situated interaction to reach cultural values and social classification, placing gyms into the contemporary wider field of commercial body work (either transformative or sportive) and considering their particular cultural and institutional configuration in historical terms. The book thus opens by discussing the cultural relevance of fitness gyms as related to the history of the commercialisation of body discipline, the negotiation of gender identities and distinction dynamics within contemporary cultures of consumption. The book then unfolds as a journey through the ordinary world of training in the fitness gym by means of ethnographic research, interviews and discourse analysis. Chapter 2 examines what gives shape to the first impressions that clients may get when they enter the world of the gym: the spatial organisation of fitness centres with their differential interaction patterns. Chapter 3 deals with the relational aspects of gym environments. While fitness discourse is all about body objectives and body maintenance, fitness centres are also about the management of a variety of social relations, and in particular those between clients from different social backgrounds, and between trainers and clients. The role of trainers as experts, task and emotional leaders is underlined, as well as the continuous negotiation of expert knowledge on fitness. Chapter 4 looks at the fitness workout as it happens in a variety of gym scenes, considering how expressive behaviour during physical activity is organised. In particular it looks at the motivational logic which fitness participants are invited to embrace and display, contributing to the triumph of self-competition. Chapter 5 deals with the local organisation of involvement in training, and at the framing of involvement as "fun". It thereby considers the seriousness of fun experiences and explores how they get translated into articulated projects of body modification that offer second-order satisfaction. Fitness enthusiasts in particular are studied and compared with novices and irregular participants in order to show how motivational narratives change in the course of fitness participation. The chapter reveals that motivations to join and motivations to stick with training may change greatly, stressing the transformational role of local practices. Considering body ideals more directly, Chapter 6 deals with the cultural value of the fit body on the backdrop of gender identities. Here, drawing on both expert discourse and gym-goers' motivational narratives the notion of fitness as promoted by keep-fit exercises is explored as against health and beauty. Chapter 7 looks at how body-mind/self dualism is articulated within fitness culture on the backdrop of particular visions of urban, desk-bound patterns of work. In particular, it shows that the meanings of fitness are related to normative values about the body and naturalness as well as the self and authenticity which provide themes that can be deployed to legitimatise body transformation. The conclusion deals with how a bottom-up approach to keep-fit practices in the commercial gym may help us critically address consumer choice and global cultures of consumption.

1
The Cultural Location of Fitness Gyms

As a dedicated, closed space for working on the body, the gym has a long history, stretching all the way back to the *gymnasium* of the Greeks and the *palaestra* of the Romans. The line of continuity with such millenarian tradition was still somewhat strong in the first half of the twentieth century with the diffusion of physical culture and the development of body-building gyms devoted to muscular growth, prevalently frequented by men often tied by strong sub-cultural relations. However, since the 1970s there has been a marked increase in the number of exercise premises presenting themselves in a new guise. They have addressed an increasingly large, mixed public. They have shifted the notion of the gym from a sub-cultural passion to a mass leisure activity, intertwined with pop culture. They have articulated health promotion in an increasingly commercial, individualistic manner. As is apparent, today the term "gym" is associated with that of "fitness" and even increasingly replaced by neologisms like "fitness centre" or "fitness club" which, as some clients and trainers claim, better convey the specific mission of this institution. To be sure, gyms reserved solely for typically masculine competitive activities – such as body building, weightlifting, boxing or the martial arts – still exist, but they are increasingly marginal with respect to the large number of premises that find a minimum common denominator in the idea of fitness. Fitness gyms aim to absorb whatever body technique, transforming it into keep-fit activity for the masses – from competitive sports to ancient oriental martial arts and meditation, from bicycling to Latin American dance. And while increasingly diversified, they are the core institutions at the heart of an ever shifting fitness culture.

That of fitness is in many ways a characteristically late twentieth-century story. Likewise, the keep-fit workout and the fit body are considered as the epitomes of late-modern society. While this book aims to explore how the notion of fitness is appropriated and accomplished in ordinary, contemporary gym practices, there is clearly a deep historic-cultural grounding to this. In broader terms, "fitness" seems to be a notion shaped by the encounter of two important cultural codes of Western modernity:

17

rationalisation and asceticism, on the one hand, and the quest for authenticity and hedonism, on the other. This chapter addresses the historical circumstances of the fitness gym development. As the history of fitness is spread across a number of different Western countries, I have endeavoured to provide an overarching theoretical-historical narrative, necessarily sacrificing the colour of historical detail. I have thus looked at how the fitness centre became shaped differentiating itself from other types of clubs and other types of gyms that spread in the West from the end of the nineteenth century, hinting at how it relates to commercialisation, the state and social differences. I thereby consider in some detail the structural elements – within consumerism, patriarchy or the class structure – which have been associated with the success of fitness centres from the last quarter of the twentieth century to today. While early forms of fitness workout, such as aerobics, have typically been associated with dominant views of femininity which reproduce women's subjugation to beauty ideals, the fitness boom in more general terms has been branded as a middle-class pursuit: the pursuit of body efficiency and secular moral salvation. Both ways, keep-fit workout and fitness gyms have been strongly associated with the transformation of the body, physical activity and sport into commodities. Commodities which under the veneer of liberation command further engulfment into the world of commodity consumption. While elements of these critiques do capture elements of fitness culture as commercial culture, a crude critique of consumerism masks as much as it unveils, and ultimately objectifies fitness. Porous and ever shifting, the boundaries of fitness culture find in the gym their main institutional setting of reproduction. This chapter sets the background for a deeper understanding of the complex institutionally sustained interaction mechanisms which support participation in fitness centres, with the objective to account for fitness as ongoing lived culture.

1. The commercialisation of discipline

Fitness centres are creatures of the present. Yet, to understand their cultural location they are best conceived as modern, and indeed late-modern, creatures. Their development and specificity as institutional formations must be placed in a longer-term context with the help of notions which have contributed to theories of modernity and late-modernity such as "discipline" and "commercialisation". In a broad historic-theoretical perspective, the rise of the commercial fitness gym is part of a long-term historical process in which techniques of body discipline linked to the birth of the nation state and the capitalist economy have slowly extended from work, punishment and education to the spheres of recreation and leisure, and have increasingly been organised via commercial relations.

Different authors – classics such as Marx and Weber as well as, more recently, Michel Foucault – have all stressed the importance acquired by disciplinary techniques and body rationalisation in the development of modern institutions, such as barracks, factories, prisons, schools and hospitals (see Sassatelli, 2001; Turner, 1987). These institutions put the body to work under regimes of positive control: through finely calibrated, detailed body work, physical abilities are modified in terms of growth and disciplined expression rather than conservation or repression as was the case in monastic institutions. In barracks and in factories, for example, the individual body is disciplined to become more useful – movements are deconstructed, measured and reconstructed in order to be better co-ordinated with those of others, and be of service to the institution.

With the development of a scientific and instrumental approach to the body, and the relative consolidation of expert discourse on gymnastics, disciplinary techniques extended to the fields of recreation and leisure (Vigarello, 1978; see also Rabinbach, 1990; Ulman, 1971). In eighteenth-century France, for example, physical techniques aimed at increasing utilitarian physical performances via a rigorous and systematic exercising of the functional capacities of the body were added to noble pursuits such as dance or archery, which required a containment of emotive expression and the turning of gestures into a spectacle symbolising status. Not only in the organisation of work, but also in recreational fields, new physical techniques were thus developed which were marked by an ethic of utility in which "active" and "productive" modalities, "linked to the economic sphere, but transferred to private lives, become more and more prevalent" (Pociello, 1981, pp. 37–9). The appearance in such fields of a regime of positive physical control is initially characterised by institutional or collective aims. For this reason, the type of gymnastics which developed in the nineteenth century, both in Europe and the USA, was aimed at strengthening the public spirit of the "masses" and creating better "citizens". Indeed, recreational physical exercise and gymnastics, organised directly by the state or by philanthropic élites outside market relations and as a form of education, was an expression of the bio-political aims of nation states, of their need to govern populations as an economic, political and even military resource, preparing the "people" to "take their place" in the social order. The origins of gymnastics are fully inscribed in this logic, and are thus very different from that of sport in the strictest sense. Many sports, whether team sports (such as rugby or football) or individual sports (such as athletics), took place in schools reserved for the bourgeois élite, where they often forged the "character" of future political and economic leaders, teaching them the ethics of fair play between equals, as well as self-control and leadership (Arnaud, 1987; Bourdieu, 1978; Elias and Dunning, 1986; Gruneau, 1983; Guttmann, 1978; Park, 1994).

Integration in well-ordered groups rather than competition among individuals was the ethos of gymnastics. This is evident in the spread of gymnastic festivals during the nineteenth and early twentieth centuries in Western countries such as Germany, Sweden, France, Britain and the

USA. While coded by gender, this phenomenon was aimed at both men and women and was fuelled by progressive ideologies (Chambat, 1987; Defrance, 1976). In more general terms, a variety of explicitly political aims – the promotion of nationalist ideals (Vigarello, 1988), the maintenance of social order (Hargreaves, 1987; McIntosh, 1963), the control of sexuality and deviant consumption (Whorton, 1982), social reform (Defrance, 1981) – marked the spread of gymnastics. Controversially, the bio-political deployment of gymnastics reached its peak with the totalitarian regimes in the first half of the twentieth century, including Nazism in Germany and Fascism in Italy, which often sought to promote their ideologies, control the population and ultimately get better soldiers through mass physical education. The use of gymnastic festivals and public displays and the pervasive workings of gymnastic associations during Nazism are well documented, and spread beyond Germany (Mangan, 2000). But also in less martial Italy, the fascist regime was keen to gain a monopoly over gymnastic and sporting activities, seen yet again as ways to produce good citizenry (Gori, 1996).

After the Second World War in Western countries, the strong symbolic and institutional tie which had been created between gymnastics and politics withered and traditional forms of gymnastics lost momentum. This left room for the development of de-politicised and individualistic, health-oriented and fun-seeking physical and recreational forms of gymnastic which were gradually integrated by the emerging commercial gyms. Physical culture and building acted upon each other, with the "immuring of physical exercise" as part of a longer, civilising trend for the enclosure of the body (Heichberg, 1998, pp. 47ff.). Keep-fit activities in the gym may be understood as inscribed in, and contributing to, the individualisation process, which matches the evolution of the bourgeois spirit (Beck and Gernsheim, 2001). They were sustained through a commercialised imperative of health (Lupton, 1994) and were related to the incorporation of more and more social strata into commercial relations. The individual needs and desires of the participants are now presented as what legitimatise effort and commitment.[1] Elements of older disciplinary techniques are taken up and organised through the market and marshalled by commercial premises, open to everyone but especially attractive to those who have time, money and interest for investing in the kind of body maintenance and body modification offered. Paraphrasing what Foucault wrote about disciplinary institutions, we may say that contemporary private fitness clubs are commercial institutions which put bodies to work through disciplinary techniques. Today's commercial gyms still provide "a specified place which is heterogeneous compared with all others, and is a closed environment": within its walls, it reproduces a "functional location" aiming at the optimum "use of the time available" and in an attempt to create an "integrally useful period of time", time, space and movement are subdivided into rigid, infinitesimal sections. Here too anything which might disturb or distract participants is eliminated, since "[t]ime measured and paid must also be a time without impurities or defects; a time of good quality, throughout which the body is constantly applied to its exercise" (Foucault, 1991, p. 151). Yet, in a much more precise sense than anticipated by Foucault (1983), the commercialisation of body discipline implies that those who are *subjected to* discipline are the *subjects of* it, too. After all they actively engage in a commercial transaction, they are the ones who pay for the time spent exercising. Targeted at clients or consumers – namely subjects who pay for a service and can always decide they no longer need it – fitness emphasises a strategic, personal dimension, and aims at being qualified as an expression of consumers' desires. The fit body is linked not to the citizen or the worker, but to the sovereign consumer, a new sacred persona characterised as autonomous and choosy.

In broad cultural terms, the fitness centre is at the crossroads of differently positioned social formations. It may be seen as drawing upon a preceding tradition of typically male, working-class informal gyms. Indeed, alongside physical education and athletics festivals directly organised by the state, from the late nineteenth century many Western countries had seen the development of forms of exercise that tried to escape direct political control. Places for physical recreation began to appear which did not aim at public health, but expressed the local, working-class men's need for working-class ways of doing exercise together, enjoy themselves, prove their masculinity and improve their bodies. A long-standing example of similar working-class clubs is the body-building gym (Klein, 1993). Comparing and contrasting body building with fitness is particularly interesting. From the dawn of the twentieth century, body building was seen as a working-class, masculine activity for body strengthening, aimed at achieving an aesthetic development of muscles (especially the chest: dorsals, pectorals and so on) by using weights and equipment (Klein, 1993). The body-building gym of today offers a "subculture of hyperbole" (ibid., p. 3). Similar aesthetically based activities were opposed to sports activities which stressed a less striking type of human being, whose muscle development was needed for resistance-based exercises like long distance running (Louveau, 1981). This more functional notion of the body was present in other historical forms of gyms, which also appear to have contributed to the development of fitness culture during the first half of the twentieth century. In the USA, for example, body-building gyms contrasted with upper middle-class athletic clubs or executive clubs with their elitism and plush surroundings as well as with more low to middle-class sports associations, such as the YMCA, with their educational goals (Maguire, 2007). Finally, as body building consolidated, stressing the masculine dominance of the gym world, new forms of exercise emerged, notably after the contestation years, which brought to the gym yet different forms of engagement with the body: they mixed exercise with dancing, popular music and fashion, and opened it to women especially from the

middle classes. Aerobics indeed rose in the early 1970s in the heavily commercialised leisure culture of the USA. This form of gymnastics marked the
entry of popular music in the gym, and potently combined pop culture,
dance and physical education. Spread by cultural icons such as Jane Fonda,
aerobics was largely designed for women aspiring to have a harmonious,
slender appearance. It contributed to the feminisation of the gym, shifting
gym culture and preparing the way to the fitness boom of the late 1970s
and early 1980s.[2] Despite its fashioning as a leisure industry, fitness is still
largely inspired by rationalisation and far away from the kind of body expression, which is typical of the anti-gymnastic movement (Bluin Le Baron,
1981), new trends are still emerging. Initially marginal, but increasingly relevant as fitness culture went global and incorporated "alternative" cultural
trends, elements of body-soul Eastern techniques, such as yoga and tai-chi,
were further drawn out of their Western contexts (the yoga studio, the martial art gym), being adapted and adjusted to the commercial fitness centre
(Strauss, 2002).

Broadly speaking, today's fitness gyms have at least *three* features. Firstly,
they are predicated on the notion of *fitness*. In ordinary language, fitness
largely means the ability to perform physical work satisfactorily; it resonates
with nineteenth-century evolutionary theory – with the leading idea of
Darwin's theory of natural selection being expressed in terms first coined by
Herbert Spencer as the claim that among competing organisms "the fittest
survive" (Park, 1994). Sexual attraction and the capacity of mating is in
many ways an under-text of today's fitness culture: even though it rarely sur-
faces in actual gym settings, it is quite often important in fitness commercial
discourse (see Chapters 3 and 6). Even more prevalent is the functionalist
outlook of evolutionary theory though: fitness is largely defined by official
bodies – from the World Health Organization to the Council of Europe –
as the capacity to face the physical demands of everyday life adequately
and without undue fatigue as well as a number of physical capabilities conducive to good health in its broadest sense (Oja and Tuxworth, 1995). As
gymnastic knowledge became legitimatised in medical quarters, and sedentary life does not work clearly as a benchmark for ordinary general fitness,
fitness has been increasingly defined via medical measurement of exercise
performance – such as the capacity of the heart, blood vessels, lungs and
muscles to function at optimum efficiency in response to a fifteen minutes
run on a treadmill. Fitness is thus strictly associated with being physically
active on a regular basis through organised exercise. As a result, the term fitness refers to both *training* in the gym (and the different exercise techniques
which are described as keep-fit devices) and the *physical condition* which such
training produces (such as energy, agility, slenderness and tone which define
a fit body). An ideal body condition, fitness is thus brought back to specialist work to be performed in a typically commercial institution, the fitness
centre. The latter presents itself as the most rational and legitimate place to

obtain such a body ideal. In this light, while the notion of the fit body is continuously shifting, the gym continues to be at the core of culture and cult of fitness: it works as the key site for the negotiation of its meanings (see Chapters 6 and 7).

Secondly, fitness gyms are indeed built on the provision of *structured variety*. The boom of the fitness industry has been matched by an equal growth in the range of workout options available. The 2007 *Time Out London Guide to Health and Fitness* list of popular workouts includes: aqua exercise, boxing training, cardiovascular machines, circuit training, combat-style workouts, core stability workouts such as pilates, exercise to music such as step and aerobics, free-weight exercise and indoor cycling including spinning. Leaving behind monolithic exercise salons devoted entirely to body building or aerobics, commercial fitness gyms are increasingly becoming integrated centres for physical exercise where it is possible to try out ever-new combinations of gymnastics and dance, yoga or martial arts. As the *2007 Time Out London Guide to Health and Fitness* suggests "over the last decade, the exercise industry has begun a process of exploration into what might be termed 'fusion fitness'. That is based on the idea that training methods from different cultures have similar objectives. At the heart of both ancient Eastern and more contemporary Western techniques is a desire for efficient, effective and aesthetically pleasing movement, together with the cultivation of flexibility, co-ordination, balance and internal energy" (p. 20). Despite their differences, most gym seems to play on variety and novelty to attract clients and keep them interested – they provide a protected environment in which each client is invited to choose between a range of physical activities presented as valid alternatives, and invited to construct a specific, personal training programme. The mixing of techniques is becoming more common among both male and female gym-goers, even though on average a gender division of keep-fit activities still holds in fitness gyms: there are few women in the weight rooms, slightly more women than men in rooms with cardiovascular equipment and predominantly women in choreographed exercise-to-music classes; men are prevalent in free-weight exercises, dominate the isotonic machines areas, and when they get into classes they prefer options such as spinning which make use of equipment (see Dechevanne, 1981; Dworkin, 2003; Sassatelli, 2000c). Aerobics is still typically a female preference (but see Loland, 2000 for male aerobicisers), while body building is, as mentioned, a more masculine technique. Yet, we must notice, both choreographed aerobics and body building involve a minority of the fitness public. In Italy, for example, only around 10 per cent of fitness participants only do body building, and only 12 per cent do mainly aerobics – the others engage to varying degree in multiple activities within the gym (Sassatelli, 2000c). Such a trend is being reinforced by the popularity of hybrid techniques – in particular spinning, combat-style studio classes or Western hybridisations of yoga – which mix male and female trends. These techniques show the current *dual* direction of the fitness industry towards *excitement*, on the one hand, and *relaxation*, on the other: to incorporate simulated activities which draw on the domestication of combat, conquest or competition to provide excitement; to include soft, body-soul techniques and pampering spaces (jacuzzi, saunas and so on) to provide relaxation. Both directions are aimed at broadening the clientele by catering for the whole life course of a prospective client.

Finally, fitness gyms reframe *discipline as fun*. When addressed to the masses to be educated gymnastics was indeed a disciplinary affair framed as duty. It is not surprising that bodywork geared to the achievement of physical capital is painful – after all in many cultures the pursuit of beauty, especially female beauty, is historically associated with sufferings of different sorts (from the corset to plastic surgery). Health also requires, we are now told, quite a bit of discipline (from regular sleep to limited food intake). Indeed, what is surprising is precisely that keep-fit exercise has become fun. This has clearly to do with the fact that bodywork has moved from the public to the private sphere, via the prevalence of the cash nexus. Fun is presented as a fundamental aspect of fitness: despite the fact that exercise demands concentration and causes tiredness, the focus is on leisure and enjoyment, rather than physical effort. As suggested by one of the most popular Italian exercise manuals, fitness gyms place emphasis on the "pleasure" of training and on the "absence of competition", while "old gyms were exhausting places, fitness centres are more gentle places, where you can do exercise in a more relaxed manner" (Castiglione and Arcelli, 1996, p. vi). The late-modern gym not only offers "the possibility of dedicating oneself to many different activities" but also the opportunity of participating in activities that are "neither sporting nor aesthetic"; they are indeed linked to the "search for physical well-being: these days, one goes to the gym to feel better and to be healthier" (ibid., p. vii). Both in Italy and Britain, gym brochures typically emphasise the "relaxing atmosphere", the "enjoyable environment", the "friendly staff" and the "enthusiastic trainers". Gym members' self-evaluation forms for training typically start by asking clients whether they "enjoy" their gym. "Enjoyment" and "fun" are taken as a measure of the success of the gym – for example, five out of eight items in a major global chain's Customer Satisfaction Questionnaire distributed in Britain in 2005 relate to pleasure, fun, involvement and enthusiasm, and the remaining three are on difficulty, safety and trainers' attention. Fitness magazines in the USA, UK and Italy similarly stress that "having fun makes exercise more effective"; they are full of tips to help readers make every exercise session "fun and easy", and suggest going to the gym with a partner or listening to one's own favourite music. Not surprisingly, time spent in the gym is defined by enthusiast gym-goers as "time for oneself" and an occasion to "let the body express itself", even though movements are far from casual and time is strictly managed by the instructor in exercise-to-music classes or by clients' reciprocal control over turn-taking in the machine area.

2. Commercial culture and bodywork

The phenomena collected under the banner of fitness have been the object of a notable amount of hype in public discourse, and have often figured fleetingly in social and critical theory as examples of the late-modern or post-modern condition in increasingly commercialised societies. Understood as a symptomatic manifestation of consumer culture, the fitness boom has been envisioned through extreme rhetorical cliché, peppered with hyperbolic images and passionate moralism. Gym culture is criticised as the incarnation of the vices of our era fuelled by the advertising industry: materialism, super-ficiality and standardisation, hedonism, dissatisfaction and even personality disorders. However, a chorus of voices has countered this rhetoric, not least the fitness industry itself which celebrates fitness training in the gym as an opportunity for self-realisation and happiness for all. In an endless swinging of the pendulum, fitness celebrators provide apologies for keep-fit workout in the gym as a global panacea for body, mind and relationships, while fit-ness detractors provide apocalyptic readings featuring gyms as the epitome of the emptiness and isolation of modern people. The development of fitness activities has either been celebrated as democratisation of sport embracing sections of the population that were traditionally excluded from organised physical activity (such as women) or it has been denigrated as being the tri-umph of consumerism (which subjugates women to traditional visions of femininity under the guise of a liberation). The mixing of physical, sportive activities with popular culture, music and fashion has either been feared as the twilight of heroic, character-building sport, or saluted as an opportunity for less stringent, health-oriented, physically active diversion.

Similar dichotomies often correspond to disciplinary specialisations in the study of sport and physical activity at large. Physical education, med-ical practice and, to some extent, leisure studies have typically played the celebratory tune, stressing the physical benefits of the fitness workout, its emancipation potential and even its psychological paybacks. In contrast, within sociology, history and gender studies there has been a tendency to view the fitness boom in a negative light, stressing its commercial nature and its disciplinary functions. As a result, fitness training has been considered an illusory and narcissistic response to a heavily standardised, profit-seeking industry and the perpetuation of heavily gender-biased images of the body.

It would be foolish indeed to deny the role of commercial images in promoting certain body ideals. Contemporary advertising has made full use of the human body to promote the most diverse goods and services, often reproducing gender biases (Wernick, 1991) and certainly working on hyperitualised images of gender (Goffman, 1979). What is more, advertising messages have contributed in turning the body into a public place, stressing the shapes, sizes and texture of its parts, representing both body maintenance routines and sexual arousal, playing with fantasies of body transformation and opening even its invisible interiors to public scrutiny via the fictional representation of medical practice and the arts (O'Neill, 1985). In all societies, certain physical characteristics are publicly celebrated and associated with high status, but they are also very often acknowledged as exclusive to the privileged or the fortunate. In contemporary consumer culture, a youthful, slim, toned, efficient and dynamic body has become a powerful image, being presented as both a matter of individual will and proof of personal and social success. In such circumstances, advertising images which urge individuals to do whatever they can in order to acquire an enviable physical appearance have become an obvious target for critical thinking, and fitness has often been read under such a stigmatising rubric.

Christopher Lasch has notably maintained that in consumer societies the rewards for constant, disciplined work on the body are no longer either spiritual salvation or wellbeing, but an improved, more marketable physical appearance (Lasch, 1979; see also Glassner, 1992; O'Neill, 1985; Turner, 1984). Lasch's argument was anticipated by critical approaches from Marcuse to Baudrillard (see Sassatelli, 2007). Jean Baudrillard (1998, pp. 129ff.), in particular, considers that "the body" has become "the finest consumer object", subject to "managed reappropriation": both "capital" and "fetish", "there is deliberate *investment* in it (in the two senses, economic and physical, of the term)" (see Bourdieu, 1977 for a different rendering, and Featherstone 1992 for a subtle reprise). The French theorist envisages elements of "puritan terrorism" in all this – "except that in this case it is no longer God punishing you, but your own body, a suddenly maleficent repressive agency which takes its revenge if you are not gentle with it ... if you do not make your bodily devotions". Such investment in the body is "narcissistic", dealing in growth, development, liberation, reappropriation. And yet, the body "is not re-appropriated for the autonomous ends of the subject, but in terms of normative principle of enjoyment and hedonistic profitability", and this normative veneer of enjoyment redoubles alienation being reduced to consumerism: "from hygiene to make up (not forgetting suntans, exercise and the many 'liberations' of fashion) the rediscovery of the body takes place initially through objects. It really seems that the only drive that is liberated is the *drive to buy*".

These now classic considerations resonate with recent works that consider investment in self-presentation via consumption as a disease of the will brought about by contemporary consumerism (see Baumann, 2007). Broadly speaking, in this view the de-politicisation and secularisation of bodywork has opened the door to a purely materialistic and ultimately vain search for physical perfection. Fitness is thus presented as a primary example of how activities aimed at caring for and transforming the body have become, as Susan Bordo (1993) maintains, "a project at the service of the body, rather than the soul", directed at purely "physical enemies" such as "fat" and "flab" rather than at gaining self-realisation. Advertising images are indicated as the prime culprit – they encourage us to pursue whatever ideal appearance might be the order of the day and make us feel inadequate in order to boost the sales of a variety of goods and services for body transformation and maintenance. In this light, fitness is not very different from plastic surgery, beauty treatments or slimming pills; it is nothing more than a body modification technique which exploits the plasticity of the body's outer shell and momentarily fills an inner void. Looking at advertising, Bordo groups together different commercially driven body transformation techniques, such as dieting, exercising and plastic surgery, as manifestations of the same ideology of body plasticity and freedom of will. Such ideology is connected with the "social mythology that ours is a body-loving, de-repressive era"; yet, she reckons, "we may be obsessed with our bodies, but we are hardly accepting of them" (ibid., p. 15). For women, exercise helps fight flab, with the toning of the female body being a response to masculine ideals of self-restraint. These ideals go hand in hand together with a general instability of the contemporary self and schizoid cultural demands for both self-denial and self-indulgence: "the slender body codes the tantalizing ideal of a well-managed self in which all is kept in order despite the contradictions of consumer culture", and its demands for both self-denial and self-indulgence (ibid., p. 201). Movie and music stars are powerful icons to imitate: just like Madonna's sculpted body "has no history and conceals the material sufferances to maintain itself" offering an endless possibility of renovation (ibid., p. 275), John Travolta toning up his body for his performance in "Staying Alive" betrays a materialistic simulation of classic male beauty: "consumer culture unfortunately can even grind playfulness into a commodity, a required item of this year's wardrobe. For all its idealisation of the body, the Greek culture understood that beauty could be 'inner' " (Bordo, 1999, p. 223).

These interpretations have met with considerable success, even though they are akin to forms of textualism which have been widely criticised as unable to grasp the lived social experiences of consumption. Consumers are not simply bombarded by advertising images, they have to decode them and will do so in different ways according to locally situated contexts of consumption (Sassatelli, 2007). Likewise, to identify commercial discourse or consumer culture with its most visible surface, advertising, draws a biased picture. How we experience the body, manage corporeal identity and participate in social rituals as embodied subjects is, to a great extent, mediated by consumer culture. But consumer culture cannot be reduced to a collection of ideological items in advertising images, rather, it should be understood as lived culture, unfolding via situated interaction in specific institutional formations that have their historical depth and their material set-up. As lived culture, consumer culture is made by living, embodied agents. A well-toned, muscular body has arguably become a hegemonic body ideal, and gender specifications certainly enter potently into this. Yet commercial images of the fit body cannot directly explain what happens in fitness gyms, how bodies, spaces, objects and relations are locally organised, and how fitness participants – both producers and consumers – actively contribute to an ongoing negotiation of the very body ideals which are at the core of the fitness phenomenon. Experimental exposure studies in social psychology continue to show that the vision of very muscular or very thin models have an immediate effect, and indeed a detrimental one, on both men's and women's body image (Dittmar, 2008). Yet, social psychology has also shown, through direct interventional studies, that actual participation in fitness activities assuages body dissatisfaction and ameliorates self-perception and body image (Burgess et al., 2009; Halliwell et al., 2009). This highlights to a gap between images and practices that stresses the relevance of situated interaction for the qualification of experience. The local organisation of experience is indeed crucial to understand how clients may get involved in fitness, and why they may consider that it is a solution to their needs (see Chapters 4 and 5). Looking at consumer practices rather than commercial images also offers a more nuanced picture of fitness culture, a picture aspiring to account for the different, varied experiences of fitness participants, including embarrassment and dissatisfaction, contradiction and disaffection.

Putting less emphasis on gender and focusing instead on class, Jennifer Smith Maguire (2007) has taken fitness culture seriously as an institutional formation. She chooses to consider fitness as an industry, suggesting that "participation in the fitness field is bound up with producing subjectivities which are *fit to consume*, in that they locate the production of meaning, identity and relationships with others in the process of consumption, and producing bodies which are fit to be consumed by others as visual representations of individual's identity, social position and subjectivity" (ibid., p. 192, emphasis added). Yet, Smith Maguire's is a supply-side book which looks at the fitness business as constituting demand. In her case, as in far too many others, what consumption means is taken from a rather static view of commoditisation and a perspective largely derived from producers. While consumers' subjectivity seems to be at the heart of her argument, in fact she looks mainly at how expert discourse from personal trainers and the fitness media shape normative views of fitness. Participants' reasons and meanings are essential, and consumption experiences cannot be left out of the picture or used impressionistically as "a means of sensitization to the ways in which the contemporary health club industry is constructed" (ibid., p. 75). To address subjectivity constitution, the ordinary mechanisms which help producing consumers through consumers' own practices must be given priority. These mechanisms are precisely what my research on fitness has been about (see, for example, Sassatelli, 1999a, 1999b, 2000c, 2003). In particular, in the present book I dissect which kind of embodied dispositions are produced through fitness training, and I consider them in the context of both the variety of body maintenance/modification techniques and the leisure and sports activities which are available on the market. This allows for a consideration of the continuous process of boundary marking through which fitness as lived culture is accomplished. Rather than offering broad theoretical injunctions, I shall provide an exploration of the ways in which fitness culture and its core consumer institution, the fitness gym, may be seen as characteristic of contemporary consumer culture. I start by considering how the main scene for the consumption of fitness, the fitness gym, is organised through clients' and trainers' co-production.

To be sure, market relations are crucial for fitness culture in so far as the fitness workout has boomed through commercial contexts such as fitness and health centres. Yet, just like affects and money are often mixed, market relations are never purely instrumental and profit oriented (Zelizer, 2004). In particular, the purchase of services or durable items, which require complex evaluations and whose actual consumption is diluted in time, thus continuously shaped by use, is strongly mediated by social networks of trust (Di Maggio and Louch, 1998). In the case of the fitness industry, promotional culture goes hand in hand with gym instructors' and personal trainers' professionalism, stressing genuine vocational qualities (see Chapter 3). A trend towards standardisation in international fitness chains and towards the diffusion of McDonaldised fitness is countered by clients' preferences (O'Toole, 2009). And clients do matter in commercial fitness. Largely influenced by promotional culture, fitness gyms put into practice disciplinary techniques of the body but attach a new meaning to the ideals of plasticity and utility. As suggested, commercialisation has changed the institutional framework of bodywork, with meaning being attributed to body transformation by "consumers" who work for themselves. Still, reference to self-care often assumes the character of a duty. As Baudrillard indeed suggested, the capacity to accomplish one's own duty towards one's body is related to status, and I would like to add, to character demonstration, or the realisation of normative selfhood. In other terms, fitness consumers are far from the sovereign consumer. But they are asked to be emotionally, physically and cognitively active in the pursuit of fitness. Much of my research into fitness has had to do with the negotiation of a rather demanding vision of consumer sovereignty as it happens in fitness gyms. I therefore could not consider that fitness participation be simply explained by one or more socially instigated motives, nor reduced to a functional appendix to a much larger gender or consumer capitalist order. Prioritising consumers' experiences, local settings and situated social relations helps in offering a roundabout picture of fitness culture as lived culture.

3. Gender and body ideals

Barry Glassner (1992, pp. 122–3) has maintained that:

> Perhaps the single greatest force that keeps men working out is insecurity. This is evident in those who exercise chiefly because they're afraid of heart disease. But almost all avid male exercisers are engaged in a passionate battle with their own sense of vulnerability. Herein lies an important distinction between men and women. For both, the key motivation to exercise is improved self-esteem, but the genders differ on what they believe produces these benefits. When surveyed as to why they exercise, women talk of accomplishment, beauty, affiliation with others; men say they're motivated by the chance to pit themselves against nature or other men and to confront physical danger. In other words, men seek to prove to themselves and others that they can survive.

Such a diagnosis points to the role of gender, gender distinctions and relations in the understanding of fitness. Often stemming from feminist concerns, and in line with a tradition of studies attentive to the gender bias in sport and physical exercise (Theberge, 1991), much research on fitness has considered it functional to the reproduction of hegemonic notions of femininity and masculinity. By and large these studies have concentrated on exercise techniques – such as aerobics and body building – which, as suggested in the Introduction, contributed to the early commercialisation of physical recreational activity. They have tended to focus on extreme phenomena whereby training becomes an attempt to escape from eating disorders, is a surrogate of personal and social realisation, and even becomes a true profession as with successful body builders. Such phenomena, while important in themselves, give a biased picture of contemporary fitness culture. Today, keep-fit training is a set of recreational but fairly ordinary practices which are very much part of everyday culture. At its core are less strenuous and more health-related exercise techniques which for most participants conjure up more reassuring and less extreme images.

Many early studies positioned aerobics under the rubric of women's domination in consumer, patriarchal societies and aimed to expose the extent to which participants incorporate oppressive forms of femininity. Aerobics was a predominantly female pursuit, often incarnated by significantly feminine icons, and it is therefore no surprise that a considerable amount of research has concentrated on the representation of the slender female body. The global success of Jane Fonda's aerobics video, for example, was interpreted as proof that women are still victims of a patriarchal regime which forces them to take an obsessive interest in their appearance (Dinnerstein and Weitz, 1998; Kagan and Morse, 1988; Morse, 1987). Women exercisers would thus spend their time in the gym exclusively for the benefit of the "male gaze" and with the effect of reproducing an alienating, commercially promoted ideal of the female body. On a similar line, other works, such as those of Gisèle Amir (1987) and Nichole Dechevanne (1981) in France, and Moya Lloyd (1996) and Joseph Maguire and Louise Mansfield (1998) in Great Britain have stressed the fact that the preoccupation with fat, associated with aerobics, can be compared to the obsession of women who suffer from eating disorders, and that continual self-observation during exercise does not free women's lives, but makes it more difficult for them to accept their own bodies. They also maintain that the growth of aerobics reinforces normative standards of femininity and once more tends towards the segregation of women's sporting activities.

Despite their critical thrust, such studies on gender and aerobics have portrayed a rather deterministic view of the reproduction of femininity and of the role of commercial institutions, such as gyms, in the process. They stress that bodywork is often conducted in the service of femininity, and consider femininity as defined by relatively narrow dominant beauty standards which may even command the obsessive, self-isolation of extreme exercise and diet (Spitzack, 1990). This overlooks the fact that women, like men, are different and that in doing voluntary recreational exercise they participate and contribute to the ongoing transformation of body and gender ideals. When dealing with empirical material, the majority of these works are largely confined to discourse, using sources such as fitness manuals, magazines and videos while neglecting gym-goers' actual activities and the meanings they attach to them. Thus, for example, we get interesting, if partial, textual analyses of women's fitness magazines, which suggests that the discourse of empowerment therein articulated is false given that rather standard views of beauty take precedence over health (Eskes et al., 1998). But in textualist approaches the voices of the fitness fans remain unheard, with the result that the analyst's reduction of their aspirations to ideological control has in itself all the characteristics of an ideological claim.

Notably, doubts concerning such interpretations have arisen from within the feminist literature itself. Ethnographic approaches have surely contributed to this, complicating the scenario. An early ethnography by Pirkko Markula (1995, p. 429) stressed the fact that "the critical voices of those who practise aerobics may change the development of dominant practice" and show that even the ideal of "curvaceous muscles" associated with aerobics is a "hybrid" between traditional, sensual feminine images and a stronger, more androgynous image. Fieldwork conducted in Canada showed that women stress the pleasures of workout, and its collective dimensions in particular: women commonly list the dance-like quality of exercise-to-music classes, its non-competitive atmosphere and moving their bodies with the group as one (MacNevin, 1999). Not only is commitment to fitness a socially sanctioned practice that stresses personal accomplishment, it can also be a rare opportunity for a woman to care for herself in a life otherwise devoted to the needs of others. Still, by and large, feminist approaches highlight that while women are no longer so patently excluded or invisible in sporting domains, new feminine physical activities such as aerobics may become ghettoes that reproduce the gender order. Thus, contributing to a collection of studies on women's corporeal experiences in sport (Bolin and Granskog, 2003), both Pirkko Markula and Shari Dworkin have suggested that women prefer cardiovascular exercise because it allows them to gain a masculine quality – strength – without transgressing traditional norms for feminine physical appearance which prescribes toned bodies rather than bulging muscles (see also Kenen, 1987; Lenskyj, 1994). Although many participants in both Markula's and Dworkin's studies rejected the unrealistic images of women featured in fitness magazines, these authors stress that aerobicisers admitted to constantly comparing their own body shape to others and to coding health mainly through thinness. They also avoided resistance training due to fears of a lesbian stigma and of being seen as a threat to men. Aerobicisers are described as yet again accomplices in constructing the female body as smaller than men's.

As the epitome of muscular masculinity, body building, both at amateur and professional levels, has also been read through critical gender theory. For example, many authors have maintained that men return to a traditional source of masculine identification, such as increasing muscle mass, precisely when they are faced with the gradual erosion of their power in the public sphere (Courtine, 1991; Ewen, 1988; Gillett and White, 1992). However, in this case as well, ethnographically based studies have been more subtle, both considering the variations in muscularity as concretely pursued (Monaghan, 1999) and showing that body building is related to the creation of sub-cultural groups where a complex and partly subversive femininity, or a traditional and yet sexually ambiguous masculinity, were reproduced. Alan Klein's ethnography (1993) on Californian body builders, in particular, showed that body building is associated with the typically masculine attempt to try and compensate for physical, cultural or economic disadvantage with muscles. But it also illustrated the economic, sexual and personal contradictions of body builders, the incompleteness of their search for masculinity, and the role of homosexual imaginaries and relations for the body-building underworld. Gay culture, muscular growth and gym practices have long been associated. They have even become the subject of popular best-selling books such as *Muscle Boys* written by San Francisco-based personal trainer Erick Alvarez (2008). A perspective on the world of female body builders and of its contradictions is provided by Maria Lowe's (1998) ethnographic study. According to Lowe, while women seem to challenge gender distinctions by deliberately increasing their musculature, during competitions they have to show their femininity by wearing jewellery and adopting ultra-feminine postures (see also Aoki, 1996; Bolin, 1992; Guthrie and Castelnuovo, 1992; Mansfield and McGinn, 1993; St Martin and Gavey, 1996).

Thanks both to a post-structuralist shift in feminist thinking and to empirical approaches sensitive to participants' meanings, a number of recent studies on aerobics and other forms of recreational gymnastics have offered even more nuanced pictures of physical activity, considering it less the locus of hegemony and more as a site for the negotiation of new and old visions of masculinity and femininity. Many of those studies are about women and fitness in the USA. Debra Gimlin's (2002) study of women's aerobics classes in the USA suggests that for many, "aerobics reduces the 'embodiment' of identity by illustrating the positive character traits that are elsewhere taken as incompatible with a flawed body. The willpower and determination implicit in participation in aerobics become more salient components of the self and the imperfect body becomes less problematic" (p. 56). Maxine Leeds Craig and Rita Liberti's (2007) study of women-only fitness gyms in the USA shows that clients and staff work at feminising the gym not only "through the continual monitoring of weight, size and body fat and in celebrations of weight and size loss" but also by sustaining "non-judgmental, non-competitive sociability (which) prevented any member from demanding that other members keep pace with the rhythm" (pp. 685–6). Leslea Collins' (2002) study of feminist aerobicisers shows that they develop a number of "strategies of distancing both to downplay uncomfortable aspects of the practice and enhance the feelings of empowerment and enjoyment which they derive from aerobics" (pp. 105–6).

Many of these studies implicitly start from the idea that expert, official or commercial discourse on fitness is important, but does not coincide with situated practices. Fitness discourse is a kind of normative repertoire which practices translate, negotiate and articulate through important variations. These variations are, in turn, taken up and reworked by fitness professionals in a continuous consumption/production dialectic. Such perspective well summarises the thrust of my early ethnographic study in two Florentine gyms (Sassatelli, 1999a, 1999b, 2000c). In that study, I showed that, while fitness gyms organise fun and satisfaction, they also harbour quite a bit of consumers' dissatisfaction and frustration. While expert discourse as well as commercial images are often reconciliatory, actual consumer practices are more commonly *disputed* – with participants having to work hard indeed to find their way through the fitness world, not always managing to transform the received, official meanings in ways that appear beneficial to them on all accounts. Body ideals of the slim, fit, toned body are negotiated and adjusted by regular gym-goers who, very often, learn to accept and even embrace what they originally thought as defects, shifting their goals from pure, and very detailed, body modification to a vision which places emphasis on self and willpower (see also Chapters 5 and 7). If, for many people who get quickly disaffected, fitness gyms appear daunting and in fact disempowering, for those who continue going, they provide a space to negotiate, rather than simply absorb, idealised visions of the body including its gender coding.

Studies on commercial forms of gymnastics and gender have fulfilled an important function, drawing attention to gender and physical activities beyond narrowly defined sports, showing the relevance of gendered body ideals and placing exercise in the context of wider social and political issues. However, with a few exception they tend to give only tangential consideration to the local organisation of training in fitness centres. On the contrary, working as an ethnographer I could start from the spatiality of the gym, as well as gym etiquette, relational codes and interaction patterns. This has allowed me to consider taken-for-granted social arrangements which are often overlooked, such as the sheer fact that these institutions are, so to speak, machines for the celebration of variety: they typically bring together aerobicisers with weight lifters, and reflect differently nuanced physical ideals trying to accommodate all. Instead of focusing on one single activity in depth, I have appreciated the hegemonic role played by the notion of fitness, its centripetal force of attraction of a variety of physical activities. I have thus problematised fitness as a specific historical and institutional construction (see Chapter 6), looking at how different activities are organised in the gym, how new activities are introduced and how gym-goers orientate themselves in such a complexity with the help of instructors and trainers. There was the need to address fitness as a constellation of exercise activities which takes place in specialised institutions such as the fitness club promoting the ideal of the fit body. Most sports may be drawn into fitness, adjusted, as it were, to its style. This style is therefore to be investigated, by considering what happens in the gym with two main cognate set of practices as a background: sporting activities, on the one hand, and body modification techniques, on the other. This book thus refuses to take a few steps which are as misleading as they are prevailing in the literature on gender and fitness: to talk of fitness training abstracting from the whole field of physical activity, to consider it as just one amongst other techniques of body transformation and to consider one of the genders more closely rather than gender relations. On the contrary, it specifies what makes fitness different from sport, athleticism in particular (Chapter 4). It considers the extent to which fitness entails a specific view of body transformation which is often predicated against other body transformation techniques (Chapter 6). And it explores in the name of which specific, normative view of self keep-fit bodywork is accomplished (Chapter 7). My work starts from the consideration that most fitness centres attract both men and women, and to a degree they even ask them to work together, encouraging both to try different exercise techniques in order to vary and continuously innovate individual training (Chapters 2 and 6). As most of the commercial fitness centres are mixed environments, it is important to address both men and women and the way they manage to share the gym space, partly reproducing, partly challenging received gender identities and differently engaging with the surreptitious sexualisation of their bodies (Chapter 3). I have thus taken gender seriously, but I have considered it as a relational, process-like feature emerging from the embedded, composite and shifting interlocking of masculinity and femininity (Connell, 2002).

4. Distinction, taste and social structure

As with most other goods and services, fitness consumption can be seen in terms of social stratification via a map that assigns participants to external categories such as class, education or gender. Data about demand for fitness in Italy, for example, show that around three quarters of those who are engaged in general physical activity in the gym are women and have an average (40 per cent) or average to high income (36 per cent); added to these statistics are body builders, who are mainly men (62 per cent) with an average (41 per cent) or average to low income (41 per cent) (Sassatelli, 2000c). On a more global scale, the increasing participation of women and the over-proportionately middle-class nature of commercial gym participation are confirmed by US and UK data. In the USA, 57 per cent of fitness club members are women, and of all members 73 per cent have incomes of more than $50,000 compared with only 40 per cent of the population managing a similar income level (Smith Maguire, 2007). In the UK, the 2007 National Audit of Fitness Consumers found that 55 per cent of gym members are women, and here again those from the lower income group are under-represented: 43 per cent of all gym members are earning more than the average gross annual pay compared with 24 per cent of the total UK population earning more than the national average (*The Leisure Database Company, 2008*). Age is certainly an important factor to consider: in all three countries club members are more likely to be young or middle-aged.

Still, these general profiles do not fully grasp the contemporary fitness gym and its specificity. We need more precise instruments to consider what characterises fitness compared both to leisure and sporting activities with fitness potential (from swimming to dancing) and to body transformation techniques (such as massage, cosmetics and plastic surgery). This is especially so, given that the majority of these activities and techniques tend to be relatively more prevalent among the middle classes, particularly the new middle classes and within those, women (Sassatelli, 2000c). If we turn to a recent study of class and consumption in Britain by Tony Bennett, Mike Savage and associates (Bennett et al., 2009), we may start to consider some of the structural mechanisms that underlie fitness participation. While differences between social groups in terms of class, education and to some extent ethnicity in participation in particular sports are not great (Warde, 2006), there appears to be a significant interaction effect between class and gender both in sport and exercise participation (Bennett et al., 2009, p. 160):

> Women who are in paid employment are more likely to do exercise. Those in white-collar occupations go to the gym or do daily exercises more often than working-class women; and this is accentuated among women in higher-professional occupations. Only 26 per cent of women in the worker-professional and managerial occupations never do exercises, compared with 69 per cent of women in routine occupations. Attending the gym is also more influenced by being younger and better educated than is doing sport. Younger, middle-class women, then, are particularly prone to do routine, "ascetic" forms of exercise.

Referring to "asceticism", Bennett, Savage and associates move in the footsteps of Pierre Bourdieu's work on *habitus* and distinction and on his early intuitions on gymnastics. In *Distinction*, Bourdieu (1984, p. 213) pointed to the middle-class, feminised nature of "the cult of health", "associated with an ascetic exaltation of sobriety and controlled diet" evident in gymnastics as "training for training's sake" (see Chapter 7).

More precisely, in his well-known essay 'Sport and Social Class', Bourdieu (1978, pp. 820ff.) suggests that the whole range of sporting activity should be considered in terms of supply providing an "explanatory model" of the way in which the corresponding demand is produced, of the way in which people "acquire a taste for sport, and for one particular sport rather than another", or "more precisely the principles which guide individuals in their choice of different sporting activities".[3] Bourdieu is essentially interested in the distribution of sports practices among different social classes. He claims that gymnastics, "the ascetic sport par excellence" – in which the attempt to "cultivate the body appears in its most elementary form, as a health cult" – responds to an "attitude towards the body", a *habitus* which is typical of the petit bourgeoisie (ibid., p. 838). With slightly different emphasis, and shifting attention to another section of the middle classes, the new middle classes or cultural intermediaries, these suggestions have been taken up by other researchers. Mike Featherstone, in particular, maintains that those who work in fields which require a capacity for representation and self-presentation, such as mass media, advertising, marketing, public relations, fashion and services, have developed a "performative emphasis" on the body. In other words, they have become profoundly aware of its symbolic value. Fitness gyms arose in order to "respond" to their inevitable "sense of insecurity, alienation and embarrassment towards their own body", as they are places where the body can be transformed in a specific way, and where, at the same time, by concentrating on themselves, participants can be freed of the stress brought on by everyday commitments (Featherstone, 1982, p. 18ff.; see also Ewen, 1988; Glassner, 1992; Le Breton, 1990).

These broad suggestions are very helpful to afford a critical perspective on fitness activities and fitness gyms, to ask questions about the structural relations of power which are inscribed into contemporary gymnastic practices as body practices that help consolidate the social structure. Yet, if we want to remain truthful to Bourdieu's early indications, if not methodology, we should explore fitness more in-depth: rather than just on structural mechanisms which may be grasped via objectified supply-demand relations, we should focus on lived cultures, or the actual, situated organisation of practices through which supply and demand are mutually organised. Bourdieu (1978, p. 821) himself observes that his explanatory model "would fail if it could not take into account the different perceptions which subjects drawn to diverse groups have of recreational activity". And to grasp such perceptions we need to get into the detail of practice, into that domain of the "infinitely small" which Bourdieu (1983) recognised that Erving Goffman had magisterially uncovered. In this book, I have thus considered fitness as a relatively separated (sub)field of practice, with producers and consumers, but I have enriched the concept of field with attention to the local organisation of practice and to consumers' contributions to ongoing activities.

A perspective on interaction and embodiment, on local relational codes, on carnal, emotional and cognitive mechanisms realised in situ, appears today as key to the study of much consumer culture. In the case of fitness, in particular, the actual mechanisms of participation and the embodied interaction order of keep-fit activities is complex enough, and productive enough, to deserve attention. A perspective on locally realised practical mechanisms is needed to complement the emphasis on structural ones for at least three reasons. Firstly, classical structural explanations are by and large far from exhaustive. Stratification studies on the frequency and loyalty to fitness centres conducted in the USA show that three main social determinants combined (age, sex, education) explain around 20 per cent of the variance in fitness participation, leaving almost 80 per cent unexplained (Park, 1996; see also Stockdale, 1989). We need sources that help us to understand what happens in the gym, as what happens in the gym may actually account for some of the unexplained. Secondly, and related to this, one of the major characteristics of these environments is a very high drop-out rate, showing clearly that in order to attend a gym you need more than a general class profile. A wealth of well-established quantitative data highlights the fact that irrespective of demographic profile or the goals which are set in relation to physical activity, more than half of those who begin a fitness programme give up after three to six months (Dishman, 1988; Robinson and Rogers, 1994). If classical socio-demographic determinants are even less able to explain why clients continue to train, reasons given by clients who abandon physical activity include the

repetitive nature of the exercises, the impersonal relations between participants and the difficulty of feeling relaxed during training, or having hoped
for a quick solution to one's problems, and consequently risking injury or
losing enthusiasm (Le Unes and Nation, 1996). Indeed, as a result of the productive experience of participation, I shall show that motivational accounts
for joining a gym are typically quite different from those explaining exercise
adherence (see Chapters 4 and 5). The latter relate more to the social organisation of gym environments and training practices than to objectified body
ideals, more to participants' fitness *habitus* than to their external, class-based
habitus.

A focus on the apprenticeship of practice, and on the local modulation of
habitus has been central to Loïc Wacquant's(2003, see also 2005) Bourdieian
study of the boxing gym. Such a focus is indeed crucial to understand fitness
culture as well. Cast as industries which entice and reproduce middle-class
demand, fitness centres can be seen as rather perverse phenomena which
will not help in the fight against a more general obesity trend in the whole
population. "Is fitness good for us?" – asks, for example, Jennifer Smith
Maguire (2007, p. 204), providing an epitaph for fitness:

> For the majority – and in particular for those lower down in the social
> ladder who are more likely to be inactive and overweight – the answer
> is not, both because a lack of capital and suitable consumption prefer-
> ences make participation unlikely, and because the private provision of
> fitness facilitate their public provision. The commercial fitness field repre-
> sents the commodification and reproduction of the problem: the already
> deeply entrenched class-based stratification of health and health-risks.

It is very apt to point to the stratification biases of a trend which, like fitness, is predicated on a universalistic and individualistic discourse. Fitness
does indeed contain elements for the reproduction of social distinction (see
Chapters 2, 5 and 7). But, if "hidden entry requirements such a family tradition and early training, or the obligatory matter (of dress and behaviour)
and socializing techniques" are crucial for elitist sports such as golf, skiing,
tennis or riding (Bourdieu, 1984, p. 217) locally realised matters of etiquette
and interaction are crucial to grasp the predicament of universalistic and
individualistic places like a gym. We thus get to the third reason why a
focus on locally realised practical mechanisms is necessary: to grasp the
power of the interaction order, its creative potential in the acquisition of
specialised dispositions which may or may not concur with broader social
boundaries. In contrast with this, Smith Maguire appears to choose a rather
structuralist and functionalist option, which starts and concludes with class
reproduction leaving very little space to explore, so to speak, what is going
on in the middle, namely how fitness training is practically organised and
external *habitus* is actively and indeed creatively negotiated via lived fitness

culture even in heavily commercialized settings. When middle-class needs are posited as both cause and effect of the phenomena collected under the banner of fitness, the result is that how fitness is practically organised in ordinary, embodied practices is largely left out of the picture. As suggested, such a supply-side perspective allows little for the contingent, concerted and contested nature of consumers' interaction.

In this book, I have tried to consider that the fitness gym, the main institutional setting which organises keep-fit activities, is inscribed in the class structure, but cannot be reduced to it. Likewise, typically organised through commercial relations, fitness practices cannot be reduced to the market. This amounts to a recognition that consumption is more than the cash nexus. And, despite its assonances with "destruction" (Wilk, 2004), consumption is indeed a creative domain, articulated with, but relatively separated from, domains conventionally indicated as structural. If income is recognised as a very poor indicator when dealing with the middle classes, the very idea of the middle class has been shown to require the inclusion of consumer as well as occupational identities (Crompton, 1996; Savage, 2000).[4] Buying a gym membership cannot be equated with participation in fitness activities in health centres and fitness facilities, nor with the quality of participation or experiences. As the sociology of consumption has shown, consumption cannot be reduced to economicistic notions of demand (Sassatelli, 2007). Consumption is a set of situated social practices through which people negotiate meanings, identities and relationships, including power relationships with producers and/or ideological relationships with expert discourse or commercial images. The local organisation of experience is crucial – we should consider the mediating role of consumer practices in defining taste and the reflexive accounts that people provide on it, rather than considering individual *habitus* as purely homologous to class *habitus*. With a structuralist notion of taste as the determinant variable there is the risk of failing to appreciate the extent to which practising fitness may provide clients with more and more varied motivational accounts, and a new disposition towards the self and the body. Nor would we be able to grasp the predicament that clients face when they drop the gym after a few sessions. Structuralist notions of taste would be too insensitive to locally generated meanings, whereas fieldwork research which focuses on participants' practices has proved useful to show that gym-going is not motivated by a single motive, static across gym careers and uniform across participants (see Crossley, 2006; Gimlin, 2002; Sassatelli, 2000c). And while expert discourse as well as commercial images are often reconciliatory, practices are disputed, with participants having to work hard indeed to find their way and thereby transforming the received, official meanings.

Following this line of thought, it becomes clearer that in fitness, as in many other cases, a logic of distinction can provide only an external view of practice – it charts, so to speak, the reciprocal relationships between competing institutions or worlds of practice, not the meanings which are important within them. For example, studies on body building reveal that those who practise this activity rarely go to fitness centres, and prefer specialised gyms. Body builders prefer to avoid fitness gyms because they see them as institutions designed to satisfy the exercise needs of middle-class professionals (Klein, 1993; Mansfield and McGinn, 1993). However, these studies tell us more about the relationships between body building and fitness than about the meanings associated with the latter. Fitness gyms are relatively mixed environments, and what is more they typically play on variety – they are perhaps more the creature of an increasingly complex class structure which blurs the possibilities of distinction and emphasises individual choice than the epitome of class belonging. Indeed, the economic barriers to attending a fitness gym are relatively contained. The initial cost is extremely variable due to commercial club stratification and the role of non-profit business. However, the minimum cost is definitely less than that required to practise other trendy physical recreational activities such as skiing, golf, cycling or tennis (Le Unes and Nation, 1996). In contemporary urban environments there are not many other institutions where one can find people from extremely different socio-cultural backgrounds – from surgeons to school students, postmen to housewives, factory workers to university teachers – spending their leisure time together. The characteristics of this being together and the kind of interactions that take place in gyms may thus help us understand how distinction is lived out in everyday life, perhaps even through its local, partial irrelevance.

All in all, this book aims to go beyond approaches to fitness which consider it functional to commercial images of the body, commercially mediated norms of masculinity and femininity, social stratification and the distinction requirements of certain sections of the population that occupy a particular position in consumer capitalism such as cultural intermediaries. These grand theoretical perspectives forget that cultures are grounded in the ordinary accomplishment of materiality and practice. They resort almost exclusively to determinants external to the field of fitness practice (gender, class *habitus*, consumerism) and consider consumers' meanings and actions ancillary to, and largely determined by, producers and the fitness industry. This book instead seriously considers the idea that "fields" or "worlds" of practice – to use either Bourdieu's or Becker's terminology – are relatively separated realities, which develop their own internal meanings and dispositions, rewards and frustrations and that consumers actively participate in the consolidation of such fields. I will show that fields or worlds of practices such as fitness gyms generate *habitus* and forms of consumer capital that can become relevant beyond the field. In the case of fitness, a relatively new sub-field, the barriers between producers and consumers are, for example, still low, and both meanings and competences acquired as consumers may be transformed into a professional career even relatively later in life, as many biographies of gym instructors and personal trainers in fact shows (see Chapter 3). More broadly, positioned at the crossroads of a variety of discourses and practices – sport and leisure, medicine and health, commercial culture and fashion – the world of the fitness gym is continuously in the making through participants' articulation of its significance and boundaries.

2
Spatiality and Temporality

"Fitness work out! You can save your heart, have better sex, improve your body and get back your good spirits" was proclaimed in 1995 on the April cover of *Salve*, one of the first Italian health and lifestyle magazines, echoing a global mantra that is repeated over and over again in countless fitness texts. Expert discourse, whether consolidated in a fitness manual or spoken by gym staff and trainers, explains that exercise is good for the body, helps to prevent illness, increases strength and vigour and maintains one's figure. Gym instructors and trainers characteristically claim that exercise is useful to "correct faulty postures" that the body "has acquired over the years", to "eliminate" superfluous "fat", to "tone" and "harmonise" parts of the body. Fitness discourse, especially as fixed in exercise manuals, is indeed a catalogue of detailed advice on how to perform bodywork, elicited by the spectre of body degeneration and complemented by broader lifestyle tips (notably on food, drink and posture) as well as heavily moralising considerations on motivation, character and selfhood. Such discourse is addressed to the individual, typically called into being as an isolated consumer by texts which play on the body-self relationship to sustain individual motivation. Fitness discourse is all about individual transformation and epiphany – work on your body to get a better, more authentic self. Yet, if we take a look at fitness workout as a practical accomplishment, rather than as a discourse, we discover that certain social arrangements are crucial to sustain whatever individual process might be in place. This is clearly the case in the core fitness institution, the fitness gym. Entering fitness gyms, we are confronted with the sheer surprise of a well-organised living culture: chaotic and yet orderly, changing and yet stable, sweaty and yet clean. The individualising nature of fitness discourse pales against the gym's necessity of providing meaningful conventions for the co-ordination of a variety of ever shifting people in a relatively small, but rather complex, space.

On the understanding that lived cultures are best grasped naturalistically in so far as they present themselves to us as ongoing practices, I started by focusing on the immediate environmental resources that fitness gyms bring into play in order to succeed as specialised institutional formations. Hoping to understand fitness participants, we need to examine what the situated interaction rules are through which the spatiality and temporality of the fitness centre is sustained. These are underlying social features of gym environments which are typically taken for granted and yet provide the basic sense of reality to the place and the activities therein. While fitness discourse is marked by reference to "nature" (see Chapter 7), fitness gyms are in many ways artificial environments. Their interiors are often quite carefully planned, equipment is to be used in certain ways and spaces are organised quite obviously to facilitate specific courses of action. In this chapter, I will show how training is sustained within the gym environment by the articulation of space, time and interaction. The gym is, to a large extent, a transformational environment, which has to help clients filter their social identities and get them in the right mood for training. The spatiality and temporality of the gym is meant to allow training to be presented as fully useful and purposeful. Spatiality and temporality are inscribed in the materiality of the fitness centre, its environmental organisation. The fitness centre guarantees relatively rigid ceremonial rules in specialised areas. Ceremonial rules are implicit scripts for participants to show, through body demeanour, glances and speech, their mutual respect or relative social position. They are crucial for the projection of local identities in interaction (Goffman, 1967; see also Elias, 1939; Garfinkel, 1956; Simmel, 1917). They are inscribed deeply into interaction patters, being often tacit and implicit, as well as embodied as forms of taste and distaste, as postures, feelings and mood.

1. A transformational environment

Following the fitness boom in the late 1970s and early 1980s, fitness gyms have been remarkably successful in presenting themselves as specialised places uniquely endowed with the capacity to provide all that is needed to get fit, healthy and beautiful. To this end they offer a number of body transformation techniques and organise them in a complex web of spatialities and temporalities. Fitness centres are different and varied, and play on their peculiar spatial arrangements and diversified service provision to position themselves in the fitness market. In Italy, as in Britain, they range from huge commercial clubs, located in wealthy and central parts of large cities, with a wealth of equipment, a swimming pool, sauna and beauty salon, to small local gyms, often much less business oriented and situated in sub-urban areas, which concentrate on a more direct relationship between clients and instructors. In an early study of the fitness market in Paris, Olivier Bessy (1987, pp. 84ff.) showed that fitness business and managers have been able to play on at least four different kinds of internal resources: "space", "equipment", "activity" and "trainers". In her recent contribution on the fitness industry in the USA, Jennifer Smith Maguire (2007, pp. 80ff.) portrays club stratification as the result of the interplay between two internally complex variables: "services" (of which price is largely a function, and personal trainers the ultimate resource) and "personality" (defined as the "feel" of the club, of which the ideal clientele as well as the physical décor are key elements). Linda Spielvogel's (2003, pp. 45ff.) study of fitness clubs in Tokyo shows the relevance of the urban/sub-urban divide: in Japan the fitness trend started in Tokyo with urban and especially very central clubs which remain often more expensive, innovation driven and with a variety of amenities not directly related to fitness (lounges, bars, boutiques); they were only later joined by sub-urban clubs that remain less expensive, but more informal and less glamorous.

Whatever the chosen taxonomy, fitness gyms rely on the articulation of material arrangements with social relations and cultural symbols to provide a world which can be perceived as uniquely dedicated to fitness. Fitness gyms present themselves as different by playing on the same variables, and we may identify some typical space-time arrangements. Access is via a hall with various gate-keeping arrangements which mark the passage to what then may thus seem a somewhat private and specialised world. The exercise areas are functionally differentiated according to the different exercise techniques performed, with class exercise rooms clearly marked out from individualised machine exercise areas. In most premises, exercise areas are formally unisex and they are rigidly separated from the dressing rooms. The latter reproduce the usual male/female distinction and allow clients to prepare for exercising. There is an increasing trend, especially in the commercial sector and in the upscale end of the market, for the development of large fitness centres that offer a pool mainly for aqua exercise, and a number of aside services, sporting plush relaxing or conversation areas, coffee shops or restaurants as well as massage rooms, saunas and beauty salons, and even providing babysitting and dry cleaning services. Still, even in the USA, smaller, non-commercial premises are important, with YMCA/YWCA, university-based clubs and municipal recreation facilities amounting to a 30 per cent share of the fitness market (IHRSA, 2006). What is more, whatever the club type, the exercise spaces are of the essence. The articulation of a particular sequence of actions that stress the exercise as the focal activity is at the core of fitness experiences. The spatiality of the fitness gym, in its turn, helps time spent training to be presented as totally useful and purposeful, its effectiveness being guaranteed by different interactions set up in each specialised area.

To emphasise bodywork, and to present itself as uniquely designed to provide the best workout, the impact of a fitness gym needs to start from its very entrance. Halls have a remarkably important role in gym culture: they set the tone of the place relative to the specific position that it occupies in the wider fitness provision. It does not come as a surprise that gym staff indicate that the first impression provided by halls is crucial for clients' self-selection, and the attitude of frontline staff is an important part of it. This is part of a larger cultural trend: the leisure industries have placed increasing emphasis on sensuous experiences as related to spatial organisation and on frontline customer care to add value to their products (Pine and Gilmore, 1998).[1] Halls are often decorated with posters that work as tacit self-identification devices for (different) prospective clients. Rules of entry are more or less strict and reflect different management orientations – typically more stringent in upmarket, exclusive clubs oriented towards client retention and looser in international fitness chains oriented towards sales promotion. Downscale gyms may have little space to provide a proper hall, but in all cases, entrance features are important. From the very beginning, through the use of various architectural devices, lighting and decoration, every premise defines its own environment and creates what managers, instructors and clients call "style" or "atmosphere".

A brief inventory from my fieldwork experiences illustrates the variety of styles enacted by marshalling entrance arrangements. For example, BodyMove in Florence is a small, inexpensive and markedly understated club, mainly frequented by low middle-class and middle-class young and middle-aged women who are friendly with the few but hugely popular exercise-to-music instructors. Its entrance is a simple glass door that leads onto a tiny lobby, adorned with photos and messages from instructors as well as clients themselves, directly facing an artificially lit aerobics room. Rather than playing on size, elegant décor and comfort, BodyMove looks very much like a converted garage and plays on informality, sobriety and a sense of community to mark the passage into its world of training. This contrasts with the entrance halls in larger, upscale clubs or exclusive chains, like Shape, again a Florentine gym. Shape is a luxurious gym, fairly expensive, with large and bright training spaces full of equipment, providing a wide range of physical activity and beauty treatments to a mixed male and female clientele coming from a wider range of ages and backgrounds. One enters Shape via a large revolving door into a small, dark room, with no photos or decorations, which provides for an experience of detachment from the external world. This small room, in turn, opens onto a huge foyer which leads to a long, narrow corridor, at the end of which one may half-perceive a natural light illuminating the wide exercise spaces. The foyer is decorated with images and fitness tips in glossy posters. Just by the rather pompous welcome desk there is a café area and fashionable clothes on display. Even at first glance, Shape appears as comfortable and professional in comparison to smaller premises, often characterised by an informal atmosphere created via the more direct participation of clients in the environment set up. Shape and BodyMove were the two extreme cases of the fitness provision in the same middle-class neighbourhood that I studied in my ethnography in the mid 1990s (Sassatelli, 2000c).

Women-only studios that are typically organised around some specific technique, like aerobics and pilates, often resemble small informal gyms such as BodyMove: the entrance is less grand and clearly marked out, the exercise spaces are more directly accessible and the restricted clientele is played upon via the elicitation of an informal community in the form of, for example, a space for clients' announcements. This contrasts with the characteristic hall of international fitness chains or, even more so, the classic entrance to exclusive clubs. For example, in 2007 the branches of one of the biggest fitness chains in two large metropolitan contexts, such as Central London and Milan, used entrances characterised by modern-techno design, large spaces, stairs and lights, as well as a cornucopia of glossy posters that show well-toned bodies and stress the health and beauty benefits of exercise while alluding to improved self-esteem and fun. It is especially in these large sales-oriented chains that images of the fit body are put on stage, captured in posters as a desired condition which is just behind the polished but fairly accessible doors of the fitness centre. On the contrary, keep-fit spaces inside university sports centres as well as local fitness gyms – to mention the two sites which I have observed in Norwich at the turn of the millenium – very rarely deploy similar images: they are typically unadorned, very straightforward and packaged with a sporty feeling.

A more subtle approach to the display of body ideals is also sported by upmarket clubs. Wellbeing, the West London branch of an upmarket British chain, downplays visual images of the fit body in favour of a more allusive, but conspicuously wealthy and sophisticated, atmosphere. Only past its spacious lobby, through a well-staffed reception desk and an electronic gate, may you have access to a members-only relaxation and social area which prelude to the real gym, which itself is completely separated from those additional amenities. Situated in a residential neighbourhood, this club offers a variety of "family" options, which are especially geared to the working mum. Even more so, Aquarius, an exclusive club right in the centre of Milan which counts among its varied clientele an assorted mix of managers, professionals and models, plays on spaciousness, designer décor, a few minimalist posters that avoid the typical mass-fitness chain aggressive body display, and more than anything, on privacy: the entrance leads to a large reception room with a characteristic game of light and stairs, the reception room is overstaffed and the whole of the luxurious gym space – studios, saunas, swimming pool, massage rooms and so on – lies beneath beautiful closed doors that show nothing of the many amenities and training options which are listed in the glossy leaflet at the desk.

To a degree, a fitness gym's clientele, and its degree of diversity, is a function of the gym's precise location in urban geography, of its managerial culture and its market positioning. Clients' diversity is especially evident in international fitness chains that occupy a middle-market position and in sales-oriented premises where client turnover is fast. But the clientele shifts during the day in most gyms, and the degree of clientele diversity follows certain recognisable temporal patterns. Each of the gyms I visited would allow for much further research on the local organisation of temporality. On the whole, though, the fitness gym has to come to terms with the fact that training is often squeezed into work day schedules. Lunch-time peak hours are busy with people working in offices especially if the premise is located in a busy administrative district. Mid-morning and mid-afternoon gym hours are often the prey of housewives, students or the retired as well as of clients employed in flexible jobs. Afternoon peak hours, immediately around 5 pm, tend to be more busy and characterised by an increasing variety of people, especially if located in both residential and working neighbourhoods. In the evening, the gym's fauna is mainly made up of regulars and fitness enthusiasts. Training scenes in these marginal time slots are, by and large, more complex. The fitness centre is less crowded, but, in a sense, fuller. You may find most of the aficionados who may be thinking of a professional career in the fitness world, the couples who make a date out of their fitness night or the gym buddies who help each other on a regular basis.

Rather than insisting on these fairly stereotyped vignettes, I shall try to account for what constitutes the fitness gym core participation experience – something that can be read in the spatiality and temporality of the gym starting from the role of gym entrances. As suggested, despite their differing features and their function as positional tools for gyms in the fitness market, halls always work as a decompression chamber which introduces clients to the world of training. They always and fundamentally work as passing devices, helping clients to enter the spirit of the keep-fit workout by framing gyms as specialised places, as a little "world apart" (Berger and Luckmann, 1966; Goffman, 1961) following their own rules and protected from the outside. They help incomers to get the impression that, as the noise of the street recedes, they are in a different reality, away from the hustle and bustle of everyday life, doing different things and focused on other concerns.

Once through the hall, lobby or reception area, many premises have either a long corridor, or a bar, stairs, set of doors, columns and plants or just a billboard with notes from staff and clients – something which further separates the actual exercise spaces from the hall, while typically allowing for the training bodies to be gazed at. Judging from observation in a large number of fitness premises both in Italy and Britain, the more exclusive the clubs are, the more private the set-up is. Aside services are also foregrounded in these clubs, which insist increasingly on pampering and relaxation. This is true especially of downtown premises in large cities, and more in Britain than in Italy – suggesting that where the logic of total provision typical of the large shopping mall is longer established and indoor socialising spaces are of the essence fitness centres may become markedly multifunctional. Yet again, spatial division within the fitness centre works to stress that whatever happens in the gym is different from everyday reality. We shall see this difference has to do with the transformational nature of the bodywork which is conducted in the gym.

As suggested by John O'Neill (1985, p. 109), advertising messages have contributed to the transformation of previously private habits into "public places": "the body and its most self-involving conducts are required to be as visible as possible, as all our bathroom, bedroom, and toiletry commercials witness" (see also Amir, 1987; Bordo, 1932; Featherstone, 1982). Such a trend has been reinforced by the development of reality TV, with shows that play on intimate relations or plastic surgery. Still, in everyday life, as opposed to the media, bodywork is hardly ever on stage and we are rarely encouraged to put our body on stage when we or professionals attend to its transformation. We do have to prepare our bodies for a number of occasions, yet typically we do that in rather private, even secretive, ways. In everyday life, there are rather private spaces for performing body decoration, cleaning, maintenance and transformation, both within the home – notably the bathroom and bedroom – and in commercial spaces – ranging from the hair salon to the nail shop, from the beauty salon to the plastic surgery clinic (see Gimlin, 2002). The fitness workout enjoys in many ways a different status, not only in the broad commercial imagery which draws on a number of Hollywood films that include training scenes, but also in actual practice.

To argue in this direction, we may look at the gym through Norbert Elias' (1939) theory of civilisation. Elias suggested that in the historical development of the West, a particular "civilised" bodily conduct has become the norm, with the shame threshold for natural functions, body fluids and body care becoming higher and higher. Body control and self-control have become "all-embracing" but also "more complex" and "highly differentiated" with spaces for the "controlled de-control of emotions", such as sport and a variety of "pleasurable" and "exciting" leisure pursuits, being organised to substitute for what is "lacking" in everyday life (Elias and Dunning, 1986). In these spaces of controlled de-control particular rules for the display of bodily conducts (that is, moves and glances) and conditions (that is, fluids and noises) are followed to domesticate the expression of the suppressed. We may add that forms of glamorisation of display further contribute to control by presenting images of appropriate display. Indeed, the fitness centre is a place where not only we are invited to listen to our body in prescribed ways rather than take it for granted, not only strenuous bodywork is carried out with a display of cheerfulness divergent from everyday reality, but also bodywork is put on stage, and in many ways glamorised through the very management of spatiality and interaction.

Fitness gyms are not so closed in on themselves as are boxing gyms (see Wacquant, 2003, pp. 29ff.). They have the feel of mainstream urban culture, rather than that of a sub-cultural site like the body-building gym (see Klein, 1993). In the frontal interstices of training – the lobby, the bar, the relaxation areas – people engage in small chat about everyday life as much as they discuss training. Topics of light conversation in these accessory areas may range from family, to work, to politics. Yet, the fitness gyms are organised to provide protected training spaces: they typically present the exercise spaces as both public and bubble-like environments where one can relax usual forms of body control, while making it work in different ways. To this end, they articulate the private/public division in quite complex ways, recreating inside themselves a more private, backside area – the changing room – which helps frame the workout as a performance. The activities that take place in the changing room are typically organised as part of a much broader sequence such as: undressing, dressing, exercising, undressing, showering, grooming and dressing again. The relevance of changing room practices will vary from one client to another. Yet the time spent there is, for everybody, an important part of their experience in the gym. In the changing room, individuals must negotiate, both symbolically and practically, their entrance into the world of fitness training and their return to the outside world. There, clients find themselves caught between everyday life as defined by their social identities, and the fitness world, with its formally universalistic emphasis on enthusiastic bodywork.

One does not go straight from the street directly into the world of exercise. Each health and fitness club provides segregated spaces where the transition from what clients do in everyday life to what they are required to do in the gym is facilitated. Indeed, changing rooms contain those transformation practices that allow the gym to be connected to the outside world on its own terms, as a space dedicated to well-organised bodywork. Decoration contributes to the cognitive function of the changing room. In many premises the area immediately outside it is filled with information, posters and images of the exercising body, while changing rooms themselves are rather unadorned, as if to offer, via tacit sensory features, a space to perceive the specificity of the place, a moment of concentration before switching into the fitness mood. Again, in most clubs I have visited both in Italy and Britain, changing rooms are often situated after the main exercise spaces, in the most internal part of the gym. In unisex clubs they are the most visible, official sign of an underlying male/female duality in what is a rather promiscuous, even though subtly gender differentiated, environment. Male and female changing rooms often stand side by side or opposite each other, with a number of posters, leaflets and decorations that stress the difference between the masculine and the feminine. In some other cases, men's changing rooms are closer to the entrance or to the weight room, with the women's being further inside the gym and possibly closer to the beauty salon. While there may be opportunity considerations at play related to architectural constraints, the prevalent location of the changing rooms is telling. The incomer will have to go through training spaces before changing and starting a workout session – this allows for forms of surreptitious spectatorship that helps in leaving the everyday world behind and get into the fitness mood. Simultaneously, fitness workout is to some degree on stage – not only portrayed in posters but also performed quite overtly in front of a flux of incomers and outgoers. The fitness gym may thus appear, more neatly, as a transformational environment where the work necessary to transform the body is glamorised, sweat becomes iconic and fatigue is no longer a self-effacing task behind-the-scenes but a publicly embraced achievement. Of course, gym etiquette, which deals with how to tame the sweaty, grunting, drained body into a polished, joyous strenuousness, becomes of the essence. As essential are the different definitions of the body which are organised within the gym in its complex spatiality.

Changing rooms have a crucial role in introducing the world of exercise, sustaining the transformational quality of the gym. However, they also become the "backstage" to the exercise areas, which as a result are reframed as "frontstage" (Goffman, 1959), despite the fact that potentially embarrassing, preparatory bodywork is conducted therein. This produces ambiguous outcomes: on the one hand, the changing room facilitates entry into the exercise areas as protected spaces dedicated to training and preparation of the body for everyday reality; on the other, it allows the exercise space to be perceived as a potential stage, with the workout becoming a performance for the consolidation of individual identity. Thus preparation for training may have a dual significance – you may want to look good for different reasons. Vanda, a woman in her thirties who confessed to me she had switched to a more upmarket club after training in an informal premise with the hope of "meeting nice people", is keen to "look good" in the exercise spaces and even uses uncomfortable support bras and tights that must remain hidden. For Vanda, who spends much time idling around the centre, other directed self-presentational concerns govern her gym style. In most cases though, clients seem to prepare to observe themselves at their best in the mirror. As Leo and Barbara put it, "looking good" during training when exercise often commands intense self-observation "makes you feel better" and "motivates you to work-out" (see Chapter 5).

2. Liminal subjects

The act of undressing, as much as that of dressing, places the individual in a delicate ceremonial position. They adumbrate a transformation whose meanings are potentially unstable – witness the fact that when at the gynaecologist's the doctor typically leaves the patient to undress in private and examines her body only when nudity is reframed as a medical necessity by the occupation of a specific position on a specifically designed medical chair. Even in highly structured passage rituals, the attributes of those who undergo a transformation are necessarily ambiguous – they are "liminal"

subjects in that "they find themselves between and within the normal circumstances designated to them by law, custom and convention." (Turner,
1969, p. 95).[2] The liminal nature of the changing room is obvious, too:
clients find themselves between what is relevant in the training spaces –
the gym core – and what is relevant in everyday reality. Liminality is furthermore stressed by the organisation of fitness gyms. A typical fitness gym
changing room does not resemble other private spaces, such as the bathroom, in which the individual has full control over those who enter. Nor
a classical backstage, such as team sports changing rooms, where shared
meanings help govern the situation. This is clearly connected to the fact
that fitness centres articulate universalism and individualism – clients from
different walks of life are encouraged to come and go according to their own
daily routine and preferences. Certainly fitness centres organise activities so
as to cater for different categories of people at different times of the day,
and self-selection intervenes in homogenising the clientele. But especially
at peak hours in the gym there are so many different courses, activities and
people that as a result the changing room is rendered a somewhat hazardous
place. Participants can feel naked, not so much because they actually take
off their clothes, but because undressing happens in a ceremonially unstable
situation. The ongoing, unpredictable coming and going of different people
in the changing room and the lack of synchronisation between clients when
changing leads to ambiguity: liminality becomes reflexive.

Changing room practices are fundamental for most fitness participants,
even though in some cases they try to minimise the time they spend there.
This is partly a function of the changing room being a place where it is
difficult to relax (Sassatelli, 1999b). Some of the dissatisfied clients I have
interviewed as well as the disillusioned gym quitters indeed mentioned
their difficulties to adapt to what they perceive as "crowded", "unfriendly"
or "intimidating" changing rooms – places where, says Maria who has
stopped going to the gym after gaining a substantial amount of weight
following pregnancy "you feel obviously looked at ... what I fear the most
now, it's not training, as I know I can do my routine pretty well, it's
my naked body being exposed as it is: just a fat naked body". Changing
rooms are not so much anti-structural spaces where the normal conventions of everyday life are subverted. They are rather ambiguous places,
whose interaction resources are highly unstable and where the cultural
de-classification which preludes transition is typically experienced individually. Clients deploy a mix of different *risk-management tactics* which are
more typical of public spaces than of private situations. These are ceremonial tactics which help clients limit the danger of being exposed to
ridicule for characteristics that may be salient, out of place or otherwise
embarrassing.

Self-absorption is probably the most prevalent tactic. The majority of clients
undress facing a wall or a mirror, avoiding the gaze of people nearby and

blatantly concentrating on their activity with a distant face that suggests contacts will be perceived as disrespectful. The success of such a tactic in removing the dangers of ceremonial exposure is limited, especially as it co-exists with more active tactics such as overt display or the promotion of an interaction team. In the first instance, a client appears to perform her activity as if on a stage, making comments, looking for people around, and generally trying to control other participants' attention by drawing it to herself. In such a case, far from being dedicated to exercise preparation, the changing room becomes the place for the display of backstage activities which are normally hidden and intimate. More typically, however, making oneself the centre of attention helps to promote informality and elicits support from other participants. In this case, those who initiate a verbal exchange tend to solicit a trusting complicity, typically evoking physical exercise as something that officially defines their presence in the gym. Here is a changing room scene from my field notes from BodyMove, Florence:

> The changing room is crowded now that the women who have finished training with Meg are coming in. We have no space. Vera, the middle-aged psychiatrist who I talked to yesterday, is there. She is all excited, looks at the person next to her and with great indifference to her total nudity, then she says something about how tired she is: "I deserve a slice of a chocolate cake now, don't you think, it's been tough". The women around her, some younger some older, all regulars at Meg's class, quickly start a conversation, they busily continue to attend to changing, cleaning, using creams and so on, but now they joke together partly self-mockingly, partly pleased on the pains and rewards of training. I squeeze a bit more into my narrow space, and I notice Rosa, she has come with Libera, her mother, this is her first time. She is waiting for the class to start, looking somehow embarrassed by their intimacy. She has come in with a bulgy gym outfit on, and only changes her trainers.
>
> (Female changing room, Florence January 1995)

The development of what one might call a *backstage team* often occurs around very popular classes that are attended by a relatively stable group of clients. Going at regular hours, in specific days may thus become, for many clients, a risk-management tactic that simultaneously works as a moti-vation device. Augusto, who has resolved to go to the gym on his doctor's advice after a "heart scare" says that "being with people who look famil-iar" is helpful to "keep going", to get over the "boredom" of training and the "embarrassment" of the changing room. Indeed, the creation of local teams, both in the changing room and in the exercise spaces (see Chapter 3), fosters complicity and informality, the possibility of sharing mean-ings and developing mutual recognition. Still, it also promotes relatively exclusive groupings which might make other clients feel excluded or distracted.

Part of the changing room ambiguity rests precisely on its two-way, asymmetrical and unsynchronised transformation practices. We get a mix of *change-in* and *change-back* practices: some fitness participants prepare for training, and the gym strives to offer them the symbolic and material toolkit to get into and perform training; others change back into their normal clothes, thereby liberating themselves from the mindset needed for physical exercise. This stresses the liminal nature of changing room practices – while before training clients are supposed to distance themselves from their social roles and obligations and get into the spirit of fitness which is locally provided, washing, dressing and grooming are a demonstration of cultural competences in returning to the outside world. The change-back practices allude to clients' specific identity requirements beyond the gym. Ethnographic experience suggests that regular clients and fitness fans spend relatively longer in the changing room. Different change-back routines, for example, are often perceived by regulars as the natural option for an adequate return to external reality and the final touch to a good training session: "to take a shower and get dressed properly is necessary if one wishes to go back to the office looking decent" says a middle-aged medical doctor, while a well-to-do mother of two considers a "simple routine", entailing the succession of "a shower plus applying cream all over the body, a precious reward for hard workout".

Not every regular client is comfortable with elaborated changing practices though. Contrary to a diffuse stereotype, quite a few women in particular seemed concerned with cutting down preparation time, partly "not to make a big deal of the gym". This is consistent with what Maxine Leeds Craig and Rita Liberti (2007) have shown in their excellent work on women-only gyms in the USA: one of the features of these gyms that is most appreciated by clients is the fact that, unlike conventional gyms, they "provide minimal dressing rooms and no shower and women wear clothes that could be for shopping at home or in a casual workplace" (ibid., p. 683). In their view, this makes the scene more comfortable to women whose bodies will not fit into fitness wear that is designed for slender, younger women.

As in-between places, changing rooms both filter and respond to clients' gender and professional status. This results in a remarkable variability as to the kind of changing facilities provided by different fitness premises. It is especially the large, often very luxurious changing rooms afforded by upmarket health and fitness clubs which invite elaborate pampering practices: activities conducted there include showering, applying creams and deodorants, combing hair, applying makeup and so on. Not surprisingly, these facilities are deemed most important by people whose ceremonial requirements in everyday life are most stringent – such as professionals. Anna, a stylish, professional woman in her late thirties from Milan, offers an example of her shifting outlook on fitness premises as she moved away from her penniless student years into her successful professional persona:

> Q. So your way of keeping fit has changed over the years?
>
> A. I have always trained somehow. I went regularly to the swimming pool when I was a child and a teenager, a city council one, quite a good swimming pool, with good trainers, even if it was crowed, but then you didn't care. Then, as I turned thirty, my job became more demanding, my body was changing, and I went to several gyms, doing a mix of low-impact and yoga. Now I do pilates, with a personal trainer, once a week, in a very good place. It's like you get accustomed to nice places, with all the comforts, large, private changing rooms, and a sauna, and you get the money and the status now, while you never get the time to relax. I am not that kind of person, but I guess that my old swimming pool would look different to me now, I have become picky, I wouldn't like to fight for a place, or queue for a shower.

On the other hand, students, lower middle-class participants or working-class fitness enthusiasts generally describe the small, even tiny and uncomfortable changing rooms which are provided by informal gyms or low-market premises as "straightforward", "no-fuss", "simple" and "all that you need" as opposed to larger ones, which seem "posh", "pretentious", "fussy" and above all "useless". Far more than what happens in training spaces, the changing room is symbolic of class-based stratification within the fitness market, it spells out the positioning of each gym and works as a self-selection device for the clientele. But what the changing room is about also relates to how participants may be able to look at the spirit of training. Elaborate changing practices stress the seriousness of training, and one's own commitment to it. Thus, coming from different walks of life, the women studied by Leeds Craig and Liberti (2007) liked to avoid gym-specific outfits and long preparation also because they were keen to downplay ability and training performance in favour of a heavily feminised sociability made of non-threatening support, the pursuit of "niceness" and the suppression of competition.

3. Structured variety

Through the management of space, different fitness premises suggest what may be adequate gym preparation by putting different emphases on what is required during training. Fitness workout in the gym diverges from body demeanour in everyday life: men and women are encouraged to drop external body definitions to get into the world of training and there is the need for adequate exercise preparation. However, the transition from the changing room to the training spaces is structured by the articulation of different exercise techniques in different spaces and time slots. Again, the spatiality of the fitness centre contributes to the exercise areas being perceived as what really matters, with time spent exercising being presented by many instructors as "quality time" – perhaps just 20 minutes, yet concentrated to the point that the short duration is compensated for by high intensity. Training demands and often obtains from clients the demonstration of a willingness to concentrate, more or less without interruption, on the training body. To boost concentration, the spatial organisation of exercise areas is arranged through the separation of different body techniques.

Contemporary fitness gyms offer a range of different exercise techniques which may be roughly divided into two main types: individual training with various machines (isotonic and weight-lifting equipment focused on the strengthening of specific body parts or endurance equipment focused on cardiovascular efficiency) and group training (focused on endurance as well as toning and flexibility, including free-body choreographed techniques such as aerobics, equipment-aided techniques such as spinning, and postural exercises often carried out in small groups such as pilates). As suggested in the previous chapter, each technique has a different historical genesis – strength training with free weights emerges from the century-old tradition of body building with its links to puritan body discipline, muscular masculinity and the American dream of individual success embodied by figures such as Arnold Schwarzenegger (Green, 1986); endurance exercises reached the masses through aerobics, a group exercise-to-music technique which was primarily related to women who sought a slimmer body and a more active self and became a hit especially thanks to Jane Fonda's videos (Morse, 1987). From this point onward music has become an integral part of fitness training more in general, being central to exercise-to-music classes. We may add to this that the latest tendency in the fitness industry is the introduction of a third type of activities of a different, less "sporting" type. This is the so-called "wellness wave", where the activities offered are mainly about wellbeing (such as spa-baths, saunas and the like) and relaxation (such as in some yoga combinations). Therefore wellness concentrates on enjoyment and relaxation, on balance between the body and mind. Many fitness gyms, especially large commercial chains and upmarket clubs in metropolitan contexts, incorporate some of it (see also Chapters 6 and 7).[3]

Whether they are the latest fitness craze or a long-established exercise technique, individual and group training entails quite different spatialities – space and interaction management differ greatly and are therefore organised in separated territories. Despite the fact that fitness discourse on training is mainly structured around body objectives (toning, losing weight, building muscles, getting a better posture and so on) the main spatial division in the fitness centre is between group and individual training, with wellness areas occupying, when present, a third, different space, often framed as a "treat" after training. Gym etiquette requires that gym-goers sustain the official focus of attention, namely the workout they are performing. In group and individual training, clients concentrate on their workout by following openly different ceremonial rules, either by acting in unison with others, or by ignoring them. The territorialisation of both collectivisation and individualisation of training helps by providing a clear perception of the exercise rhythm.

Group exercises are typically conducted in dedicated areas of the gym: the spinning room, for example, which is often a rather small room crowded with bikes; the aerobics studio where, at different times, a variety of exercise-to-music instructors lead not only classic aerobics sessions but also a variety of classes such as step, pump, pilates, low-impact, stretching and so on. Large premises have several studios and may dedicate one or more of them to postural techniques, body-soul combinations of fitness with yoga, or to martial arts and combat techniques. This further spatial separation inserts further complexity in the fitness centre, which allows for a variety of participation patterns and increases both the flexibility of the institution and its alienating potential.

Whatever the specific technique, the various forms of group gymnastics are structured in such a way that the instructor demonstrates, both visually and verbally, the movements to be completed, and continually urges the participants on, encouraging them to do their best.[4] The instructor adopts a fundamental role in class by setting the rhythm, counting the repetitions as they are performed and, what is more, choosing the accompanying music – something which is an important feature of each and all classes. Even in pre-choreographed classes, where instructors just apply a branded, standardised exercise format, their role in interaction is crucial. Crucial is what is perceived by clients as their "personal way" of interpreting their role (see Chapter 3). In group exercises, instructors are considered unanimously fundamental by clients, and many of them try to organise their training schedule in order to work with the particular instructor they like. Clients are supposed to arrive as the class starts and stay for its duration. Each client will have to try and reproduce the movements proposed by the instructor. A shared focus of attention and synchronisation are of the essence – while it does not entail friendship or team spirit, it is a major interaction and ceremonial requirement which allows few distractions and affirms the reality and importance of the workout. Regular participants in a class may not identify themselves with the rest of the grouping, partly because class composition is largely shifting. Yet, they will typically recognise and acknowledge the presence of other regulars, and will try to keep to specific positions inside the classroom. The spatial element of keeping to a routine appears to be essential for regulars in all the gyms I have studied. In their words, regular gym-goers try to get in early, so that they "get the same spot in the class", they "like to be close to the trainer and the mirror, to see every movement very well", they "avoid the last row, it is so distracting to have all those people in front of you". Indeed they are helped in this by the fact that an apparent feature of the newcomers is their difficulty with gym spatiality: small details in a class – such as the distance of the mat from the step or the position of a step facing the mirror – may cause difficulties which disrupt the normal course of training. As a result, newcomers often opt for back or interstitial positions and must be given special attention by the trainer. Such a dynamic does not always lead to a harmonious happy ending. Some regulars complain about classes which fill with too many people because newcomers are "disruptive"; some newcomers find the special attention they tend to receive from the instructor "embarrassing", others find it "insufficient". As it is evident, there is always a strong element of contingency in a fitness class. For trainers the management of this contingency is an important part of the job, and they may develop elaborate ways to self-monitor their responsiveness to it (see Spielvogel, 2003; see also Chapter 3). For clients, the capacity to feel part of a fitness class as well as to look at oneself in the mirrors that reflect a broader group image of mimesis (of the instructor) and co-ordination (among participants) are crucial features of group-training participation. Regular clients are typically more reflexive about this, while tending to perceive training as an involving, taken-for-granted routine (see Chapter 5).

In contrast, machine-based workouts are highly individualised and individualising and a crucial feature of machine training is the capacity "to put one's own body to work together with the machine", as an enthusiast declared.[5] The flexibility offered by machine exercise, including the freedom to go and train whenever one feels like it, is paid for by the absence of a shared focus of attention with a class and the motivational help of a class leader. Typically, in the machine area clients are isolated and spread out across its different sub-zones of cardiovascular workout and isotonic machines. Cardio equipment – such as steps, bikes and treadmills – are typically the shop-window of most fitness centres, often occupying large areas close to the entrance. Arranged in rows placed in front of a window or, increasingly, TV screens, these machines are designed to be used by clients on a self-service basis: each client can set up the machine, personalising it to their weight, self-assessed level of fitness, desired workout time and so on. But it is mainly the machines' geometry that stresses individualisation and limits sociability – something which is reversed in some women-only fitness chains where machines are set in a circle and women exercisers are engaged in small talk by an exercise leader that stands in the middle (Craig and Liberti, 2007). Self-engrossment and the selective removal of sociability are emphasised by many clients who spend a large amount of time with cardio equipment. They typically choose to plug into one of the channels available, or listen to their MP3 player. Contrary to class exercises where collective attention is channelled on mimetic exercises, individual training with aerobic equipment is often a multi-media, multi-focus experience, where body and mind may be separated, and different senses are stimulated. "Jogging," says Robin, a young American who is studying for an MA in London, "is quite boring, and may be dangerous and dirty, I really hate that. Here I manage quite a bit of running, I can focus on MTV as well as get my MP3 player, you know, I can keep my mind occupied, and my legs just run. I may occasionally take a look at myself, but otherwise there's not much to worry about, just keep going and fill your ears and eyes with stuff." Occupying one's own mind while training helps project an impression of self-absorption that is functional to the individualisation of space, and allows the introduction of mimetic fantasies, something that several gym-goers reported. For example, Mike, a middle-aged university professor from London, considers that he could not train without his MP3 player. He plays "only music which I consider strong and fast…I get upset if halfway through the album there is a ballad, though I guess actually this gives me a useful pause to slow down in a 40 minute session. I try and close my eyes and, in effect, dance which must look a bit odd to others" (see Chapters 4 and 5).

Reliance on fantasy is less possible with isotonic and weight-lifting machines, which are typically used in a sequence, for limited repetitions each. Here, the workout requires much more attention to both one's own body to check posture, and to other participants as equipment is shared in fairly unpredictable ways and used in turns. Turn-taking in the use of machines is especially pressing with anaerobic equipment – it allows for elements of sociability, but also accounts for tension among clients, who may go so far as to adjust their fixed training sequence in order to avoid contacts. The gym instructor, rather than accompanying the client, performs a mainly introductory role in both aerobic and anaerobic exercises with machines. Gym instructors here are in charge of an induction session, during which they demonstrate the correct use of the equipment, leading novices around the gym, designing a training sequence based on their expressed objectives, correcting posture, advising on the number of repetitions to be completed, the weights to be used and so on. After this first session, the instructor will take a back-seat role and clients will be expected to train and use the exercise equipment on their own. While the instructor remains typically on hand and, occasionally, will walk round offering small talk and advice to clients, the continuation of the exercise depends on each client's ability to isolate themselves from others and focus their attention on the workout using the machine as benchmark and stimulus. Mutual expression of "civil inattention" (Goffman, 1963a) punctuated by courtesy in turn-taking and an overt representation of self-absorption in exercise performance dominates in this individualised territory which appears to accommodate many different individual exercise goals and a variety of individual training schedules.

The organisation of different techniques in spatially differentiated areas helps project the idea that the fitness gym is a comprehensive place, that it contains a well-organised variety. Indeed, that it provides *all that is needed for fitness*. Managers are keen to structure variety in time and space so as to offer what Luca, the manager of a well-established, upscale fitness centre, defines as "a fulfilling experience, a 360 degree fitness workout". Increasingly fitness training draws on cognate areas – such as sports, martial arts and dance – to provide different blends of aerobic and anaerobic, free-body and equipment-based exercises. As Shawn, an Australian-born personal trainer who works in London, claims, "now things have got quite complicated and in my opinion they don't need to be necessarily this complicated. There are so many different types of trainers now...In the gym I work in every single trainer is doing something a bit different." The continuous introduction of new techniques and the role of trainers, both as gym employees and as self-employed personal trainers, in pushing innovation and differentiation forward is clearly a feature of today's fitness industry. "You get a new fad every year, most come from the US, but it's also a feature of the fitness industry as such – each of the best instructors everywhere offer their special workouts, trying to imagine new ways of getting people involved", says one of the key fitness entrepreneurs in Italy.

An impression of variety is reinforced by trainers who insist that all clients are expected to find or discover "their own way" to train, and to do so by using the various alternatives available. In their manner of speech, preference for different techniques is presented as a "personal choice", as a selection from a range of valid techniques of what is "best for each person". When a trainer proceeds with the "fitness test" on a new client, or when the gym staff approaches a new client with the fitness application form, trainers and staff emphasise both *variety* and *equivalence* of activities: most typical is a litany suggesting that the vast assortment of techniques are all finely tuned to fitness, albeit differentiated to cater for individual needs. Although different in terms of the individual resources they call forth and the physical qualities they promote, the activities of a fitness gym are portrayed by trainers as "equally good" and "positive", effectively "available" to each client to ameliorate their bodies. In the gym, the possibility of choosing among different techniques is concretely underlined by some apparently obvious *minutia*: all techniques are easily accessible; their place on the timetable varies over the week; small notices in the hall promote new techniques or machines, new options are the object of much promotional attention and so on. Above all, the selection and/or combination of different techniques is symbolically supported by all of them being presented as close substitutes, that is, sound, guaranteed alternatives. In this way, the fitness gym seems to offer a wide range of "safe options to choose from": different possibilities, all valid and useful, which each participant must evaluate according to their own personal needs.

The many activities, spaces, techniques and instructors available in a gym may be perceived differently by different clients, as a function of their participation. Some of the quitters I managed to talk to also stressed the gap between what they perceive as their simple, straightforward needs and what they consider as an unnecessary "show of equipment" and a merry-go-round of "exercise fads". These clients appear to perceive more acutely as artificial and alienating the concentration of slightly different and ever changing body techniques in what remains for them a difficult territory. Clients who attend irregularly or limit their participation to one single technique, often feel "insecure" and unable to command the surrounding environment, perceiving variety as puzzling. They often shy away from most spaces and limit themselves to one area of the gym. Libera, a middle-aged clerk who regularly follows just a couple of classes of low-impact aerobics a week, maintains that she really avoids machines. Explaining her feelings, she reckons that in her gym "the exercise machines are always occupied and, on top of all that, I'm not too sure how to use them. They're in another part of the gym and, really, I never feel at home there. I always pretend that [the machine area] doesn't exist." Libera's attitudes reflect the persistence of a gender division of keep-fit activities and spaces (see Chapter 1).

Still, in the fitness centres I have visited, women had started to participate in machine activities, although to varying degrees. And exercise-to-music group activities were a feminine province to which men were increasingly drawn. When they worked in a class, in general, men preferred pilates and yoga combinations or indeed spinning as opposed to the most choreographed options, such as aerobics, which remain feminine at their core. But, by and large, regular male clients often suggested that exercise-to music is also "important" and "classes are fun". Similarly, regulars among women did a variety of exercises with the machines, even though more often of an aerobic variety such as pedalling on a bike or stepping on a stepper, while avoiding exercises with a strong iconic masculine connotation, such as free weights or weight-lifting. As for men, though, the general perception among female clients was that "machines are useful". The verbalisations of two regulars from Florence well illustrate these points:

> First, I do power-building exercises [with weights] and then exercise in a class. I keep my body in fairly good shape and don't have real problems with putting on weight, even though initially I found it a bit difficult because it's a more feminine type of exercise and centres around co-ordination, but I find it really useful because it's aerobic. You do more movements and you need to concentrate more.
>
> (Civil servant in his late thirties)

> [With machines] you work on a different muscle group every day, so you work on every muscle in the body. I don't want to be either too thin or

too muscular... You see someone who's quite thin and you look her up and down, and I don't want people to look at me like that, I want to have muscles.

(Clerical worker in her early thirties)

These verbalisations open the way to a discussion of gendered body ideals (see Chapter 6). But they also help us figure out the role of variety. While irregular clients or, even more so, quitters consider variety confusing, regular gym-goers typically come to master it (see Chapter 5). As we shall see again while exploring successful initiation, dedicated clients are generally quite familiar with the different activities and areas in their gym. They are normally the first to take advantage of innovations and they feel relatively in control of the gym environment; even when they are not interested in new techniques, they typically relish the gym because it makes an effort to be "varied", potentially "rich in new and diverse activities" and, therefore, always "stimulating". The rigidity (of movements, schedules and so on) of each specific body technique in the gym is matched, for these clients, by a horizon of combinatory freedom. Enthusiasts insist on the possibility of using relatively rigid elements of training in a multitude of different personal combinations, describing their combination as something of a "personal achievement".

4. Complexity and contradiction

In many ways, the gym is an institution that *trains participants to train*. By and large, the organisation of quite a complex articulation of places and activities, interactions and identities is geared to push clients to concentrate on training, attain some functional distraction, try out many different work-out techniques, choose what they like and *keep going* (see Chapter 3). When clients enter the fitness centre, they have to learn to distance themselves, at least partially, from their external roles and social obligations; ideally, they must concentrate all their attention on what is relevant inside the fitness world. This may entail a partial, official filtering of those social attributes which should not interfere with training – including class, gender, sexuality and ethnicity. The fact that training preferably requires a "uniform" which is essentially defined by each specific physical activity suggests that within the confines of the gym, the relevance of broader social differences between clients are, at least formally and temporarily, suspended. True, gym outfits not only reflect the dynamics of fashion but also negotiate wider social identities as defined by gender and class. Yet, in most cases, clients will somehow adapt to, or even take advantage of, the exercise-specific requirements – with, for example, some of the few male participants in choreographed exercise-to-music classes daring to wear brightly coloured cycling shorts. When outfits are markedly in contrast with external identities, such as in the quoted example, this may even entail the negotiation of participants' gender identities (see Chapter 6). Leo, a heterosexual professional in his thirties with a passion for acting, claims that only through step-aerobics training, for which he has resolved to use a fitting black unitard, has he learnt to appreciate different facets of his otherwise traditional masculinity:

> not just muscles, not just strength, but also somehow the beauty of co-ordination and dance, which is strength and power, but combined with grace...not typical of a male, perhaps, but then, you see, ballet dancers do this and have the strongest bodies, very masculine.

Most clients, especially those who take training seriously, tend to highlight the symbolic importance of changing into gym-specific clothes. Changing into gym outfits works as a "clue" or a "key" (Giddens, 1984a, pp. 376–9; Goffman, 1974, pp. 560–76) to training, helping people get into what they describe as "the right mood" for the exercise. Not surprisingly, the majority of clients' descriptions of their gym experiences include a detailed list of micro-activities carried out in preparation for workout. For example, Libera, the previously mentioned middle-aged clerk who shies away from machines, believes that in order to enter into the "spirit of the gym", one needs to be in the "right frame of mind" by allowing for exercise preparation: "You have to take your time," she says, "I always go on a quiet afternoon. I like going there on foot...and undressing slowly, as if I'm preparing for an important job I have to do...and I have my outfits and all". Carmelo, a middle-aged surgeon who follows a rather demanding strength and cardiovascular routine, is adamant:

> To train properly you have to leave all your problems behind. When you arrive and you undress, you're already beginning to distance yourself. Then you take your time to change and you're ready for the gym...maybe that's why when I had to stop training [owing to injury], I looked nostalgically at my [weight-lifting] belt.

As these words underline, gym outfits – trainers, sports bags, leotards, workout pants, t-shirts – manifestly work as a *fitness identity toolkit*: they help clients enter the world of training with the right attitude, they are both a catalyst for fitness enthusiasm and a reward for fitness participation. Yet, the reliance on objects which are most typically purpose-made commodities has a sociological significance which goes well beyond their role in the fitness world. These objects draw clients into a commercialised world, where fitness participation may be mediated by the purchase of a variety of commodities. Thus, they may draw people in a spiral of consumption, which stretches well beyond outfits to include equipment, supplements, magazines and so on. To be true, this spiral may not be related to actual participation. On the contrary, some leavers, especially among the wealthy, suggest that they "have bought all that is needed" for fitness, and nevertheless did not manage to stick to training. For them the gym outfit clearly has become "sterile ownership" (Simmel, 1990), an object that has remained useless, whose meaning is typically attached to a sense of disillusionment and distance, perhaps to be reappropriated in everyday life and put to purposes other than gym-going.

Yet to say that the provision of dedicated outfits is merely functional to the generation of business would be a very crude, functionalist dismissal of how fitness participants go about their practices. I have met with clients who buy fashionable gym items, some use them to show off body improvements, some consider them a reward for their capacity to stick to a training programme. But on the whole, I have met with as many people for whom fashion considerations are secondary to training discipline. Furthermore, for many clients evocative items are not necessarily the latest fashion in sportswear. For example, Lindsay, a middle-aged lecturer who after a rather active youth now trains twice a week doing low-impact aerobics at her university sports centre, says that she has

> bought nothing, really, just for my class. I sort of bought – only after a while – nice trainers, but I use them also elsewhere and then I just wear an old fashioned pair of leggings which I love much and make me go back to my youth ... what counts is that you enjoy yourself and that your class becomes a routine, you do not need expensive outfits for that. I like this class because there is very little of that fashion show-off that people associate to aerobics, you know ... Fitness is fashionable nowadays, it's like you must enrol in a health club if you are to be cool, the right kind of person, but training is something else, you do it for yourself rather than for showing off, and I like to play it down, like the outfit, the gadgets, because it keeps me down-to-earth, normal ... just fitness you know.

The words of this client delineate one of the central contradictions articulated by the fitness gym. The fitness gym is caught in the wider paradox characterising Western consumer culture – *commoditisation* and *de-commoditisation* are constantly dialectically intertwined in so far as subjects perform their identity through commodities as different from commodities (Sassatelli, 2007). In consumer culture, commodities have been given the fundamental role of objectifying cultural categories, of tangibly fixing meanings and values (Miller, 1987). Yet, we must come to terms with consumerism, to signal our distance from commodities and our being in charge, autonomous and authentic. Thus, very often, consumption is about the selective appropriation of meanings from the world of commodities, it may involve gift relations, sacralisation, sobriety, recycling and so on. One of the most interesting findings of my fieldwork, and which became clearer and clearer as I went to different premises and learned the fitness biographies of a variety of participants, is that motivation is achieved via open negotiation with commoditisation and consumerism. Individual motivation is something that most clients as well as instructors consider at the core of fitness. It is what makes people train, which in turn legitimates the auspicial body changes and bears witness to the moral superiority of the fitness devotee (see Chapter 7). Even gym instructors and personal trainers, who clearly have a role in mediating between standardised production and individualised consumption, need to present themselves as professionals – they may thus offer advice on fitness commodities, but do so by taking some distance from the process of commercialisation, emphasising neutrality and vocational qualities (see Chapter 3).

The complexity of fitness gyms may be further appreciated by looking at another challenging paradox: the fitness gym is typically a commercial, universalistic institution which plays on *inclusion,* yet training needs individual motivation, something that may reintroduce hierarchies, differences, exclusivity and ultimately *exclusion.* As we shall see, there are basically two levers which can be marshalled in order to keep a balance between these two tendencies: relationships and bodies. Considered as webs of relations, gyms appear to be institutionally organised so as to facilitate involvement in training while providing secondary benefits and aside motivations via various forms of light sociability (see Chapter 3). For example, both in the changing rooms and during classes, it is quite common to notice that regular participants form cliques that exchange friendly comments. The formation of a gym team, fleeting as it may be, may work very well as a resource for continuous attendance as it helps combat boredom and anxiety. Those teams are typically locally generated, and contribute to the impression that the gym is a place where you can find a broad variety of people who work together on their fitness independently of their external social roles or their gender identities. Still, teams may introduce hierarchies or closure which alienates prospective clients, newcomers or simply those who are not their obvious members. Gym staff have a crucial role in managing interaction among clients, facilitating a relational tone that keeps exclusion at bay while providing a sense of inclusion and reward for successful participation. As suggested, in the frontal interstices of a fitness centre, that is, the margins of exercise areas, corridors and foyers, we may find clients talking about matters which have nothing to do with exercise. These exchanges typically occur between regular clients, loyal to a club, and appear to provide these clients with both a sense of ease in, and attachment to, the place (see Chapter 5). However, such exchanges remain marginal in the emotional economy of the gym which is on the whole characterised by rather detached forms of courtesy. Inclusion in gym activities is itself quite paradoxical as it must provide, as many clients say, an experience of detachment (see Chapter 4). As a keen gym-goer such as Marica exemplifies:

training is not just about keeping in shape but also about relaxing and forgetting everyday worries that go along with work and sometimes with your relationships with other people. Coming here is like retreating into a little corner of the world where no one bothers me, where I don't have to take anyone else into consideration, and where I can concentrate wholly on my training.

The body – its training competence, on the one hand, and its looks, on the other – is also invested by such a dynamic of inclusion/exclusion. Clients who get fitter and know their training routines well may actually experience a heightened sense of identification with fitness, the gym and its environment, acquiring more central positions in training scenes. Still, as we shall see, official hierarchies are excluded in the fitness gym. Although class options are often offered at various levels – "beginners", "intermediate" or "expert" – providing the instructor with a relatively homogeneous audience which helps in managing contingencies and in treating all clients as equal, these categories are not strictly enforced. The management of incentives as to training achievement, whether in terms of exercise performance or more characteristically of physical goals, is a crucial element of fitness culture, which nevertheless has to be carried out without excluding potential clients who may not be as well endowed or proficient (see Chapters 3 and 6).

Finally, a third paradox is articulated in the practical organisation of training: fitness training is justified as the most rational and effective way to transform the body, yet involvement in training is of the essence (see Chapters 4 and 5). Keep-fit practices harbour a daunting contradiction between *ascetic rationality* and *hedonistic passion*. The various forms of fitness training are presented by trainers and expert discourse as the most "rational" instrument to keep fit, take care of the body, get slim, toned, healthy and so on. Fitness training is accounted for as a rationally instrumental activity which deploys disciplinary techniques of the body, but it does not take place in a coercive, compulsive and hierarchically organised institution. Gym spatiality and temporality is coded also through elements of popular culture, such as notably pop music and fashionable sporting clothes, which stress leisure and recreation, something that is furthered by the cheerful, welcoming attitude of gym staff towards "clients". This is what qualifies fitness gyms as compared to disciplinary institutions such as the prison or the factory (see Foucault, 1991). Indeed, as a commercial institution, the fitness gym addresses the individual as a consumer, rather than the citizen or the labourer as a member of a population. As it is clients who pay for the time spent training, it is up to them to judge the value of fitness. Thus, while it is not possible to stay in the exercise areas without at least showing some commitment, gym staff tolerate quite a bit of interstitial play with training. By this I refer to the fact that people are not only institutionally encouraged to create their own personalised training programme, but they are also allowed to make use of the gym and its activities in a fragmentary, constantly changing and at times undisciplined manner. Alessia, a young postwoman who has been exercising in shape for a number of years, clearly illustrates this point:

> no one pesters me. I do whatever I want, if I want to do weights then I do, if I want to follow classes how and when I want, that's what I do, even just for half an hour and then I don't want to continue; but when I used to go swimming, I had to swim for two or three hours because it was competitive, and you couldn't just leave. Here you've got room for choice, and no one's imposing anything on you.

The margins of freedom left open to the individual, provided their interstitial play is not disruption of the training scene, help to reframe the keep-fit practices as leisure. The elements of rationalisation in fitness can make the workout quite dull and dry, which fits badly with the fact that going to a gym is, after all, an activity to be practised in one's own leisure time. Thus, fitness gyms must also provide hedonistic incentives, stressing emotional involvement, pleasure and fun (see Chapter 5). Involvement and fun are also, as I shall show (Chapter 7), related to the "natural" quality attributed to keep-fit activities in the gym, a naturality that contrasts markedly with the clearly artificial, precisely planned and continuously managed concentration of a structured variety of elaborated body techniques in one single, indoor place.

3
Interaction and Relational Codes

"Become a member of a club", urges the brochure of a major British fitness chain for the 2007 annual joining campaign. The list of benefits provided by membership includes fitness classes, spas, pools, massage services, bars and the "improvement of social life". The concept of a "club", which is increasingly associated with commercial fitness gyms, certainly suggests intense sociability as a key element of the institution. Indeed, as the notion of the fitness centre consolidated, gyms increasingly presented themselves as sociable places, where one can meet people and spend some pleasurable time with others. As noticed by Nick Crossley (2006), with membership figures above 10 per cent of the population, "fitness gyms are a significant form of association in contemporary society". Crossley's work on fitness training, based on his own participation in a club belonging to a major UK fitness chain, stresses the role of social relations and networks among clients, especially regular, long-term gym-goers. For Crossley, much of the success of a gym has to do with the development of a proper club atmosphere, which provides vital relational incentives to clients. Crossley recognises that social networks are important mainly for enthusiastic gym-goers who attend at regular times and focuses his analysis on evening attendance at circuit-training classes. As he suggests, clients who tend to "make a night" of their gym attendance, spending a few evening hours in their club weekly, will also tend to look for a full leisure experience that may start with training together and end with a late beer in the pub.

While this kind of warm, close friendliness is certainly an important aspect of gym attendance for a few clients, fitness premises are, on the whole, much more varied emotionally. Frustration, embarrassment and anxiety are indeed common experiences among those starting out, and feeling comfortable does not come easily. Fitness gyms are open an average of 12 to 14 hours a day and cater for different patterns of attendance, including quite a number of gym-goers, especially those who train around lunch-break or immediately after work, who adopt a rather instrumental, training-oriented attitude which allows for little sociability. They deal with many different clients, including many who do not attend regularly. Probably more prevalent in sales-oriented clubs than in those which aim for customer retention, a shifting clientele is a feature of most gyms. New customers are encouraged to join, and the gym staff are typically asked to monitor that they get involved in training and are not left out. Gym staff – trainers, instructors, receptionist, managers – all work hard on the social tone of the gym trying to deal with some of the contradictions of fitness training organisation. Indeed, *sociability* or a sociable sociality (see Simmel, 1917, 1950) in the gym does not come spontaneously; on the contrary, it is largely the result of collective work, performed by clients (with the result that a certain clientele will, to a degree, define the tone of a club) and by trainers (whose job in many ways is relational and emotional). Above all, fitness gyms are individualistic environments where clients can and must "concentrate" on themselves and on the exercises their "body" is performing. They are also formally open to a broad clientele and, as a result, joining brochures are keen to stress the gym's capacity to adapt to every individual need and to cater for every individual objective, illustrating this with a wealth of images glamorising individual workout and achievement. Such an institutional blend of individualism and universalism is not particularly conducive to sociability, to the point that it may frustrate clients, especially those approaching from previous athletic experiences in team sports. As a result, the role of the gym staff in the promotion of cordiality is crucial to present fitness as a leisure pursuit and the gym as a club, transforming clients into members: "some people will get a lot of fun out of sweating for their routines," says the President of the Italian Fitness Federation, "but most will need a nice environment, with nice faces, smiles and enthusiasm, in order to continue training. We do work at it, we try to help clients feel at home and socialise a bit."

1. Anxiety, individualism and sociability

Going to a fitness gym often means finding yourself in close proximity to relative strangers as you put your body and its physical potential *on display*. In the gym, clients are often among a rather unpredictable mix of men and women from a variety of backgrounds, with different bodies and training abilities, often having to deal with people that they would not have otherwise regularly met. While fitness magazines are full of cheerful training scenes with beautiful, fit people working out together in an enthusiastic atmosphere, actual gym scenes are much less glamorous. Training may be a rather intimidating experience, especially for new gym members. Even for experienced gym-goers, going back to training after a long period away may be threatening. As Davide, a middle-aged Italian who has been living around Britain for many years, describes: "going back after four years has been a killer. No stamina and it seemed like all those people were looking at me, I just had to remember their faces would eventually become normal."

The uneasiness which accompanies the first encounter with the gym has been mentioned over and over again by clients and trainers. The gym can be perceived as being "a strange place that wants to put you together with everyone else and yet you are alone. It can be frustrating, because when you're exercising, and afterwards in the changing rooms, you're actually alone", says Chiara who has indeed stopped going after what she considers a negative experience in a couple of Florentine gyms. As suggested, fitness training is often sought after as a remedy to a *misfit* experience, but gym environments can indeed heighten a sense of not belonging, resulting in high drop-out rates. Quitters mentioned three particular aspects: the *look* of their body as compared to better looking, fitter people; their poor *performance* with exercise equipment and training techniques; and their sense of *exclusion* from the social scene.

Consider again Maria, the London-based mother of two who had been a fairly regular gym goer for a couple of years but now, after a bunch of magazines and a couple of free trials, concludes her gym days are over. Time constraints are a concern for her, but most of all she reckons it is too difficult to "face the mirror" now that she has put on "a lot of weight": "when you have had a good body, then that's hard, and I know there is no going back...having fought for too many years with my weight, now I take it as it is and try to walk a bit more. Going to a gym only makes me feel bad about it." Valeria, a secretary from Bologna, plans to do some exercise to recover from injury, but will not go to a fitness centre. She is thinking of joining a swimming course. She wants to be in good shape, but does not want to do anything too demanding. The gym seems fussy to her. She visited a couple, even had a free trial on which I met her, but there were "too many things to do" and "too many different types of exercises with glamorous names". She is looking for something straightforward, uncomplicated, not a "fancy place with lots of people that in one way or the other will take you time to adjust to, but a straightforward type of exercise that I am familiar with".[1] As these accounts suggests, it is not physical activity, more or less organised, which may be rejected as such. It is the fitness centre which may not be perceived as a good answer to one's own needs, but in fact a threat to one's own project or self.[2]

On the whole, a measure of anxiety seems to be a well-recognised feature of fitness gyms. Vicky, a London-based personal trainer who specialises in pre- and post-natal training and weight loss, puts this down to the "very competitive market" in which fitness centres operate, with the consequence "that there is a lot of marketing and promotion":

> people are put under the light and it can be pretty overwhelming. I think that many customers feel the need to prove themselves because they are showing themselves off to others. There is an intimidation element...yet they also have the potential to become good social environments [for clients].

Indeed a friendly and welcoming atmosphere seems to be crucial in helping gym-goers to overcome gym anxieties. Valentina, a fitness instructor who looks after the clients in the machine area in a local gym in Bologna, says:

> You keep your clients mainly through the human relationships you manage to develop with them. Sure they trust you if you know about muscles and offer good exercise tips, but the psychological element, helping them to face their objectives with some balance, is fundamental, and the friendly atmosphere is vital, most people need that.

To be sure, different gyms deal with initial anxieties and uneasiness in different ways, providing more or less emotional support to training. Shawn, an Australian-born personal trainer who works in London, claims:

> You can see huge differences. You just have to go to Club Tavistock over the road and then you can look at Get Active down here. Club Tavistock is kind of a pretty place whereas Get Active where I go is where people work hard and I would say is a proper gym. It's more of a community feeling in the gym that I am [enrolled] in, whereas it's much more commercialised over there. They have a cafeteria over there, we don't have that. Club Tavistock is a chain of clubs ... The main difference between my local gym and the chain gym environment is that my gym has a stronger community feeling about it. It's like comparing McDonald's to a local bar, or like comparing a franchise with a small shop. The turnover is massive in big fitness centres whereas in local gyms they can have members for 30/40 years.

To an extent, anxiety is a function of the diversity of the people that you might find in a gym. The degree of clientele diversity is itself a function of the specific location of the gym in the urban context, its managerial orientation and its market positioning (see Chapter 2). While diversity appears to be overtly relished by clients, positively enforced by trainers and even celebrated by fitness discourse, it may indeed be quite daunting and tends to be collaboratively managed by fitness participants. The management of diversity is achieved essentially in three ways: by *discretion*, by *self-selection* and by *partnership*. Opting for discretion, for example, many participants consider it appropriate to deploy external symbols of status in rather inconspicuous ways. Discretion is a key element of interaction in the gym, something which I shall consider more broadly later when dealing with interaction during training (Chapter 4). Self-selection is also crucial. It evidently operates systemically in that different times and different types of exercise tend to attract clusters of people with similar daily rounds and external responsibilities. Off-peak attendance is a special tactic within a general tendency on the part of clients to exploit the gym's temporality and its shifting clientele over the course of the day. Going off-peak when there are fewer people reduces exposure. From her Norwich experience, Lindsay says she prefers this, not only because she may have "the changing room all to herself", but also, and more fundamentally, because "it's nicer to train when it's not so crowded". The key to this is that clients may see people around them which helps motivation, and yet avoid direct contact which may be threatening – they may get the benefit of group training, while obtaining enough individual attention. Lindsay continues explaining that she does not like it "when it's just two people and the instructor", but she wants to go at her own pace, in what she defines as an "airy group", with no difficulties as to sharing space and facilities, and with the instructor able to see what participants are doing. A final tactic relies on the establishment of partnership among clients. To face the gym and its varied fauna, clients may consciously adopt what a fitness buff described as "tandem strategy" (that is, going with a friend, relative or lover). Several novices have admitted that they find it useful to start going to the gym with a friend, and mention the fact that this has enabled them to both cope with and avoid skipping classes. Jenny, a Florentine, claims that "you feel more relaxed when you're with someone [that you know]. You know there is someone who you can talk to while you change. It becomes more of a group activity in the sense that you can say to them, 'oh come on, let's go and work out'." Jenny continued to go to the gym even when her friend quit, and she has now moved from a tandem to a much looser gym-team tactic: going at regular times, she finds a couple of other women she has got to know and whom she enjoys be there while training.

A number of gym-goers both start and continue going with a friend or a partner – this not only helps overcome initial anxieties, but also helps "overcome laziness and stick to it" making gym-going a "pleasurable experience". In my experience it is especially people who have a negative attitude towards the gym and towards themselves or those who are worried about regular physical exercise that tend to start with a friend. The company of a friend provides an initial boost that helps divert the fear of being exposed to strangers who are more at ease in the place. Sandro, a painter and decorator who has been going to a local club in Florence for over three years, admits:

> In general gyms are inhibiting! I started because there was another guy here, and together we encouraged each other. I had my hang ups, he had his...the shock of going to the gym for someone who has a poor physique is terrible. This friend doesn't come with me any more but I feel at ease...if you've been going somewhere for a long time, you feel more at home. It's the others that are just arriving, but I was here before, so it's as though I control the situation. The tricky bit is being the newcomer and thinking that the others are all there judging you...I like it here, there's good atmosphere, people do aerobics because they need to or they want to, and not to be seen.

Sandro's story illustrates that joining with a friend may be a help, but also that even a very anxious client may eventually feel at ease going alone. For Sandro, continuous attendance has meant not so much the development of a lively gym sociability, but rather the appropriation of exercise techniques and the transformation of his body. He claims that although he "can't make friends" in the gym, he now feels fine: the place is more familiar as he "know[s] the manager who is very nice" and he "know[s] the routines", having developed a sense of "control" on how machines and his body respond. Now that he has got enough exercise competence to feel comfortable on the scene, and an obvious level of fitness that demonstrates his competence, the superficial but friendly relations he has developed with trainers and managers in the gym are all he needs.

Tandems or gym partnerships are not the most common occurrence in the fitness gyms I have studied. They are considered demanding by many. They appear to run against the individualisation of daily rounds characterising late-modern urban living. And, more specifically, they seem to be a distraction from what is, after all, a form of exercise geared to rather individualistic goals. Many gym-goers report that they have been encouraged by friends to join a particular gym, but then suggest that they ended up following their own schedule "for the sake of convenience". Amy, a university student who has been a keen gym-goer for years, explains: "I prefer to go alone. Going with other people never works out. You're forever tied to their needs and it gets complicated trying to fit everything in." Going alone also helps maximise one's own time in the gym. Roberto, also a university student who organises his day around his training, explains: "when I'm training, I'm something of a loner and I think that's necessary if you want to concentrate. Plus, of course, I don't want to stay in the gym for three hours. Some people are in there for the entire afternoon but I want to be in and out in an hour and a half." Marica, a secretary in her late twenties who has gone to the same gym for nearly a decade, says that she likes the place as she knows many people, but she values her "independence" and the fact that she can "concentrate" on her "specific" and "individual routine": "I don't like tying myself to arrangements, like when people say 'let's meet up and go together' – I like to be free, I feel more relaxed. I'm not interested in training together with loads of other people because everyone has their own agenda. I follow my own individual programme and I think it's better that way."

While many clients go to the fitness centre alone, there is a general emphasis on the importance of a sociable atmosphere. What Simmel (1950; see also Goffman, 1982) called "acquaintance", the fleeting reciprocal acknowledgement that helps people feel at home in a public place is certainly important for regulars. More specifically, courtesy is the fundamental relational code in fitness environments, promoted by gym staff and regular clients alike. All fitness gyms are relatively restricted environments, which demand a high degree of co-ordination between clients. Courtesy is crucial in maintaining an orderly, clear, even if fairly irrelevant, interaction among equals – the polite client will allow another to maintain a close physical distance whilst, at the same time, maintaining an emotional distance – they will acknowledge other clients' training needs while pursuing their own training. Thus, in an aerobics class, a participant in the first row will move a little to one side to allow those at the back to see the mirror, another in the machine area will move from the machine they are resting on as another client approaches to use it.

Gym etiquette entails a tacit agreement on discretion or "civil inattention" (Goffman, 1963a) when others demonstrate their self-engrossment in training combined with a positive, even supportive, respect for the routines of the others around. This allows for some anonymity, and is perceived by clients whose bodies are flawed as the possibility of "looking funny and yet not caring about it". Besides discretion, gym etiquette also entails the recognition of the other, which may even amount to fleeting forms of sociability largely coded via what may be defined as a "positive attitude". A positive attitude is made up of courtesy, small talk and non-judgemental encouragement. As Cristina, a high-school teacher who has been looking for a satisfactory gym for some years, says, it is important that "there are no long faces when you're training" but, instead, people who "could, perhaps, even give you a hand". Even the most training-oriented clients consider that having "friendly people" around is important: in their terms it is "very pleasant to exchange a few words from time to time", "someone making a joke about a particularly difficult exercise" can even be encouraging and "familiar faces around you, with a nice attitude, help a lot". Positive exchanges at the margin of training can even give way to vicarious relational experiences, as Federica, a secondary school pupil who has just started training, suggests: "I really enjoy myself when I'm waiting for a lesson to begin, listening to everybody chatting about their problems. It's fun. I like being there and listening." And this is true also for men's changing rooms – a mature university professor just returned to the gym after many years confessed the pleasures of fitness training were more in the "eyes" and the "ears" than in the "muscles" for him – you may end up "straining your ears" to overhear telephone conversations in the locker room or take delight in "following the sweat beads on the woman's breast across the room" while pedalling on a bicycle. As I shall show, gym etiquette prescribes that the listening and the watching be carried out discretely, channelling interaction to facilitate concentration in training while offering some surreptitious gratification.

Surreptitious gratification is indeed part of the gym environment, and this is particularly true as sexuality, officially excluded from the scene, comes into play. As suggested in the previous chapter, in many ways sexually laden gender divisions which are dominant in many everyday life settings are confined to the changing room and may be ignored, at least officially, during training.

The gym is all but a dating agency: training spaces are defined as places where the body should lose its sexual connotations, thus becoming more of a tool for exercise. While bodies are on display and often move at the rhythm of popular music, while clothing may be revealing, and movements and postures certainly stress carnality, the fitness gym is very different from a night club or a disco. As happens in the formal context of mixed working environments, training operates on official body de-sexualisation and its surreptitious sexualisation. The de-sexualisation of the body is in some ways more an interaction device to facilitate training than a precise description of reality. Some sexualisation does come into play, albeit subtly, during interaction and follows the dominant heterosexual pattern which may be encountered in external, everyday reality. In the gym you may thus find half-hidden glances, hesitant innuendos and flirtatious comments being made half-jokingly in the interstices of training.[3] As a participant observer I have witnessed countless of these, but mostly I have witness the air of embarrassment when they got out of hand, became too obvious or insistent.

Clients do have different views on similar occurrences, partly depending on whether they consider the gym as a place just for training or an opportunity for socialising. In Mauro's opinion, the presence of "women in the gym makes it a more sociable place and people are more inclined to think about something else apart from exercise". Anna and Sandro, on the other hand, believe that an all-female or all-male gym would allow them to avoid this sort of "annoying distraction." Thus, while flirting is officially excluded from the gym environment, among clients there is also the recognition that a gym is a place where one can meet others who one may be attracted to, look for a fling or a partner or, more often, just eye up good looking people with whom one has no intention of forming a relationship with. These motives are more readily available for those who spend lots of time in the gym, at fixed hours, so that the gym become a relevant place for socialising which uses up a remarkable proportion of people's free time (Crossley, 2006; see also Unger and Johnson, 1995).

Sexualisation and responses to it in the complexity of a unisex fitness centre are largely a function of a *gender-activity matrix*. For example, among men who participate in exercise-to-music classes I have indeed found concern for the way they were looked at. They often feel comparatively marginal to the scene and less proficient with the movements. Their masculinity may be called into question. While trainers work hard at avoiding this, they may feel to be in a feminine space, especially as they join a class. Nina Loland's (2000, pp. 122–4) study of Norwegian men and women participants in choreographed aerobics classes indeed reports a number of men being concerned with their properly masculine looks to the point of wanting to participate without being seen. She also mentions that they liked to participate while looking at women, who, on their part liked to be looked at by men or other participants, but covered certain body parts which they considered unattractive. If we move to the more masculine area of the gym, where weight-lifting isotonic equipment is used, we may observe the reverse: women appear less confident here, and many reported the feeling of being looked at as more dangerous, as if their femininity was revealed in potentially uncontrolled ways. Subterraneous sexualisation thus goes hand in hand with the evident, if officially downplayed, gendering of activities. Thus, in the female-only environment of the changing room I have witnessed women making fun of men's clumsiness with aerobics, and reproaching them of "boasting strength with the machines, but being out of breath in a sec while doing aerobics". And chatting with men engaged mainly in machine training I have heard that certain positions were "good to look from the back at the girls running on the treadmill", a type of activity which was qualified as "what girls mainly do, if they come close to a machine, they do not like to lift weight, it's too hard". These claims also reflect the endurance of gender dichotomies in the rendering of the "fit body" in fitness commercial images (see Chapter 6), which may work against a less obvious gender division of exercise activities as promoted by trainers in unisex gyms.

On the whole, surreptitious sexualisation in fitness gyms is gendered in fairly dominant ways: while some of the men I have interviewed reported that nice-looking girls were a plus of their gym and few of them overtly complained about women looking at them, women were less into voyeuristic glances on men, they were more concerned with, either pleased or indeed disturbed by, men's glances. Thus, trainers may actively work to keep sexualisation at bay. In a training scene at Shape, for example, the step aerobics teacher intervened in defence of her female-only class, scrutinised by two middle-aged men who were standing at the side of the room just watching, and directly invited them to participate and to "make an effort". To start with, the two unfortunate men justified themselves by maintaining that they wanted to "try out" a new activity, then they quickly moved away and finally one of them decided to take part in the following lesson. The pressure of the unisex character of fitness thus appears to work slightly differently for the genders – both men and women are encouraged to take up both traditionally masculine and feminine activities which may pose a challenge to their masculinity or femininity, but the female body appears to be open to more direct sexualisation. The development of the women-only gym partly responds to the anxieties that this may generate (Craig and Liberti, 2007).

If we go back to courtesy as a dominant relational code in the fitness gym, we may see that it works both positively and negatively, both facilitating and limiting contacts. In the fitness gym, contacts are typically managed as an aside to training. For regular clients this institution also provides the scene for more significant bonding – it's "a place where people can meet on a daily basis" generating reciprocal expectations, or "a gathering point for people who are getting to know each other" and provide each other with a sense of continuity. Gym bonding is an important source of motivation while training, but it may also become demanding. Going to a gym, like every other leisure pursuit, takes time and competes for time with other activities. Those who invest more time in the gym are more likely to make it into a sociable occasion, one where gym-based friendships assume greater significance. Gym bonding thus may become a source of social pressure, with regulars allowing themselves to monitor others' participation to the point of telling them off for their absence.

Despite its role, gym bonding tends to largely remain an accessory to training, stressing that the latter is the official aim of the institution. Not surprisingly, such bonding is typically bounded to gym attendance. As Crossley (2006, p. 37) notices about gym bonding, "group members who stop going to the gym for whatever reasons, very quickly drop out of the social activities of the group". This is what makes fitness gyms a rather weak form of association, if one at all.[4] Thus, while in many ways gym relationships are what allow the time spent in the gym to become proper leisure time, the gym leaves little room for the development of close friendships or the affective immediacy which characterises anti-structural spaces and communities (Turner, 1967). Still gym bonding is particularly important for certain forms of training (such as circuit training or body building) (Crossley, 2004; Klein, 1993; Lowe, 1998), for special temporalities (such as evening attendance) (Crossley, 2006), special publics (such as women-only classes and gyms) (see Craig and Liberti, 2007; Dworkin, 2003; Gimlin, 2002) and in general for regulars. For regulars, gym relations perform important functions. They help clients face training and its hardships, provide some distractions and translate the bodywork into a leisure pursuit – something which is relatively light and detached from external duties and relations. Regular gym-goers learn to value these forms of courtesy to the point that their accounts take up and subvert the impressions of gym quitters. Marica, for example, describes the gym as a place where "you're alone and free from everyday worries" and, at the same time, "with lots of other people" with whom you can establish "a relationship that is warm but superficial".

Gym etiquette and gym bonding help positively define the social world of fitness centres for regular clients. They are definitely listed among the "pleasures" of training in their accounts of sustained practice (see Chapter 5). The fact that clients' conversations are mostly confined within the gym, even though they may involve a variety of small chat topics, allows them to create a world apart where they can detach themselves from their external personas. Some clients do precisely appreciate the light, undemanding quality of gym relationships. Betty, for example, calls people she knows in the gym "buddies" yet she would not mix these with her "friends outside the gym": "I know a few people down at the gym to say hello to, have a small chat around training, a joke with, but it doesn't go any further than that." The affable exchanges and the undemanding acquaintances made in gyms become a pleasure in themselves as they have a "release" and "escape" quality. For example, Bonnie, a middle-aged housewife who has been going to a local gym for over four years, maintains that the gym has "an anti-depressant effect. There are these kind, pretty girls here...it's a way of escaping, of lightening up the day: you've got no obligations or anything, and people are really kind." Precisely because they are confined and in many ways light, casual and carefree, gym relations are important because they form a real alternative to usual, external relationships that are typically tied to work, kinship or long-term obligations. Even a self-defined loner like Roberto explains that he has "learnt to appreciate the idea of a casual acquaintance a bit more, seeing so many people pass by makes you appreciate this, that you just meet someone as they're passing is an enjoyable experience in itself". In the gym, courtesy also helps bringing participants' differences in as "nice" and "small" diversions. Many clients have stressed that in this health-orientated environment, it is not important, at least officially, if someone is a professional or a manual worker. I've often come across clients who suggest that one of the most "interesting" and "enjoyable" aspects about going to the gym is the chance to meet people from all walks of life. Amy, for example, explains that "you find a lot of different types of people in a gym and that's good". "Actually", she adds, "it's one of the things I like the most!"

Courtesy, gym etiquette and gym bonding facilitate interaction by channelling distractions around the execution of prescribed activities, making them functional, in many ways, to training. The point of gym sociality is rarely the development of strong friendship ties – after all, as Glenda, a middle-aged physiotherapist maintains, going to the gym "isn't like going out with friends, it's an individual thing". This may produce some frustration in clients who have only just started going, especially those from a team sports background, who may feel disillusioned to the point where they stop attending because the environment does not offer a "real" group experience. Donata, an accountant in her mid-thirties who has decided not to renew her three-month trial subscription, believes that "with sporting activities, everyone is in a team", but in the gym "that group dynamic does not exist", people "do not work together" and things "get boring". The individualistic nature of fitness centres is sometimes regretted by regular clients who have put effort into developing their social life in the gym. Let's consider Mauro's story. He is a civil servant who has been going to the same Florentine club for almost three years and is adamant that "doing something for your body" and "making friends" should be reconciled. He claims he has tried to "break" the "individualistic nature" of the gym, but things have "changed only a bit": "I thought I could make new friends, communicate and at the same time do the physical exercises you had to...I got to know people. It took time but I made a few friends, some of whom I even go out with, but it was mostly owing to the effort I put in. The gym environment itself hasn't changed." The institutional priority of the gym is individual training and the gym remains, to quote Mauro's insightful observation, a place "where you go to exercise and then you leave again, in and out. Even though you may meet nice people, there aren't many people there who are really interested in making friends."

2. Commercialised courtesy, individualistic universalism

Clearly, with its different spaces and services, long opening hours and shift-ing clientele, fitness centres allow for a variety of ways of interpreting their sociability. Gym-goers clearly indicate that a friendly environment is impor-tant, that some human contact is important, but how they are to interpret this is quite varied. For some clients, gym-specific relationships are an impor-tant consideration, to the point that gyms may become a source of social capital (that is, a place to meet acquaintances which may be helpful for other external needs such as getting information about a job) or a place which offers nice background distractions and indeed a pastime (such as when the stories of other clients become a source of entertainment, something to keep up with). For others, going to a gym will never be like going to a café or a social club where the whole point is to be with other people. For these clients, while it is nice to see friendly faces, the gym remains the place to go if you want to be on your own. Gym sociality is therefore pulled and pushed in different directions by different clients, and the clientele of a specific gym greatly contributes to its actual relational content.

Still, gym staff are asked to work at gym sociability, qualifying it in specific ways: courtesy and gym bonding are promoted by trainers with the objective to include new clients, keep old clients motivated and in general provide a social environment conducive to training. Trainers are particularly keen to make sure that gym sociability does not exclude new clients, and believe that it may work as a loyalty building device. Valentina, the fitness instructor from Bologna that we have encountered earlier, clearly illustrates this:

> We organise quite a few social events, evenings out in a disco, at a restaurant, but also here in the gym – like last month we did a wine tasting evening, which was a great success. We also mark festivities, like Christmas, doing a Christmas tree and have little presents for members. [This gym] is small, we can get to know the members, they can connect with each other and with us, so they really feel at home. And there are also those old clients, who come just to take a shower, have a chat, and then go...these are people who come just to spend an hour with people they know.

Sociability in the fitness gym is demanding for a trainer; it is indeed an important part of a fitness instructor's job. The work carried out by instruc-tors and trainers – as is the case with other service workers – requires quite a lot of emotional labour and a measure of controlled personal involvement

(Hochschild, 1983). Again, in the words of Valentina, this may extend well beyond the workout scene:

Q. So you end up going out with your clients?

A. You must foster participation, for sure. Indeed, at certain times of the year, I may end up having six nights out just to go out with the people from the gym, like [one night] the step group, then the women from the circuit training. It's part of my job, but you do it with pleasure, it makes work easier and more enjoyable.

Q. What do you talk about in these occasions?

A. You always speak about the gym, gym gossip, gym workouts, petty arguments in the gym, incidents, all that gym stuff.

The picture offered by Valentina points to the role that gym staff plays in channelling sociability through commercially mediated relations. Considering the relational codes, the fitness gym lives through a rather unstable combination. By and large, gyms are officially aimed at individualistic goals such as the attainment of a fitter body, yet they are organised in accordance with universalistic principles. Like many consumer places, they combine universalisation with individualisation and, as such, they promise to treat everyone as a specific, even special, individual. Such a combination allows for economies of scale, with large numbers of clients using relatively small places in relatively orderly ways, yet it also generates frictions and contradictions. Gym instructors and personal trainers are typically called in to keep such frictions at bay, managing the relational predicament of the gym by adjusting the mix of universalism and individualism to the specific occasion. Thus, while instructors may try to encourage sociability among participants by organising an evening out with a favourite class, during the course of training they have to keep everyone focused on keep-fit routines. As suggested, too much chatting with one classmate may exclude other people and disrupt training. Instructors must not only be polite with every client, but they must also keep an eye on situations where small groups of gym buddies disrupt the scene for the whole training group. Clearly it is a delicate task, which is normally dealt with by the instructor with jocular and ironic comments, especially since these groups are usually made up of gym veterans who get part of the satisfaction that keeps them going from such exchanges.

An infinite number of scenes in the gym will therefore show us how complicated the client-instructor relationship is. It is imbued with different meanings and potential conflicts partly because everyone can adopt different roles. The best-loved trainers seem more able to juggle these roles, stressing their own expertise and, at the same time, their willingness to help clients.

They are able to preserve equality among clients whilst concentrating on each individual's specific needs. This was evident in my initial ethnography in two fitness gyms in Florence (Sassatelli, 1999a and b, 2000c). When introducing a new, young female client to the exercise machines, Omar, an instructor at Shape, appears to accentuate the professionalism with which he usually conducts this role, almost as though he is underlining the fact that the relationship is that of teacher and pupil rather than two people of the opposite sex. Passing by a chatting couple seated peacefully on the seats of two exercise machines, Omar jokingly comments: "You two are hardly overdoing it today!" The unlucky victims of his wit are gracefully invited to leave one of the machines they are clearly not using for "this beautiful young lady who is trying to learn". While the couple separate and return to their training with renewed vigour, Omar turns to his new client and immediately re-adopts his previous professional and detached tone. Similar scenes can also be witnessed at BodyMove. Marisa, a young, enthusiastic step teacher, tries to encourage the clients to attend regularly by telling them that "coming when you're really busy shows your commitment". She also demonstrates her expertise by highlighting the best exercises and simultaneously emphasising the fact that "everyone can learn" and that "perhaps" they could train "at home" and repeat their favourite exercises. She suggests that they should try stretching, "because you can't just build your body up, you have to stretch it as well".

During an aerobics session at Shape, a scene involving a popular instructor called Pamela clearly shows the risks that instructors run when juggling different roles. As the lesson draws to a close, Silvana, a middle-aged lady, claims her right as a "solvent gym member" to "work on her hips" referring to the fact that in the session, a particular exercise for the buttocks had been skipped. Pamela answers with emphasised politeness, both underlining her expertise ("although we've done it in a different way, during today's session we've used all the important muscles") and reinforcing the fact that her services must be offered to everybody without exception ("there are other people waiting to come in and I have to attend to them as well"). Pamela eventually allows herself to make a comment about her client saying that she is "one of those people who are never happy" and immediately turns the joke round by adding that she herself is "one of those people". Such an exchange shows the delicate nature of the client-instructor interaction – in this case, while the majority of the clients rush to leave, Silvana and a small group of regulars continue talking to Pamela, who is having trouble avoiding increasingly personal matters. She is unable to start the following lesson on time, to the obvious disappointment of the awaiting clients.

While different gyms attract different clienteles and work differently on the kind of social environment they provide, the relational codes of gym environments have to negotiate with the dual imperatives of commercial fitness: universalisation and individualisation, standardisation and personalisation. The role of the gym instructor is a particularly important and delicate one when it comes to training, something that is recognised by clients, manages and instructors themselves. On the one hand, instructors must be able to draw in each client to exercising, and they will therefore tend to change their approach according to the needs of those whom they are training. On the other hand, they have to promote their services to the whole gym clientele. When this does not happen as it should, the gym risks discouraging new clients. Cristina, a young high-school teacher, has left a number of gyms precisely because she could not stand "the instructor's little entourage that gathered round her and just stood there chatting". In that sort of situation, Cristina adds, "you feel left out". Rebuking what she considers "unprofessional trainers", she says, "the instructor should at least try and pretend that he's looking after everybody. I mean, we've all paid our money and that's his job, isn't it?!"

All the instructors and trainers that I have met with in the course of my field trips both in Italy and Britain have stressed what they call "personalisation". Whether working in a group or individually on an exercise machine, it is important that the instructor responds to the needs of all the clients considered as individuals. Even keep-fit videos, a rather standardised means to address an audience, are now increasingly oriented towards personalisation. For example, in her hit-video '28 Day Total Body Plan' released in 2004, Joanna Hall, probably the most famous fitness personality in Britain, proposes three routines that can be followed by inexperienced or advanced people by illustrating the workout together with two assistants, a young, fit-looking woman on her right and a plumper, older and slower woman on her left. Viewers are encouraged to follow either of the two according to their self-perceived level of fitness in order to adjust the training to their needs and abilities. Personalisation is an important element of what instructors define as their "professionalism" – instructors both in Italy and Britain all stressed that keeping aware of each and every client in all the workout sessions is one of the most demanding and yet qualifying tasks for a good trainer. Many examples of this may be found at the interaction level. For example, in group activities, the trainer must reinforce the impression that all clients are treated equally by specific modes of address. When illustrating the exercise they often address the group as an equal whole or the individual as an abstract participant (typically using "you" in the singular). For example, they use encouraging remarks such as "come on, you can do it", or general exercise tips such as "keep those hips raised", "remember to breathe", or generalised detailed directions such as "you must feel your spine opening up, unfolding into the ground". There are also procedures that reinforce the equality of the clients exercising on machines. Gym "induction" is one such procedure: a machine instructor advises newcomers on the sequence of exercises they have to follow, the posture they should adopt and the number of repetitions they have to complete. Even more so, machine instructors are often present on the scene and part of their job is to monitor that each client is comfortable and knows what to do.

Most of the time, in order to stress equal treatment, the instructor cannot treat clients with anything other than courtesy, and yet it is this courtesy that qualifies a relationship that would otherwise be excessively rigid, mechanical and irreverent. Fitness centres, like other spaces for mass consumption, commercialise respect for the person, and transform it into courtesy for the individual. In other words, courtesy is part of an interpersonal code which allows commercial institutions to offer every client a standard and yet personalised service, aimed at capturing some of the salient traits of a variety of individualities. Courtesy is a basic feature of the instructor-client relationship and it manifests itself in the attention that every single client should be able to receive regardless of their physical attributes or their socio-cultural characteristics. It makes the anonymity of formal equality more acceptable, the latter being balanced by the consideration an instructor has to give to the clients' requirements as they emerge and evolve throughout their training performances.

3. Trainers as experts, task and emotional leaders

Gym instructors and trainers can do a great deal to initiate clients into the world of the gym. Most clients who agreed to answer my questions maintain that a good trainer helps both in getting into the right spirit and in continuing training. The ideal trainer is someone who "helps you to identify yourself a bit with what you are doing" and who can "also give you useful advice". These words once again stress the fact that, whatever the activity, trainers have a fundamental cognitive task – that of regulating the inclusive and exclusive meanings of the clients' efforts. In other terms, they help towards "frame alignment" (Snow et al., 1986) by helping clients' expectations coincide with what is provided by the fitness centre and, conversely, stretching the interaction details of fitness provision to align with clients' attitudes. As I shall show, they describe their work also in the emotional terms of "motivation" and "loyalty" which are both portrayed as features of a successful frame alignment.

The relationship between trainers and clients cannot be reduced to a "service transaction" (Goffman, 1963a, 1982), that is, an automatic supply of benefits which is given and complete. Trainers play a very active role which requires an adequate display of knowledge. Trainers present themselves as experts and as keepers of expert knowledge. The dialogue between trainers and clients during training, for example, clearly indicates a disparity of knowledge via an asymmetrical structure similar to a medical consultation or formal teaching (see Frankel, 1984; Mehan, 1979). In verbal exchanges, the last word is generally that of the trainer, who closes with a comment that works as an interpretation of what has taken place. The recourse to expert knowledge is an important professional tool for gym instructors, something which helps in overcoming gender bias for example. A young, female gym instructor, for example, comments on the difficulty that a woman trainer may face in a machine area populated mainly by men who are building up muscles and strength: "you teach them the theoretical part of the work, you know muscles and physiology, they may know the routines, but they are not experts, like medical and technical knowledge … in the end they come to accept this about you, on your specialised knowledge and they do not see you as a woman anymore".

Loyalty to a gym is hard work for gym instructors and gym staff. Instructors in particular, both in Britain and Italy, have all stressed that exercise adherence is a major concern for them – and one which they try to solve by reinforcing their emotional centrality, on the one hand, and their role as fitness experts, on the other. In their words, they not only promote "gym sociability" and a "welcoming atmosphere", they also continually try to show their own "professionalism" and the "validity" of their "specialised knowledge". To do so, they routinely resort to a variety of characteristic moves for professionals – the use of a specialised vocabulary mainly derived from medical terminology; the display of official credentials on their cards and in the gym; the participation in professional associations and initiatives. These moves contrast with the fact that trainers are typically referred to by their personal names, or even nicknames, both on gym timetables and in actual interaction with clients. As both experts, task and emotional leaders, trainers do not make use of disciplinary power as such, that is, power which is based on establishing exclusive and hierarchical rewards and on the subdivision of individuals into non-negotiable categories. They rather work on persuasion, and must use their own body and their own emotions directly to demonstrate correct movements and correct attitude (Phillips and Drummond, 2001).[5]

As I shall show (Chapters 4 and 5), although not all clients succeed in building their own training programme, normative emphasis in fitness rests on the need for clients to consider only their own body and their own ability to follow the exercises, evaluate their own progress and find their own space inside the gym. Fitness culture is not only aimed at "an increase in the mastery of each individual over his own body" (Foucault, 1991, p.137), but also puts weight on each individual's capacity to understand – "see", "feel" – their own body and choose what is most enjoyable. In fitness centres, clients are required not only to conform to given body techniques, but also, and above all, to participate as active subjects. In many ways, even if trainers keep a strong hold on the training scene and shape the knowledge and ability of their trainees, the emphasis on clients' role in monitoring their bodies, keep self-motivated, choose body techniques and so on effectively makes them co-producers of fitness.

By attending, regular clients thus accumulate knowledge which is potentially in competition with what is proposed in the fitness centre. Even though it is trainers themselves who maintain that clients must learn to evaluate their own bodies and progress, clients' knowledge may on occasion frustrate their authority. A few voices from my Florentine fieldwork illustrate this well. An experienced fitness fan such as Anna, for example, stresses that "over the years" she has changed and refined her "way of going to the gym": "I have now learned to exercise," she explains, "I know what's bad for me and I realise immediately if a trainer is bad for me. And I don't let them get away with it, I prefer to change gyms!" One episode described by another long-standing regular, Paola, exemplifies the nature of clients' accumulated knowledge and specifies the way in which it binds trainer and client. Paola says she is "very satisfied" with her gym because she has found "well-prepared teachers", yet she vividly recalls a class where: "a substitute came to teach, and she only made us work our lateral abdominals. We [the clients] told her that we were used to something more difficult, so she made us do a series of fifty reps, but in the end we were only moving the external parts... really, someone who is teaching us has to make us move all our muscles!" In this scene it was evident that, although the unfortunate instructor was criticised, the knowledge which Paola and the other clients had acquired by appropriating the precepts of preceding instructors came out as reinforced, becoming a source of pride and belief in the validity of fitness as a precise form of knowledge. Training in classes or with machines in a gym has potential for a critical appropriation of fitness (that is, one which is not exclusively tied to the authority of a particular trainer), but also reinforces the impression that fitness knowledge is true and conclusive.

Efforts to promote fitness as a scientifically based form of knowledge have long been frustrated by the contamination by pop music and popular culture, by the limited formalisation of careers and the proliferation of famous but non-professional experts such as Jane Fonda or Cindy Crawford (Glassner, 1992; Park, 1994). Fitness knowledge is not fully consolidated in science. Nor is it esoteric knowledge which can be shared only through scrupulous observance of particularistic, personalised instructions. Experts conform to forms of knowledge which are increasingly standardised. Standardisation is, in turn, related to keep-fit experts' claims to universality and impartiality and indicates a knowledge which aims to be empirically and objectively verifiable, founded on rational-empirical grounds as much as on personal qualities. Clients who are familiar with body-soul disciplines, such as yoga, typically channelled via the charismatic qualities of the teacher, are quite vocal about this. Jamie, a Londoner who has resolved to go to a dedicated yoga studio after injury, says that she left the fitness gym and prefers the studio precisely because she can relate to one particular teacher: "It's because of my bad back, but also because the teacher here is inspirational, it's not like the usual move up, move down, the dry approach, there seems to be something human, something less standardised, more spiritual." Regular fitness clients often invert Jamie's judgement while agreeing on the description. It is precisely because fitness training is "rational" that it is a safer bet when compared to yoga: "finding a good fitness instructor is difficult, but is way easier than finding a yoga teacher, who has to be extremely good and who you must have an intense, very personal, particular relationship with". In contrast, in fitness gyms "body work is rational: I move the right muscle and then the left one, if they don't help me improve my abdominal muscles or my buttocks I'm aware of it, and I can always do it on my own" (see Chapters 4 and 7).

As much as fitness training may appear as a rationalised activity, it cannot succeed without "trust". Trust has indeed been indicated by all gym instructors and trainers I have met with, both in Britain and Italy, as the key to a good client-trainer relationship, a facilitator of both loyalty and motivation. The first and foremost concern of gym instructors, and even more so personal trainers, is to encourage clients to trust them. Here are some telling quotes from instructors:

Trust! It's a matter of trust, because you work with their bodies, it's like a medical doctor, it's very much a psychological work, to gain their trust and use it to make them work in the right way.

(Valentina, gym instructor, Bologna)

[The most important thing in the relationship with clients is] trust, competence, seriousness. A class costs 60 Euros, so people obviously want quality feedback, they invest money and want good results back. They put their trust on you, so you must plan training, and increasing difficulty based on the progress or personal characteristics of the client.

(Elena, pilates instructor, Milan)

Good, trusting relationships with clients are very important. But you should never cross boundaries. Some people don't have the ability to keep their distance and be friendly at the same time, but this is what you need to do.

(Tom, gym instructor, London)

Regular clients also use the term "trust" to stress the necessary quality of a good relationship with trainers, as these comments make clear:

It is important that you can trust the teacher. They cannot rule with an iron fist, they have to have the authority of expertise. I can't put up with someone I don't respect. If I think a teacher is good, even though I might criticise them, I immediately absorb what they want to teach, but if I don't think they're up to it, then it's much more difficult and I start to question them.

(Leo, regular stepper, Florence)

[My first pilates instructor] was a very nice person, a devotee to the cause, very motivated, who believes in what she does and does it very seriously, loving her job. This helps trust what she does, and has really helped me get into it.

(Clarissa, pilates enthusiast, Milan)

This is a good gym, you know. It's not too crowded, and there is always a gym instructor you can ask to give you advice or something... The trainers are very professional, they know their job, you know. You can trust them, and they are nice and it's welcoming.

(Minnie, regular at a downtown chain, London)

Trust in gym instructors is based on both their expert knowledge and their ability to be emotional leaders. They must get close enough to clients as people, without losing their authority as experts. While this balancing act is a key professional feature in the figure of the personal trainer, gym instructors also have to work hard at it, and at relationships more broadly. Besides being related to the demonstration of expert knowledge, trust is thus largely related to the instructor's capacity to fine tune the many personas which bear on the training scene. As experts who offer their services in a commercial institution, gym instructors are oriented towards the satisfaction of their clients. This is evident in their vocabulary. Fitness participants are indeed recurrently described as "clients". Less frequently they are also indicated with the terms "consumers" or "customers", as well as with general expressions such as "people" or "person" or gender-specific names like "lady", "girl", "boy", "men" and so on. Fitness participants themselves endorse their role as clients, using it in their relationships with trainers. They not only play the inexperienced trainee role, but also the tough client who demands value for money, lest he or she quit. They may switch to their gendered persona – for example, by stressing body parts which are "problematic for a woman". They may enjoy a joke acknowledging their sentiments as "people" – as when they relish the comment of an instructor stressing common experiences of laziness, fatigue, frustration and so on. Clearly the multiplicity of personas which can be played upon by participants is such that one of the most difficult tasks for instructors is to marshal it in ways functional to exercise involvement and adherence.

4. Professionalisation, standardisation and personalisation

To address trust as a necessary requisite to make people work out, gym staff and gym instructors typically resort to the idea of "professionalism". This notion has potently entered the fitness industry (Smith Maguire, 2007). This is true not only of Britain or the USA, which, as we know, have long been characterised by strong systems of professions comprising well-structured, vocal and autonomous professional groups, but also of Italy, which, as many other European countries, has traditionally placed less emphasis on professionalism. Courses, festivals and professional organisations are mentioned by fitness workers at all levels, and increased levels of professional credentials are considered both a career achievement and a market competitive advantage. Professions are cornerstones in contemporary society, not only for what they can tell us in terms of occupational structures, but also because they exemplify a particular relation to work and its public, which is crucial for "service" jobs. Claiming a privileged access to both knowledge and status, the members of a profession deploy a particular altruistic ideology of work which mixes rational and emotional elements that engage in a continuous jurisdictional game (of conflict and co-operation) with other professions (Abbott, 1988; Hughes, 1963). While the professionalisation of fitness is a relatively recent phenomenon, most fitness workers I have met with – both instructors, trainers and personal trainers – are quite proud of their job and professionalism is a mark of pride. This partly reflects the investment in education which trainers have to make in order to acquire credentials. Most of them have a relevant BSc in physical education, sport psychology or related field. All personal trainers, both in Italy and Britain, have taken courses with their respective national fitness federations (the Federazione Italiana Fitness in Italy or the International Health and Racquets Sportclub Association in the USA and UK). Most of them have some other complementary expertise – often in Britain this involves some kind of nutrition specialisation, while in Italy it often relates to rehabilitation, massage and physiotherapy. All of them keep well informed by attending courses, reading books, going to festivals, trying new techniques and so on. But these more or less formalised credentials and forms of knowledge are certainly not enough to describe what trainers or personal trainers do and what professionalism means for them.

To get a grasp on the meaning of professionalism for trainers, we must listen to what their experiences are, what they are really proud of and what is difficult in the relationships with their clients. Valentina's reply to a direct question on professionalism is telling:

Q. So what is for you "to be professional"?

R. To be professional is when you manage to convince people that you are doing something good for them, that you can't possibly deceive them, that you want them to feel good...I believe in what I do, therefore I am not a salesperson, I can't sell a product – well, I sell it because I believe it, but I am not a "shark", I do not tell lies. I couldn't, and I like to work here, at a local gym, because there is less competition, and sales are not a priority – too much of that works against you doing your job with passion, because you know that you can help people.

Professionals sell a service and live off the money they earn from such sales. But the value of the service is not in the money; it is in the claim that the professional successfully makes about the value of such a service, its utility and its quality. *Authenticity* or *vocation* are crucial for the credibility of the professional claim. Like other service professionals, fitness workers play on the cultivation of authenticity as much as on expert knowledge – the latter becomes alive only in the enthusiasm through which it is communicated, which in turn is witness to the truth of what is being sold (Hochschild, 1983; Smith Maguire, 2007). Not surprisingly, like other "cultural intermediaries" (Bourdieu, 1984; see also Featherstone, 1991; Nixon and Crewe, 2004) they are also the "perfect consumers" of fitness, spending much of their free time training as both recreation and an investment in their jobs, or organising their social lives around their services and through their services.

The ability to "adapt themselves to the needs of their clients" and to "make clients feel at ease" are considered the ground rules of a fitness professional. Trust and the facilitation of frame alignment require a degree of flexibility from trainers. Still, instructors working with a class or in a machine studio may be limited in many ways. As suggested by a manual advertised as a portable personal trainer for individual gym attendance: "even if some courses are excellent and there are only very few people attending them, even the most expert and willing instructors cannot follow and advise every single client who needs help" (Goodsell, 1995, p. 9). Indeed, in the face of fitness gyms' economies of scale and composite publics, the insistence in fitness discourse (from magazines to gym's brochures) on the personalisation of services makes the limits to personalisation in a standard client-trainer relationship obvious. The development of the figure of the professional trainer may be seen as a way of stressing professionalisation by allowing for further degrees of personalisation. Conversely, personal trainers, especially in Britain, are adamant that they are "health professionals" or "fitness professionals".

Let's consider the figure of the personal trainer more closely, and it in the context of the broader provision of fitness. Personal training is offered as a service in most fitness gyms, but personal training has rapidly become a successful business it its own right, based on the premise of personalisation. The 2007 advertisement of an established London-based personal training agency is instructive on this feature. "The key word in personal training is 'personal' – we read – Every person has a unique combination of strengths and weaknesses, goals and desires, lifestyle demands and challenges. The key is creating a programme that allows for all of these. That way, it fits seamlessly into your life." Playing on the meaning of fitness, the distinguishing aspect of the service is presented as the possibility of adjusting to individual needs and lifestyles. Especially if self-employed personal trainers are in a competitive and co-operative relationship with fitness centres. Danielle, who runs this established personal training agency, clearly demonstrated in her interview how the job of personal trainers may go beyond fitness centres as we know them, and may even represent an alternative and a challenge to them:

> I have never worked in a gym. I don't like the environment and don't like the personal training experience that you get in a gym or in a fitness centre. What I learnt, especially in Australia, is that you go one-to-one with your client. That would be in a studio or at their home or even outside but never in a gym. They can be claustrophobic and quite depressing places and I found that the reason why lots of clients aren't fit and end up coming to a personal trainer is because they don't like the gym and find them very intimidating. There are so many people who have a gym membership but they don't go to the gym because it is not a pleasure for them, they don't enjoy it.

Her account is an attack on the "gym environment" based on the intimidation traits mentioned at the beginning of this chapter. The services of a personal trainer are presented as important in order to bypass gym anonymity and provide sustained motivation.

Similar comments on personalisation as partly geared against the often reported intimidating qualities of the gym are not uncommon among personal trainers. They do need gyms to bring their clients to, but may also work at their clients' homes or outdoors. Personal trainers, indeed, often refer to gym-induced anxiety to explain and justify their role within the industry. Adam, a young personal trainer working in London, says "many people are actually intimidated by the gym environment and that's why they come to me. I suppose I adapt my knowledge and expertise to their needs and make them feel at ease". Anna, a top personal trainer from Milan, with many international certificates, stresses yet again that "people often need someone to trust" and explains that "a gym is not the ideal place to look at yourself and keep motivated, there are distractions and many women just feel out of place, and do not have the time, nor the desire to get into the core of a gym. Professional personal trainers can give you motivation, keep you on target and make you feel important even though you are not a gym queen."

Presently, the role of personal trainers in the gym environment is indeed a dynamic element of the fitness industry. Fitness centres vary in their degree of openness towards self-employed personal trainers. Some international chains directly hire personal trainers who work only for them, to both offer their clients the possibility of further personalisation, and to control what gets done in the gym. Some small businesses are quite open to selected self-employed personal trainers who may have developed a relationship with the manager. Some others may indeed ban personal trainers from the premises. This is the case at the local gym where Valentina works in Bologna. This small business has positioned itself in the fitness market as a welcoming, down-to-earth, local gym where all clients need some personal attention from staff. Gym staff in turn endeavour to promote a "community" feeling. Valentina thus says:

> We do not have personal trainers here, we want to keep a certain coherence, so it's the three of us, we are gym instructors and we help clients work with machines, we really know them, support them, it's not like having a trainer, but it's not that different, and you are less depended on. This is like an all-inclusive service.

A small gym with a relatively stable clientele may provide an all-inclusive service, but this becomes more difficult in large premises and highly standardised international chains. In these chains most gym instructors do not offer classes they have devised themselves, but work with standardised formats. By providing standardised exercise-to-music formats, and leaving relatively little room for instructors' creativity, fitness centres become analogous to global fast-food chains, offering fairly predictable training that may be taunted as "McDonaldised", to use Ritzer's (1993) label. In this light, standardised exercise may be seen as having a rather "dehumanising" effect in so far as it is the final globalised expression of the process of rationalisation.

Like personal training, exercise standardisation is an important trend within fitness gyms and it is the result of a complex division of labour within the fitness industry itself. The largest producer of exercise-to-music formats is Les Mills International, a New Zealand company that has launched its seven different exercise formats under the Body Training System brand name in the early 1990s.[6] Les Mills International operates with a process similar to franchise (Felstead et al., 2007): instructors must be affiliated to a club that holds an agreement to use the programmes, the club is provided with promotional materials such as ceiling banners, posters and leaflets, instructors gain qualification by participating in assessed training modules, and they teach to the rhythm of the global enterprise which quarterly releases fresh choreography for each of its training formats. As much as it is continuously changing, such choreography is globally standardised across the franchised clubs around the world. Based on interviews with trainers and gym managers, a recent research by Alan Felstead and associates (ibid.) has looked at the job of exercise-to-music instructors in Britain contrasting "freestyle" instructors who devise their classes in terms of music selection, choreography and style and "pre-choreographed" instructors that deliver a pre-packaged product. Freestyle instructors have to "map music", have to "write dancing" movements and have to "convey an appropriate image" that they create themselves. This may be very rewarding for trainers, but it is very risky for gym managers. In the mentioned study, predictability and sub-stitutability were quoted by managers as reasons for buying a Body Training System subscription (ibid., p. 200): "If you buy BTS you know what you're getting for your money – if you leave it to the instructor, then really it's a bit of a lottery"; "they are going to come in with the same music and they are going to do exactly the same thing. So if one of my instructors can't do it, I get another BTS woman in here."Clearly, as Felstead suggests, under such system of provision, instructors' power is reduced and their services cheap-ened, and so is their capacity to fine tune exercise to clients' needs. Through professional credentials for pre-packaged classes that prize standardisation and discourage inventiveness trainers specialise, but their general exercise-to-music competences are in fact restricted: "training can actually deaden rather than awaken individual creativity. A growing proportion of training and continuous professional development undertaken by instructors schools them to deliver 'one size fits all' types of class. These pre-choreographed classes are manufactured and scripted by specialized workers located far away from the point of view of delivery" (ibid., p. 203).

Felstead does not consider what is the impact of a growing trend towards pre-packaged exercise-to-music classes on clients, on their training experi-ences as consumers and on their exercise adherence. In my research, I have noticed that it was fairly uncommon for clients to be aware of the complex, varied system of provision of exercise-to-music classes. Yet, personalisation, inventiveness, personal involvement and enthusiasm were generally appre-ciated, and indeed required, from instructors in all classes and gyms. The fitness consumer may accept a McDonaldised class, but wants it delivered by a human being, and an "enthusiastic", "joyful", "authentic" one. When instructors do not convey enthusiasm, when their performance appears false and too standardised, we get one of the main reasons deployed by gym drop-outs to justify their exit. Conversely, gym loyalty is often granted on the basis of a more or less dense relationship with gym staff, trainers and instructors predicated on genuine competence and involvement.

In the gym, standardisation may thus produce quite strong contradictions, and this is evident also for fitness workers. Instructors typically enter the fitness industry because of what they reckon is a "genuine interest" or "pas-sion" for fitness, describing themselves as having been fitness "fans" or even "junkies" before seeking a professional career. All trainers and instructors I have met with brought a considerable amount of personal knowledge into their job – variously related to their interests in competitive sports, conquest sports, food and nutrition, martial arts, natural pursuits, massage, rehabili-tation therapy, dance, swimming and gymnastics, to mention just some of the relevant pursuits mentioned by my interviewees. Personal knowledge is rarely codified, resulting from a combination of different, often disparate, experiences that were initially carried out as leisure. Becoming a fitness professional entails a switch from leisure to work, thus from the pursuit of one's own pleasure and discipline to the promotion of others' pleasure and discipline (Guerrier and Adib, 2003). But it also requires an ongoing enactment of the original vocation or passion for the job. And it may require quite a bit of continuous self-work in order to come to terms with one's own body ideals and objectives (Phillips and Drummond, 2001). In the long run, this may be more difficult to sustain for exercise-to-music instructors that are discouraged to put to work their personal knowledge and yet, as opposed to machine instructors or personal trainers who train clients from the sidelines, must actively demonstrate authenticity and enthusiasm in front of a class.

We should also explore the relationship between standardisation and personalisation as the fitness industry develops along the local-global dialectic. Personal relations are important even in McDonaldised settings and transactions (see Sassatelli 2007). Different levels of personalisation, as related to different levels of service orientation and commitment to clients' integration were evident in the different organisational cultures of two US Curves franchises according to Jenny O'Toole (2009). Looking at both members and workers of these globally marketed rationalised fitness programmes for women, she observes that local culture, as effected by different location, membership and managerial orientation greatly influences how much standardisation and rationalisation are shaped to accommodate substantive needs for movement in a sociable context. However, even in more structural terms, the global diffusion of fitness gyms and fitness chains does not simply follow the logic of McDonaldisation. To borrow from Weber's well-known terminology (Weber, 1922), I would like to suggest that the expansion of the fitness industry mixes rationalised forms of organisation with charismatic elements. Just like the contemporary retail sector is characterised by two directions of development which both diverge and reinforce one another (on the one hand, the spread of discount stores emphasising price and standardisation; on the other, specialty shops and niche chains with a renewed emphasis on quality, difference and variety), so the fitness industry realises a duality, mingling standardised training and personal training. Standardisation and McDonaldised branding is indeed the other side of the coin of personalisation and personal training.[7] To a degree, these two trends respond to the need of enhancing the productivity of each premise in an increasingly saturated market. And they may work in synergy as much as in opposition, their arrangement sustaining gym differentiation. We may thus identify at least two poles in fitness gym provision: local all-inclusive gyms, on the one hand, where exercise standardisation is lower and personalisation is provided in a more informal manner, and standardised chains that complement exercise standardisation with the in-house offer of personal training services, on the other. In large international chains and upmarket clubs it is quite common to have a team of personal trainers who have undergone specific in-house preparation, and who work as a team with gym instructors and gym staff under the auspices of the management to strengthen the whole branding of the premise or the chain. The services offered by such in-house personal trainers are also, to an extent, standardised, in that the tone of the relationship with clients is in some ways prescribed.

Even in this case, however, a personal trainer is understood to offer some kind of partnership in training. Their job trades on charisma as well as on standardised qualifications. In March 2008, the issue of *Fitness Management Magazine*, a US-based online professional periodical, describes personal trainers as "partners in fitness" – they help individuals with their training as long as clients make their health a priority and enjoy their exercise programme, ask any questions as and when necessary, and remain as open-minded as possible regarding their goals, abilities and health concerns.[8] In Italy the professional magazine *Il nuovo club* (The new club) celebrated its 13th birthday in January 2006 with a special edition that featured a number of well-established fitness professionals – the marketing expert, the fitness equipment entrepreneur, the exercise-to-music instructor, the personal trainer. The personal trainer, in particular, is asked to acquire in a rather personalised fashion a complex set of competences. According to the reported Italian magazine, such a figure is "a 360-degree professional", both with a "scientific" preparation – from "training theory", to "physiology", to "occupational therapy", to "nutrition science" – and "clearly human gifts" – such as "diplomacy", the ability to "know how to listen" and so on – combined with "notions of psychology" and "motivation theory".[9] To personal trainers themselves that with a client may appear as what one of them called a "total relationship" based on both expertise and emotions. "You must create a total relationship with your client", said indeed Carmine, a personal trainer from Bologna, and thus specified:

> [a relationship] which is technical, about objectives, and schedules, which is motivational about getting in tune with the person, his needs and emotions...you must be professional, serious, precise, reliable and organised. The human relationship is very important in order to build a rapport, then when you have done so, you must give it all your attention. My clients are people who want to have an excellent human relationship, they want someone to trust, to yield themselves over completely to in order to reach their objectives.

While "personal", the personal trainer-client relationship is, however, quite bounded. The issue of boundaries is fundamental and may be best appreciated if we look at what, in their own views, personal trainers should never do in their job: they should never get too close or too personal; set inappropriate goals; bore clients and make them feel bad. Let us take a significant interview exchange to illustrate the main themes which emerge from personal trainers' experiences of their relationships with clients and what they consider to be good practice:

Q. What type of relationship do you want to establish with your customers?

A. I have a very structured programme which covers fitness and provides nutritional advice. These people pay a lot of money and I want to give them a top class service. The relationship has to be friendly because this is also about fun and enjoyment but you are essentially providing a service to them and you must keep focused and professional at all times.

Q. What is the most important thing for a trainer in their relationship with their customers?

A. I think that the most important thing is to set a clear and realistic target which responds to their motivation. In other words, it is important to give them a reason, it can be anything, but they have to focus on a certain strength.

Q. What should you never do?

A. You shouldn't give them false hopes or unrealistic expectations. Some people almost want to pass on responsibility to the fitness trainer. They have to understand that this is not about purchasing a new body but it's all about small but constant changes.

(Vicky, personal trainer, London)

As much as it is emphasised, the personal element in personal training must remain accessory to training. In doing their job, personal trainers should avoid making clients "feel uncomfortable, overwork them, make inappropriate comments", they should instead "motivate clients" and "try to make them enjoy what they're doing". The best option towards these ends is to "be friendly without getting too close" – something that trainers themselves reckon can be quite "hard".

While, as suggested, all fitness instructors must be both experts, illustrate tasks and act as emotional leaders, motivation is the very essence of the job of the personal trainer. Motivation is managed mainly in two ways: on the one hand, by playing on new and fun techniques, and, on the other, by helping clients negotiate their initial objectives. These elements are so professionally entrenched that they become part of personal trainers' official self-presentation. In 2006 Adam, the London-based personal trainer we have already encountered, advertised himself on his website as using "the latest training techniques to maximise the efficiency of your workout time, we can ensure you achieve the most from your fitness efforts... Emphasising diversity, and most importantly fun, exercise will never be a dull and monotonous experience again." The management of motivation by novelty and customisation came up in his interview as a qualifying element of his training services. He reckoned that for doing the job well, he must "try to keep ahead of the game, so I am interested in anything new, particularly with anything that comes from America. I adapt to my customers' needs, and listen to what they want and work on it together with them." Clients' initial objectives are often deemed "unrealistic" and therefore much of a personal trainer's job relates to objectives negotiation. The initial interview with a new client is very important. As in most gyms, new clients are asked to describe their sport biography, their medical biography and what they want to attain or achieve from working out. But personal trainers also offer step-by-step personalised negotiation of training objectives. "We work on the objectives to negotiate them," says Franco, a personal trainer from Milan. "If you manage to get them to start, they feel good, and then their initial objective is a bit forgotten, they learn there are other important things."

It is worth stressing that the idea that body objectives are negotiated in the gym is prevalent among all fitness participants both on the production side – personal trainers as well as gym instructors – and the consumption side. As I shall show, regular clients reckon that training may help people "get real" about their bodies, coming to terms with media-fuelled illusions (see Chapter 6). While the emphasis in fitness discourse is on professionalism and personalisation, in practice the negotiation of objectives, training variety and the management of fun are, in many ways, the core practical elements of fitness, and steer the boundary between production and consumption. Indeed, as a young personal trainer from Bologna admits, "to have a really personal exercise you have to become a personal trainer yourself, you have to train yourself, become an expert not just interested. This is why I ended up becoming a personal trainer." Despite increasing professionalisation, fitness workers' biographies stress how intertwined are the production and the consumption of fitness. Instructors and personal trainers often get initiated into fitness by practising it as a leisure pursuit, and subsequently make it into a profession – with a similar trajectory being more typical in towns rather than metropolitan contexts, as well as in Italy as compared to Britain where a more bureaucratic, institutionally enforced distinction between professionals and clients exists.

All in all, despite the role of gym instructors and personal trainers as expert, task and emotional leaders, clients are co-producers of the training scene. Training for clients may thus be creative, but it is also clearly "hard work" – not only in the obvious terms of physical fatigue, but also in relation to the playing out of different roles, the negotiation of objectives, the ability to keep focused and have fun. A number of contradictions thus harbour the world of fitness. While fitness programmes are sold as leisure, and trainers help clients to participate in fitness, for clients there is quite a bit of work to be done. Likewise, the gym is typically presented by the fitness industry as a place to relax, but, as suggested, there is a lot of anxiety present. In such a context, where does the experience of detachment from the external world, which so many regular clients report, come from? How does concentration happen? Which motivations are prescribed in fitness and why might such motivations help concentration? How is concentration coded? How is it connected to exercise adherence and competence? These are some of the questions which I shall address in the next two chapters.

4
Framing Fitness

Inside the gym, clients find themselves in a relatively separated world of meanings, with its own interaction rules aimed at facilitating relatively stable and exclusive concentration on performing structured and prescribed physical activities. According to regulars, this is a quality of fitness gyms which is much appreciated: they think it crucial that these places "push" them to exercise even when they do not feel very motivated. Clients actively contribute to the training scene. Fitness is a lived culture wherein participants, providers and clients, co-produce the scene of consumption. Amy, a young woman who has practised fitness training for many years, illustrates this point alluding to the "concentrated people" that she sees around her while training. She thus elaborates the compelling character of the scene:

> The gym is important because I would not exercise at home. I know it does me good, but if I had to do it on my own, laziness would get the better of me. Going to the gym is a way of saying: "I do physical exercise." It is a stimulating environment, which allows you to concentrate on trying to better yourself; for an hour no one disturbs you, so you exercise.

In the previous chapter, I began to look at the give and take marshalled in the fitness centre via the management of local relationships. Probably even more crucial is the management of meaningful involvement in the workouts. As a fundamental element of situated practice, the management of meaningful involvement is indeed the cornerstone of the study of any and all cultures of consumption (Sassatelli, 2007).

To understand how involvement in fitness training inside the gym may actually take place we shall consider the exercise scene and focus on the cognitive, affective and moral organisation of interaction. The scene is sustained by small, tacit rules of interaction which require close ethnographic observation to be fully appreciated. This is so because they are typically taken for granted, and yet in their humble, recurrent quality they give shape to participants' expectations. Indeed, interaction during training is carried out by trainers and clients in such a way as to limit embarrassment and boredom while pushing and pulling clients to carry out the exercise in a regime of intense visibility. Interaction rules "frame" – to use an expression made famous by Goffman – the keep-fit workout, making it clear that the ongoing activities are indeed fitness training. The notion of frame is particularly useful for understanding how physical activity catches clients' attention. Goffman (1974, pp. 10–11) used this concept to indicate those "principles of organisation which govern events – at least social ones – and our subjective involvement in them".[1] A frame is a "context for understanding" and "reference", a set of "organisational premises – sustained both *in the mind and in activity*", which orients our perceptions within that context via the deployment of "transformation rules" about what is relevant and irrelevant (ibid., 1961, pp. 27ff., 1974, pp. 247 and 39, emphasis added). Training scenes can be considered as contexts of practical understanding which define, more or less implicitly, what is relevant, appropriate and what should be valued during keep-fit exercise. The fitness frame also defines what fitness is: *how* and *why* it shall be carried out. The former is what we may call the *internal trim* of the frame, namely the relation that the participating subject has to develop with the activity. It is largely defined by a specific *motivational logic*. The latter is the *external trim* of the frame, namely the relation that the framed activity has with other, similar, physical and sports activities. It is largely defined by a specific *justificatory logic*. Let's consider the external trim of the frame first, as this allows for a portrayal which better mimics clients' encounter with the gym.

1. Sport, fitness and performance

In contemporary Western societies sports and keep-fit activities are in many ways intermingled. We may do sport for keeping fit, and we may train in a fitness gym to run a marathon. Also, training in contemporary sports activities is quite often organised via disciplinary techniques (Chambliss, 1989; Guttmann, 1978; Heikkala, 1993). In the words of Foucault (1991, pp. 136–7), disciplines are methods of intervention which obtain holds upon the body "at the level of the mechanism itself – movements, gestures, attitudes, rapidity: an infinitesimal power over the active body"; whose constrains bear at the level of the "the economy, the efficiency of movements" rather than "the signifying elements of behaviour"; and, finally, which supervise "the processes of the activity rather than its result", being based upon the "meticulous control of the operations of the body" to assure a "constant subjection of its forces" and the imposition of a "relation of docility-utility". As physical education, its forebear, fitness training is also inspired by rationalised detail and control (Vigarello, 1992). Yet, on the whole, fitness is described by participants – gym-goers, trainers and gym staff – as *different* from most contemporary individual or team sports activities. Let's explore this.

Although contemporary sports differ greatly from each other, by and large they are all customarily presented as ends in themselves. Practising a sport for some time has visible effects on the body, yet body transformation is secondary to the acquisition of highly specific abilities. These abilities in turn are released on certain occasions that are organised within the sporting world, even though they may become a highly lucrative spectacle for the masses. In sport, body transformation is thus subordinated to the style of execution, the athletic gesture and the exceptional performance. Indeed, contemporary sports activities are inspired by *athleticism*. Athleticism is a normative ideal whereby sport is conceived as a self-referential activity, whose rationale is in the satisfaction which participants feel in its performance or in the affirmation of a specialised competence.[2] Although, economic or political issues impinge on the world of sport (Booth, 1993; Giulianotti, 2005), the "sport for sport's sake" principle is sustained by the release of peak performances in special occasions – such as races, games, matches and so on – which are institutionally, temporally and spatially defined (Bourdieu, 1978; Guttmann, 1978). Body modification and training are geared to specialised performances: the athlete exercising with the competition in mind, repeating sequences of movements that reproduce the perfect exercise which will one day have to be produced, or working on a sluggish muscle whose condition impedes peak performance. The body is moulded to improve *athletic performance*, the latter being the official justificatory logic for sports activities.

Fitness, instead, is about what I call an *embodied performance*. As suggested, some clients may join a gym with an external athletic goal in mind, like playing a weekly football match with friends. This perhaps is increasingly happening, and for at least two reasons, as both Italian and British fitness managers maintain: on the one hand, fitness centres are increasingly available, and try to cater for ever wider publics; on the other hand, the anticipation and provision of external athletic targets, such as participating in sporting events, appears to sustain gym adherence and loyalty. In itself, though, fitness training is not geared to a specific performance to be achieved or reproduced to the maximum on a special sporting occasion. The refinement of movement or the individuation of specific muscles and body parts are not aimed at obtaining an ultimate better quality exercise. Performance in fitness is embodied – the ultimate achievement goes beyond carrying out the exercises, and coincides with the opportunity for body transformation and improvement. In the typical, official justificatory account for keep-fit activities the prospect of modelling one's own body dominates the exercise, to the point that emphasis may not be placed on clients' capacity to perform the exercise at their best, but good enough to work on the body. Fitness as a rather general and broadly instrumental physical quality is the paramount embodied performance of fitness training (see Chapter 7).

The differences of sports and fitness activities are expressed in these terms in official publications on sport and health. The Council of Europe, for example, defines fitness as something which goes beyond the "highly specific abilities" connected to performance typical of "athletics and sports activities", and associates it more with a "general functional capacity to deal with physical demands without excessive difficulty" (Oja and Tuxworth, 1995, pp. 6, 13). As much as it is concerned with the promotion of healthy sports practice, the Council of Europe considers that the long-term effects of physical "conditioning" are secondary in real sport, which is of necessity characterised by the "acceptance of exclusive rules" and by "competition".

Most gym-goers contrast fitness with sport on the grounds that the possibility of modifying, improving and maintaining the body qualifies the former. Mauro, for example, maintains that although one may do something for one's body by playing tennis, it is neither sufficient nor adequate as the exercise is not specifically designed to achieve a better shape. In playing tennis, "even at an amateur level", he explains, "you can't really concentrate on improving your body" and you could even "push yourself too far" in an attempt to achieve top performances. When asked to think of possible alternatives to the gym, many clients mentioned jogging or swimming, but they felt that the opportunities for physical improvement provided by such activities were far less precise and, more than anything, overly tied in with peak or specific exercise performances. To illustrate these points, here are some quotes from two quite diverse fitness novices who have previous sports experience. Cesare, a middle-aged sales representative, reports: "When I did judo, the movement techniques were oriented towards judo activities, but here they're simply oriented towards improving your physical shape, and I don't learn anything." Federica too, a high-school girl who has practised athletics since she was a child, says that she is "far from being the kind of person suited to gyms" since she "like[s] to do something to learn something". According to her gyms "are only to build muscles or to tone them, because I don't have the chance to do anything else, so at least I keep active. It may be pleasant at the time, but the exercises you learn are of no real use; it's not as if you're going to have to present them, or that there's going to be a competition in which you'll be recognised for what you do".

Thus, in some ways fitness is all training, relying heavily on rationalisation. As recalled by a Florentine fitness trainer who has long been in the business, "in the human body there are 639 voluntary muscles, and we can identify and move each one of them". One enthusiastic novice to the gym world suggested that she has learned not only to "move" but also to "see" and "feel" all the "various muscles" and to recognise their function: "bit by bit, I have managed to co-ordinate my movements, and I've discovered lots of little muscles which I've never seen in an encyclopaedia". Another gym novice, coming from a sporting past, says he "has learnt to see things differently": "As far as the body's concerned, movement is movement. It's not as if it prefers weight-lifting or doing leg exercises, so if I want to keep fit, I might as well go to the gym, where I can target training to whatever I want to achieve." Similar views are common among regular clients both in Italy and Britain – they all proudly refer to their newfound abilities to see and feel their bodies in detail.

As an early study on the most authoritative French health and beauty magazine illustrates, fitness is presented as both allowing for the greatest "personalisation of movement" and as offering the "best matching of movement with the desired effect" (Amir, 1987, p. 116). During exercise, the articulation between space, time and body is both analytical and minute, and demands not only that time be subdivided into exact and infinitesimal units, but that each movement should be assigned a length of time which matches its effectiveness. Such rationalisation is typically presented as providing effectiveness and efficiency, with fitness manuals often suggesting that their programme works in detail, and works fast: "[t]ime is money. Energy is precious. Why waste them in something futile?" (Pinckney, 1992, p. 47). In broad theoretical terms, the deployment of disciplinary techniques signals a contrast between, on the one hand, traditional legitimation claiming to reproduce ascribed differences and, on the other, instrumental-rational legitimation concentrating on the better means for achieving analytically defined goals for all.[3] The fitness gym is no exception: clients are asked to consider that a "better body" can be acquired by anyone who wishes to sufficiently commit themselves and the "rationality" of fitness training in getting a better body is presented as its *raison d'être*.

In this sense, effectiveness and efficiency act as a dispassionate justification of the gym beyond the gym. Even for the clients who cannot bring themselves to attend regularly, for those who do not enjoy exercise, for those who claim to prefer other activities, the gym is typically perceived as the most "rational" and "rapid" solution, an effective "short cut" for doing something about one's own body, something which "makes the most of the time available". "Going to a gym," says a reluctant participant such as Cristina, "is a solution which doesn't take up much time, you can do it when you're in a hurry and you see the results quickly." While, as I shall show more in detail in the next chapter, fun, competence acquisition and sociability are crucial determinants for prolonged subjective participation, fitness as a broad socio-institutional phenomenon largely rests on rational arguments, stressing efficiency and effectiveness in getting external rewards.

Clients' stories of successful initiation to the gym typically stress the role of instrumental-rational considerations when approaching fitness training in a gym. For example, Paola, who is a regular at Shape in Florence, says that she tried out fitness gyms because other activities were not "functional", "convenient" or "specific" enough. Even though initially discouraged by the first fitness gyms she visited, she continued trying to find a good one because she was convinced the gym was the "most rational" solution. In the end she found one that was really "good and involving":

> I started off with Yoga, and then I dropped it, and spent three years doing nothing... I don't have the time to go for long walks, and going to the gym is a way of getting things done in a short space of time, because you cram everything in. It was my head which told me to come to the gym, not my heart or any real desire to do it... the first experience [in a gym] was disastrous, exercise was boring and I didn't feel the slightest bit involved, [yet I knew] it was the best solution, and for a number of years I looked out for a suitable gym... [one that could] get me involved... [now that I've found it] I want to use time in the gym thoroughly – an effective lesson is one in which I'm aware I'm doing something, you're working on your body with a specific goal in mind, so you have to move various muscles.

On the presumption of the fitness gym "rationality", enthusiasts like Paola seem to have progressed from an instrumental emphasis on external rewards to an expressive involvement in keep-fit routines and a reflexive appreciation of internal rewards (see also Chapter 5). But they are quite happy to say that keep-fit exercise "works because it's specific", "the various movements are targeted at physical form, at improving this or that defect, so it's obvious they work".

Newcomers and marginal clients, on the contrary, often express their discomfort with rationalisation. In particular, the estranged clients or the gym-quitters may get to question the effectiveness and efficiency of the fitness centre, on the premises that the fitness workout is too boring to be good and that it does not necessarily suit everyone. Their stories turn successful initiation stories upside down: if involvement or internal rewards are not there, external rationality is nullified, and to keep looking for the perfect gym may be vain. Emphasis on non-competitive improvement of the body may have the effect of devaluing fitness training. Expressions of disillusionment include: "doing exercises is not very useful if you get really bored", "fitness may be for anyone, but it is surely not for me", "it takes up too much time", "you can get the same results with other things which are better because they are less boring and mechanical", because "you have to compete, you have tactics and all that". These stories often touch upon sports activities stressing their better capacity to provide for involvement and thus to allow for exercise adherence: sports such as tennis or volleyball are re-evaluated as less specific but in fact more effective means to do something for the body as they can provide involvement and fun.

To be true, competition is always somehow impinging on the fitness scene. But it is mainly seen in a negative light, officially excluded and not elaborated though official narratives of self and achievement. Competition with others may inject a dialogic, strategic element in training, but it cannot be overtly carried out. Competition is often likened with opposite, negative feelings such as pride or insecurity, contributing to creating an unpleasant and intimidating atmosphere, dissuading rather than involving newcomers. Indeed, some clients do not seem to be able to avoid resorting to competition with others to give some kind of meaning to what they are doing. Competition can be an outlook which derives from having previously participated in competitive sports activities. Some participants may dislike fitness training individualism and may be unable to feel satisfied without a more dialogic engagement with others, even through contest and competition. Others may indeed feel constantly reminded of their inferiority in terms of body capital and performance. Sandro exemplifies the hesitation and continuous adjustments that even regular clients have to face. He was at first "hindered" because he felt "inferior", and then helped by the fact that he "had improved". He now says with a certain pride: "I'm no longer the newest person here, now it's the others who have to learn from me", but then quickly suggests that it is "important" that no one should "show off their muscles" during the exercises.

These observations move us from the external to the internal trim of the frame, how the participant of a keep-fit session has to relate to the activity. In contrast to traditional sports, fitness training has, at least officially, nothing to do with a struggle for superiority – it appears as a perfect example of what Bourdieu (1978, p. 839) defines as "health-oriented sports" which "do not offer any competitive satisfaction". Official expert discourse as expressed in exercise manuals stress this point, often inviting prospective gym-goers "to refrain from competition with other participants". The advice of a successful Italian fitness manual expresses the spirit of training in the gym very well: "avoid competition with the friend you are training with, or with others in the gym: there is no prize for those who become tall and slim before any of the others" (Rizzi, 1992, p. 9). Callan Pinckney (1992, p. 26), a famous American trainer whose books are translated into many languages, invites those who wish to follow her programme "not to make the mistake of thinking that all the others are 'perfect' and you are not. Work with what you have. You can always improve."

Competition control is indeed one of the main tasks performed by instructors and trainers in all gyms I have studied. The most popular trainers are often those who take great care to encourage everyone and to appreciate the effort made even by those who have only just started, while managing to engage with regulars. These trainers seem to pay particular attention to participants who seem to be lacking in concentration or experience (see Chapter 3). Both in Italy and Britain, I have repeatedly witnessed instructors asserting the importance of non-competitive dedication. Drawn from my early ethnography of two Florentine gyms (Sassatelli 2000c), here are a couple of the little speeches that popular gym instructors have given to their classes during training:

> You aren't in competition here, you're not in a race, so don't look at those next to you. You have to try and do a little more every day... A little more effort every day and in the end you'll see the difference.
>
> (Lory, stretching and low-impact aerobics instructor, Florence)

> You're wonderful, all of you. Don't worry about those in front of you, concentrate on the exercise and what you are able to manage. You will improve, just keep going, keep going.
>
> (Pamela, step-aerobics instructor, Florence)

Such encouragement is typical when one or more newcomers join a fairly established group. This is well illustrated by the following excerpt from my field notes in the London branch of an upmarket British chain:

> Pilates class, late afternoon. I play the newcomer. The instructor welcomes me, learns my name and she gives me special attention during the whole of the class. The class is big, there are about thirty of us, with only six men. Laura, the instructor, calls most of the people by name. She addresses us in the singular, but is very wary of giving too much attention or too little attention to any of us. Towards the end of the class we use equipment. I need some but the remaining plastic cylinders are too big for me. She suggest that a man next to me gives me his, and he can take a bigger one. I say half-jokingly, "Oh! He is very good then" She replies, "He has come regularly from September, twice a week, you see what you can do!" The man smiles, and puts extra effort in his routine.
>
> (Pilates class, London, January 2007)

This scene shows clearly that instructors must acknowledge the improvement of clients by encouraging them, but avoid alluding to hierarchies in terms of performance which may introduce the spectre of competition. Clients themselves seem quite collaborative on this point, and tend to mimic the inclusiveness of trainers.

Keeping competition at bay is very important. In the gym, training is not, at least officially, practically organised via competition and hierarchy, even though in the fitness industry, exercise contests are becoming popular among professional trainers. To be true, an element of competition seems to be present in gym initiatives such as the "Member of the Month" schemes which have been introduced in many gyms, and which are especially prevalent in the chains which I have visited in London. Such schemes are all about achievement – they focus on clients' success stories, stressing the instrumental value of training (getting slimmer, fitter and so on) rather its intrinsic value (fun, fitness competence). As such they may indeed introduce forms of competition and the surreptitious possibility of establishing hierarchies of clients. In all the gyms I have visited, gym staff maintained that these schemes are an excellent way to keep clients motivated, create a community feeling and promote gym adherence. However, they were also adamant that too much competition must be avoided. Judging from the brief accounts of the justification of these monthly winners as they appear on the announcing posters in the gym, competition is too much when it amounts to internal hierarchies of bodies and exercise performances. Stressed is clients' equivalent motivational positioning. What is praised then is effort and improvement. But these are highly individualised – emphasis being placed on individuals getting better, stronger, slimmer, fitter on their own individual scale, which officially excludes inter-individual comparability. And if competition is there, it is about how good clients are at the incessant demonstration of their commitment via strenuous and yet cheerful participation in gym activities. Or it is displaced onto external sporting events.

To be sure, clients who regularly attend generally improve their own performance. Closeness and complicity, which tend to keep gym teams apart from other participants, may develop among regulars. Similar processes have already been observed by Klein (1993, pp. 46–80) in body-building gyms, where the most prominent positions are occupied by professionals and semi-professionals who train together and keep their distance from all those who have not developed similar bodies and abilities.[4] It is certainly a feature of boxing gyms as studied by Wacquant (2003). In observing a women-only aerobics class, Joseph Maguire and Louise Mansfield (1998, pp. 117ff.) have also maintained that "the more established women [in a class] get power by using exercise knowledge, a better shape and the getting of more acceptable bodies" and that they love to "show" their "enthusiasm" and their "slim, toned bodies" at the expense of those who are not so fit or cannot profitably follow the exercises and may therefore ultimately feel ashamed and powerless. A few of the regular clients I met, in fact, confessed that some of the gyms they attended were not good precisely because they were "full of big-headed people who want to show off" or who are "not very serious" and are "indiscreet". A few regulars also suggested that they nevertheless felt very "gratified" by public recognition of their abilities by the trainers, with comments or the assignation of tasks and difficulties. Still, observing training scenes in many and diverse premises, the creation of privileged, exclusive groups seemed to be marginal, and not simply because these processes concern a small minority of clients. Along with seduction or exhibitionism, competition between clients and the creation of exclusive élites generally remains discreet, and it is as much stigmatised as it is tolerated.

Clients' role in keeping competition at bay is central. During both group and machine activity, clients are likely to work together to limit competitive attitudes and performance show-off, which consequently take on a somewhat furtive character. Many regulars, despite sporting physical signs of their training achievement, comment ironically on blatantly competitive people: they stigmatise the "excess" of the "fanatics" – that is, people deemed "obsessed with results", "competitive" or "narcissistic" – in the small talk before and after training and in the dressing rooms. Similar dynamics have also been mentioned in sport psychology (Vugt et al., 1998). Indeed, the open display of a competitive attitude may be risky for clients. Paola, a Florentine secretary in her late fifties, remembers two "good-looking women" who were constantly "disturbing" the free-standing exercise lessons, "because one of them was giving instructions to the other" and they were "showing off too much", to such an extent that "the trainers tried to put a stop to it". "Little by little," said Paola, "all those who were there just to get on with their workouts cut them off, even making jokes about them." Gym enthusiasts who seek confirmation of their superiority in competitive terms often end up training off-peak, in the early morning or the late evening, when their attitude is less of a concern and they can develop a more personal relationship with trainers (see Chapter 2). For most of the day, for most clients in most training scenes – and certainly in terms of what is officially prescribed and institutionally promoted – incentives for fitness participants do not come from competition with other participants. Indeed, most clients I interviewed replied to a question on what had been for them the most rewarding occasion in the gym, referring, on the one hand, to the personalised attention and advice they may have obtained from trainers, and, on the other, to feelings of self-accomplishment for hard work or having gone beyond one's own limit.

2. Self-competition and abundance

Fitness training in the gym does not demand a denial of all challenges. The internal trim of the frame has not only a negative dimension, but also a positive one: a number of expressive devices, including direct verbal solicitation, are deployed to boost involvement and commitment turning competition on itself and replacing it by *self-competition* – a striving to better one's body and exercise performance. In the exercise spaces, clients are thus asked to enter a world where there is no competition with other participants, at least officially. This is not because everyone is or will indeed be equal. But because everyone is placed in an *equivalent motivational position*, that of making one's own performance the object of a continuous self-challenge. Like regulative rules of Searlian memory (see Perinbanayagam, 2006, pp. 64ff.), self-competition extends beyond the game, spilling off the training scene to somehow define the whole dominant spirit of the fitness gym.

Metaphors of combat have been observed as being prevalent in fitness discourse across the world – including Amir's study of the French periodical *Vital* (Amir, 1987) and Morse's analysis of North American aerobics videos (Morse, 1987). Various forms of self-challenge are paramount in health and fitness magazines whose pages invite readers to "eliminate" fat, "combat" cellulite, "defy" age and so on (Sassatelli, 2003). Trainers' and instructors' exhortations do not simply have the negative function of removing competition among participants – while gym-goers cannot openly measure their ability against that of other participants, they are expected to compete with themselves, doing a little bit more every day, improving their exercise performance, setting training goals and so on. In my fieldwork both in Italy and Britain, I repeatedly encountered instructors inciting clients to continue exercising by using images of battle. During a difficult step sequence, I thus learned that fat was "burnt" and "attacked", getting to the end of an aerobics class I was invited, as all participants, to "hold on, up to the breaking point". Machine training also requires that each participant "pushes oneself to the limits of one's own strength". Instructors and gym staff praise effort and perseverance and reinforce gym adherence: "you must tell them [the clients] that going to the gym when there are so many things to do, proves your own worth ... what's important is commitment, everything else will come of its own accord", says Mario who runs an independent well-established fitness centre in Milan.

Self-competition is indeed at the heart of the *motivational logic* of keep-fit training. By motivational logic I do not mean effective individual motivation, but the form that action must take when subjects display their motives, affects and desires (see Burke, 1962; Wright Mills, 1940; and for a discussion in relation to consumption, see Campbell, 1994). Not every participant manages to endorse it, or wants to do so. The official emphasis on clients' motivational equivalence may precisely be disrespectful of client's different capacities to actually endorse self-competition. This typically gives way to alienation from interaction and, consequently, gym drop-out. Self-competition amounts to how participants in fitness should represent, to themselves and to others, their own desire to proceed with the activity. It does not imply a stimulus to action which precedes and defines it from the outside, like the often vague desire to get fit as expressed by the purchase of a gym pass. Instead, self-competition is an emotional code through which clients can transform and reconstitute their own motives according to locally prescribed modalities, and transcend habits, desires or objectives which could project them beyond the immediacy of the exercises. It acts as a filter for subjective motivation, and becomes the form that desires and motives must publicly assume in order for individuals to pursue relevant activities on a regular basis.

Self-competition is celebrated as a major achievement by regular gym-goers that I have met both in Italy and Britain. Regulars all agree that it is essential to try and "outdo yourself", attempt to "always do better" and almost engage in "a competition with your own abilities". Self-competition is essential in order to enter into "the spirit of training". This is what Jenny says: "I like the incremental side of doing exercises. I am managing much better. You improve your ability, you do more. And you want more. You say to yourself 'if I did it every day, who knows what I'd be like? Who knows what I can do!?!'. " On the contrary, irregular clients who regretfully achieve only erratic attendance, have difficulties in embracing self-competition. Cristina from Florence is one such client, and even though she realises that "self-challenge" is a crucial motivation, she "can't be bothered that much":

> Yes, I know I'm lazy, but I don't think that's why [I don't manage to go regularly], the fact is I don't enjoy it, I'm not stimulated by the idea of doing a bit better day by day... when I work hard, all I think of is that I have to improve my thighs, for example. Some people are just aiming at that, some keep trying to do better, but basically I think it looks ridiculous, you'd never do exercises like that on the beach, so there's no point in continuing to do them better, well, there might be some point if you want to go to the beach with an attractive bottom. Maybe I can't forget it and so it all seems a bit ridiculous to me... and it's boring.

Boredom, on the one hand, and anxiety, on the other, are self-acknowledged, major sources of alienation from keep-fit exercise for most clients. In order for self-competition to define a relatively engaging and non-contradictory domain of practice, keep-fit activities are organised as adapting to the varying abilities of the participants. This is managed via a comparatively high degree of tolerance to individual failures as compared with the training scene in competitive sports (Chambliss, 1989). And happens with the tacit concession of individual deviations – such as when a client stops to have a drink or tie up their shoelace, or when another one works with heavier weights than the rest of the class. But it is also officially prescribed by, and inscribed in, training. The creation of prescriptively exclusive groups based on performance level (advanced, beginners) is not enforced and indeed it is systematically softened by the notion that "everyone" should "do what they can" and that "no one is perfect". What characterises all keep-fit techniques is what I like to call adjustability. By this I mean the fact that assigned tasks or movements are modulated and made accessible. This is true not only of personal trainers, but also of instructors working with groups. All of them, for example, apply a set of small variations on the same movement so as to personalise most exercises, especially in the case of newcomers, older people or people who start a fitness programme after injury. Indeed, as Jan, an exercise-to-music instructor in a Norwich health club told me, instructors pride themselves on their capacity to "adapt all the movements to each client". This "capacity to adjust workout difficulty is the trademark of a good trainer", she continues, adding that she "tries to keep updated precisely to look for new ways of making the moves, which work for any problem and need". At stake is not only professionalisation though (see Chapter 3), but also the broader need to fashion discipline and self-challenge as a commercially mediated, universalistic and individualistic leisure pursuit.

The very material culture of the fitness gym realises such adjustability, potentially to keep all and every client involved. Machines are designed in order to accommodate different body size, ability and pace. Both in individual training with cardiovascular equipment or weights, and in keep-fit classes or groups, emphasis is on exercise tasks that are neither too easy nor too difficult. Body sculpt, aerobics, stretching, pilates and even more strenuous activities such as step aerobics or spinning hardly ever involve extremely difficult movements or sequences, nor do they entail an impossible pace and rhythm, trainers are all very aware of clients who may be left behind, or indeed of those who need some extra difficulty. Of course, individual performances vary a great deal. But the official emphasis is narrowed down on how one improves as compared to one's own previous performance. Improvability is the other key element of keep-fit training. Improvement is presented as limitless, even though different kinds of exercise may entail different kinds of improvement. With machine training, difficulty and improvement are typically articulated on a quantitative scale, consisting of numbers of repetitions, miles, calories, minutes or weights. Group activities are based mainly on imitation of movements and generally entail an infinite series of qualitative improvements. Improved performance implies an ever increasing control of gesture, posture and expressiveness.

Movements, in fitness as in other disciplines, become fully intelligible to the self only in the repetitive repetition of the exercise. And in the case of fitness, repetition entails self-competition sustained by adjustability and improvability. These two features facilitate the exercise hold on the body – enabling the body, space and time to be closely articulated, being geared to allowing for little hesitation, doubt, inertia or opportunity to pause. They help the exercise to be incorporated, to transform whatever theoretical understanding clients may have of trainers' instructions into embodied capacities. But they also qualify how motivation is narrated to the self and to others. The dominant script is that "what counts is commitment" with the objective that clients with limited abilities may keep exercising without feeling too excluded or exposed to ridicule, while very proficient clients are reminded that their display of zeal is just a requirement. In stressing the fact that commitment counts more than results and that no performance or result will ever be definitive, such script is meant to favour the creation of an ever stimulating scene. This configuration yields to three further, important and related features of fitness training. Contrary to what happens in athletic sports, fitness gyms deny scarcity of desire, ability, honour and so on. Instead, this field of action is founded on the generation of a *pluralistic abundance*. Just like contemporary consumer culture through which it is mainly channelled, fitness culture solves the problem of competition by offering non-competitive gratifications predicated on an infinite and diverse horizon of growth. There is always something more, something else, something new in fitness, something which can be adjusted to clients' needs. The lack of challenge with external opponents and the difficulty to get one's own achievements recognised in an official hierarchy is replaced by *novelty* and an emphasis on *self-experimentation*. Coming to see and feel one's own body through the regular practise of a variety of new activities is presented as a feature of fitness gyms (see also Chapter 7). Regulars both in Italy and Britain maintain that in order to continue training when exercise capacities improve they constantly need to get new incentives and possibly try more difficult things and explore different techniques. Likewise, the trainers and managers which I have interviewed in my study all insisted that clients should consider their gym as a place where each person has to find a "personal" way of training by using the array of techniques available and by making the most of all novelties. The creation of personalised and continuously renovated training programmes is itself a major device for the provision of non-competitive satisfaction (see Chapter 5).

3. Strenuousness, glances and expressions

The fitness frame sustains not only a particular motivational logic for involvement but also a particular emotional qualification of involvement. Clients are invited not only to compete with themselves, but also to demonstrate their own enthusiasm for the ongoing activity via the *display of strenuousness*. Indeed, they declare their utmost appreciation for their own and others' "desire to work really hard". They cherish and sustain "the energy" which seems to "envelop the group" while training, or the possibility of "looking around" and "seeing" that "everyone" is, in their own way, "determined" to do the exercises vigorously and enthusiastically. In everyday life, pain, far from being positively valued, is a sign that something is going wrong. In keep-fit exercise, as in many organised physical activities, aching muscles may be reframed as a sign of success which articulates involvement and rationalisation. "Even though I have only been going for a short while, I think it's working" says young Federica, for example. "In the last two weeks," she continues, " I feel all my muscles are taut: I'm sure that I will benefit from it, because that's what it's designed for". Joanne, on the other hand, suggests that she does not "like feeling pain, but it's a clue that I am really working hard, and that the muscle here, which is aching, is getting tougher".

Self-competition as displayed via strenuousness carves keep-fit training out from the flow of everyday life as a relatively separated reality. As I shall show, proper display of self-competition requires, at least, the performance of a visible, incessant concentration on one's own movements and a discreet solidarity with others present. As such, it may amount to a cognitive and emotional device which defines keep-fit exercise as a specific reality. It may prevent the social characters of the subjects from intruding into the exercise world, but may keep them in the background, always available for use in terms of the internal logic of the exercise itself. For this reason it works like a frame which is continually being reconstructed, a real "membrane" which separates fitness activity "from a field of properties that could be given weight", steadily selecting "the way in which various externally relevant social distinctions are to be governed during interaction" (Goffman, 1961, p. 71, see also 1982). The successful management of distraction is the prerogative of the trainers and the regulars who are, indeed, the masters of the frame – while trainers master the frame professionally, regular clients end up learning not only to perform better moves, but also to handle possible distractions as furtive, limited parentheses, or as pauses dedicated to irony and joking. For them, the frame around physical exercise is thus at the same time both resistant and elastic, combining, as I shall show in the next chapter, seriousness and fun, repetition and excitement in quite a precise, distinctive combination.

Before moving onto the emotional aspect though, let's focus on the cognitive power of framing. The cognitive function of transformation rules has been persuasively stressed by Gregory Bateson. A crucial source of inspiration for Goffman, Bateson (1972, p. 161) has defined "framed activities" as spheres of action marked by "meta-communicative messages" – a message which "explicitly or implicitly defines the frame" and provides "receivers instructions or help in their attempts to understand the messages contained within the frame".[5] A meta-communicative message is therefore a message which guides the evaluation of those messages contained within the frame it has set up. Rules of expression management are crucial to testify to the supremacy of the motivational logic of fitness: self-competition. The involvement of the participants as displayed in their expressions of effort, their clear attention to the movements of the teachers, their tensed expressions, sweaty clothes, their continuing to exercise despite their own insufficient performance or physical characteristics, all contribute to reinforcing the message that "this is a fitness session". Expressed correctly, through the display of an appropriate motivational logic, the involvement of each participant in the centre of official attention is therefore an extremely important signal. It stabilises the definition of the situation. In other words, it tells others just what they need to know regarding everyone's intentions and perspectives. Participants can thus get confirmation of the importance of whatever exercise is officially prescribed, and of the momentary irrelevance of other, different worlds of meaning. Properly expressed, self-competition helps define what is relevant and ignore what is not. By inducing subjects to push their own limits, physical exercise brackets broader cultural ideals of the body onto which fitness culture itself feeds, and provides what seems to be an instrumental and individualised goal – to continue exercising to the best of one's ability. A procedural environment is created, in which what really counts is involvement in performing the activities according to local rules, and not the end results of those activities (see Chapter 5).

Training in the gym requires almost continual testimony of one's own dedication. Exercise scenes are relatively rigid and formal interaction occasions, characterised by a high degree of adherence to the prescribed expressive behaviour, even when a particular exchange provokes tension or embarrassment. In general, clients in a class must continue to exercise even when they are tired, thinking of something other than their bodies, or that they are unable to follow the proposed movements satisfactorily. The very fact that in fitness centres there is a continual coming and going of different people, the fact that everyone knows that sooner or later they may meet again and the impossibility of isolating yourself or carrying out exclusive training means that it is very important to adhere to the rules of expressive behaviour and stimulate a continual reciprocal control on their effectiveness. While it is perfectly possible to abandon the exercise scene as one pleases (see Chapter 2), it is not quite so easy to stay unless behaving appropriately, and appropriateness in an exercise scene means, above all, a demonstration of dedication to keep-fit training.

The process of framing is not only the result of participants' spontaneous orientation. While clients actively collaborate to sustain the exercise frame, the elements which frame keep-fit workout are the result of the hegemonic position of gym staff, instructors and trainers. They act so as to render the prevalent, official definition of the situation as "natural", de-legitimating other, alternative definitions. What is excluded – definitions of bodies, identities, motivations – is as important as what is included, and the negotiation of the very boundaries of inclusion and exclusion is crucial for the framed scene. During my early fieldwork in Florence, I tried out an ethnomethodological experiment (see Garfinkel, 1984) which I have since repeated in other gyms in Britain and Italy. As a client participating in a variety of group training options – step aerobics, pilates, aerobics, stretching, body sculpt and spinning – I stopped performing the required movements, and waited. Normally, after a short while, all gym instructors began asking me to either continue or to account for my behaviour. Such incitements may have continued for a while, the teacher might have come close and tried a more individual approach, but on my continued reluctance, I provoked quite stern reactions – I was quite blatantly told off, I was quietly asked to leave the room or I was resolutely encouraged to come back another day. Such experiments show how difficult it is to remain in a group which is exercising while limiting oneself to watching others, without continuing the activity or providing an explanation for one's behaviour. Trainers are the ultimate keepers of the frame. However, only rarely do they have to intervene directly in the interaction to clear up any possible ambiguities. They are even less likely to find themselves having to impose a specific course of action, and their disciplinary intervention is seen as a real incident.

Routinely, indeed, the rules of expressive behaviour which govern keep-fit exercise are maintained inter-subjectively through the tacit co-operation of all participants. Clients have a crucial role in ensuring the official focus of attention. This is also true in the machine areas, both with cardio and weight-lifting machines. While in these areas there is more room for aside exchanges, gym etiquette requires that training activities takes precedence. Co-operation between patrons takes the form of ongoing expressive micro-adjustments – a glance, a sign, a sigh, a word. For example, clients learn to adopt a visual focus which stresses physical activity as the only relevant and officially appropriate course of action in the gym.

Of the various aspects of expressive behaviour, *visuality* – that is, who can be watched, and how they should be watched – is of particular importance. Let's explore how looks can and should be directed, exchanged and perhaps controlled via verbal justification, to stress commitment to training. Looking around and watching other clients intensely is at least "dodgy", as a couple of Londoners confessed while chatting with me in the lounge of the central branch of an international fitness chain. It is certainly considered negative by most regulars although when a class is too crowded, clients may watch someone immediately in front of them who seems better able to perform the exercises. When accompanied by the continual demonstration of commitment to exercise performance, this may be a legitimate focus. However, in general, looking at others may indeed bring in definitions of the body – such as sexuality (see Chapter 3) – which are officially excluded from the scene and which may shed doubt on the observers' dedication to training. The importance of keeping this danger at bay can be seen in the interaction which follows episodes when, observing the movements of the person nearby, clients exchange glances and are unable to maintain the same facial expression or to show the same attention to the exercises. In such circumstances, if clients do not quickly look away, they are expected to exchange a reciprocal support signal, or even to verbally justify their glances. These reactions stress that sustaining one's own look on another client may be ambiguous. As it is not officially prescribed, such gaze could be seen as an intrusion of irrelevant meaning and a lack of respect. Giorgio, a well-built, middle-aged man who regularly attends evening aerobics classes among a female clientele, thus found it necessary to justify the fact that he repeatedly exchanged glances with two young female newcomers. He said to the instructor, "you can see they are new, but they're really good...at the beginning I found it much more difficult to follow all your movements".

Verbal justifications of glances may remove equivocal interpretations, as well as provide support for continuation. Thus, looking around can be a way to elicit support from participants by slightly disturbing the order of inter-action. Augusto, a pensioner who has just started going to the gym, often stands in the middle of the group in the early morning exercise-to-music class, and seeks eye contact with his neighbour, which he then tends to justify by making comments such as: "I've had it, how on earth do you keep going?" or "This step's impossible, I keep losing my balance...oh, I'm feeling dizzy: it's such hard work!" Referring to his "feelings", Augusto thus confirms the importance of the exercises, and displays strenuousness by expressing involvement despite his poor performance. He thus obtains public recognition of his legitimate participation in the training scene, in the form of supportive glances during training and acknowledging greetings after it.

Clients' facial expressions and their ability to express their own involvement through signs of a shared symbolic value – such as making comments to themselves about the effort required, or simply making "strain grunts" (Goffman, 1981, pp. 104–5) – is possibly even more important in the machine area. Here, each client carries out an individual training session which requires the execution of a sequence of different exercises intermitted by brief pauses. Demonstration of commitment to the task and emotional alignment among participants is important when using the machines because, unlike group activities, instructors do not continually illustrate tasks or suggest how one should feel, but afford general supervision after providing an initial outlook by giving a personalised gym induction. Material culture is devised towards this: the provision of individual training schedules with details of training are useful much beyond the accomplishment of specified tasks as a tool to display involvement and adherence to the exercise frame. When they are having a break, clients may remain seated at the machine which they were using, or swap it with a neighbouring client, or sometimes move around between machines. In this recuperation phase those training on machines often look around without concentrating for long on one person, adopt an expressionless or even hostile look, avoid exchanging looks with others or may give someone a distracted smile. Unlike group activity, where there is a shared centre of attention, training with machines renders individuals more vulnerable to distraction. Participants seem to oscillate between the attentive performance of the exercises and the intrusion of parallel interaction which tends to develop into micro-encounters marked by various courtesies and at times subtle conflicts. However, here too, as in the studio, when glances are repeatedly exchanged, clients feel the need to account for what is happening and again and again they refer to various aspects of keep-fit training.

4. Visuality and mirror work

The capacity to concentrate on one's own body during the exercises as well as to control one's own performance and physical characteristics are organisational demands which require quite a bit of work on the part of participants. Self-surveillance is, in many ways, one of the central elements of fitness training. It is sustained by the gym spatiality, interaction order and material culture. As conversation is largely banned from interaction during training, verbal interaction is limited and bodily conducts prescribed, mirrors become crucial. They amplify the communicative potential of any minimal gesture, glance or facial expression. They augment visibility, and a visibility which is expressively non-conversational (as participants are not typically standing one in front of the other), but in many ways panoptical (as bodies may be seen from a variety of angles, see Foucault, 1975; see also Ewen, 1988; Markula, 1995; Sassatelli, 2000b and c). The possibility of very detailed self-surveillance is especially marked in activities on Nautilus machines and the like – which display objective parameters, indicate precise muscles and impose precise positions. However, even in group activities with minimal equipment, such as aerobics or step, the task of mimicking the movements proposed by the trainer is based on the ability to observe oneself in fine detail as reflected in the mirrors which surround the training spaces. Mirrors here allow the eye movement co-ordination which is at the basis of the mimetic work to be carried out – a dialectic of movement and visual understanding which is also present in some aspects of boxing training (Wacquant, 2003) and ballet (Faure, 2000). Self-surveillance is spurred by trainers' encouragement identifying the relevant parts in each movement, with the breaking down and recomposing of movements being aimed at identifying and improving specific muscles. The amount of detail commanded by training of course varies. For example, in yoga combinations there is a much greater emphasis on "feeling one's own body". Still mirrors and watching oneself in the mirror are crucial features of the fitness training scene.

The type of visual focus which is officially prescribed centres on the use of the mirror. While themselves using the mirror to further their capacity for surveilling clients, trainers reinforce clients' self-surveillance. Gina, a popular step instructor, stresses the facilitating function of the mirror in her encouragement to clients during her lessons: "you must look at yourselves in the mirror, it is important to perform even the slightest movement correctly, and the mirror is there to help you understand what you are doing with your body". Clients may be more or less able to observe themselves, but they understand that the ability to check their movements in detail through the mirror is what may grant maximum benefit from the activity. Self-surveillance is thus naturalised as a value in fitness culture. Even gym manuals normally advise people to watch themselves in the mirror, keeping an eye on the trainer's movements:

It is not always easy to look at yourself in the mirror, but it is extremely important to get used to doing it in a way which will allow you to judge whether or not your movements are correct, and whether you are stretching yourself to the limit when performing the exercises...It is important to compare yourself with the trainer: watch your trainer's body carefully, and keep looking at your own body at the same time.

(Caplin, 1992, p. 309)

Fitness training is often described by trainers and clients as providing an "objective" perspective on the body, with a vocabulary that draws on rationalised, detached forms of knowledge on the body. Yet, visibility in the gym is best defined as *prismatic*, with the large number of mirrors symbolising and encouraging multiple angles (and agents) of surveillance. Clients face their body as reflected in a number of differently positioned mirrors, a body which is thus at the same time both farther away (objectified in its totality) and nearer (visible even where it would not normally be). Clients may be very good at avoiding eye contact, but their bodies are to be seen from countless angles. They themselves can watch their image variously reflected, look directly at parts of their own body and observe their own movements in relation to those of others. The body is never complete, nor absolutely perfect, nor necessarily lacking, since everyone of its images may always be reversed, further broken down or included on a larger scale. Only the exercise may somehow fix the reflected image, providing an anchor to the prism, and thus the feeling of "objectivity".

To look at oneself in the mirror is a practice dense of meanings. The mirror does not simply reflect the body, it reflects it through a particular visuality which is informed by expectations as to body ideals and subjectivity as well as by notions on how we must look at ourselves, when and for what purposes. The mirror has somehow to be activated through what I call *mirror work*. By mirror work, I mean the work that a subject has to undertake to use mirrors in ways that are appropriate to the scene, to fit their notions of self and to negotiate with received body ideals in a game of revelation and concealment of body details. Looking at oneself in the mirror can be daunting even in the solitude of one's own bedroom, and quite demanding on self-esteem even with one's own favourite item of fashion (see Sassatelli, 2010). But as carried out in the fitness gym, mirror work is both highly demanding and demanded.

Different from what happens in ballet studios – where observation of one's own body during training is also officially geared to a constant comparison with the best performers and performance hierarchies are related to an ideal gesture to be performed in front of the public as peak artistic performance (Faure, 2000) – appropriate mirror work entails watching oneself in the mirror and observing the trainer with the view of carrying out the exercise through self-challenge and the display of strenuousness. Fitness fans generally claim they "use the mirror a lot", making the point that this is "useful" for the exercise to be effective. When training in classes, in particular, they stress the importance of carefully following the trainer's body not only directly but also as reflected in the mirror, and compared against one's own reflection, they find it "normal" and "right" as well as necessary in order to carry out the activity. Watching the trainer is the only way of "correctly performing the exercise", says Leo, a step enthusiast, and this practical necessity somehow orientates his attendance: he likes to go to the gym when it is "not very crowded" because "it is easier to follow the teacher's movements – you keep your eyes on her and watch yourself in the mirror".

It is clear that learning to exercise does not simply mean learning to perform certain movements. It is also necessary to adequately read the meanings of these movements and the body that performs them. This means reclassifying both the characteristics of one's own body and one's own motivations mainly in relation to performing the exercises, and exploiting all the varied signals which make physical activity a sphere of highly specific relevancies. It is not surprising then that some clients describe the ability to observe one's own movements as a real victory. And in many ways it is a victory also against one's own feelings of inadequacy and ceremonial exposure. Appropriate mirror work entails also a particular fashioning of emotions. Clients are asked to observe themselves in a constructive, positive manner – one which focuses less on defects and more on assets, one which appreciates improvements rather than failures, one which celebrates one's own display of strenuousness rather than competitive achievement. The supposed objectivity of surveillance is nothing but the acquisition of a point of view which is internal to the exercise and provided by the cathartic tuning of body and exercise – removing the body from other, external considerations, and partly in competition with them. And it is precisely this which is highlighted in the comments made by enthusiasts: they reckon they learned to "move" and "see" all the "various muscles stimulated by the exercise" and to "feel" and "recognise their function bit by bit by sticking to training". As I shall show in the next chapter, they claim they have learned to look at their training bodies switching to a "positive frame of mind" which exploits the energy of the scene to avoid being let down by errors or defects.

As much as it is recommended, clients may not feel comfortable with the required mirror work, and this is very true of clients who do not attend regularly as well as newcomers. The use of the mirror remains an ambiguous practice: voyeuristic or narcissistic looks always impinge on the scene bringing in notions and hierarchies of beauty and attraction that are officially excluded. They may disturb the scene by spurring competition, exclusion and frustration. Some novices, those who feel estranged from the keep-fit scene, perceive such ambiguity all the more and, by and large, are at odds with its management. They tend to recognise that looking at the mirror is fundamental for the exercise, yet they often cannot concentrate properly on what matters in the reflected image. Donata, a disillusioned client we have already encountered, explains this well:

> Following even the smallest movements is useful...or rather, would be useful for understanding where to improve...I can't follow the lesson because I don't know the movements very well, so I concentrate on the teacher all the time, but you see all those people looking at the mirror, and you don't know if they do it because they are vain or because that's the only way to do the exercise properly – I guess both, but it's a no-win situation, you don't get those bodies if you do not look at the mirror, but then if you do not like what you see that much, well, it's hard to look so intensely.

Loretta, a young shop assistant who has been to gyms on and off for more than two years, does not like to "watch herself" while she is exercising because she thinks she looks "awkward" and "ridiculous". Elisa, a university student, who has taken over a year to feel slightly less "weird" in the gym, still prefers to "avoid looking at herself in the mirror" because it makes her feel "vain". The mirror is frightening for these clients – it may show them their shortcomings in terms of body qualities or exercise performances, but it also may make them doubt their commitment to training, as though they were not really working out hard enough, but just pretending, and being interested in "how they look" rather than "how they train". Looking at oneself in the mirror while also looking at the trainer is thus, in many ways, an expedient to code one's own mirrored image as solely pertaining to the exercise spirit. The ambiguity of gym visuality can be kept at bay only by the exercise.

Following from this, most regular clients I have met in Italy and Britain generally place emphasis on detailed self-surveillance as a requirement of effective training. Betty, a fitness fan from Florence who is always in the front row in step classes, is adamant:

> It is essential to watch yourself when you're exercising, and I always want to go in front, not so much to look at myself and say, "ooh, aren't I attractive!", but because you have to look at yourself for some of the exercises...to look at the position of your spine, your abdominal muscles. Otherwise there's no point doing exercise, because you have to be precise if you want to work on the muscles.

Similar arguments are used to account for the type of clothing worn during training, which may be minimal and close-fitting, illustrating that regulars feel strongly about fitness visuality not being inspired by narcissism or exhibitionism, but by the need to perform movements correctly (see Chapter 2). They stress the fact that in the gym, "you can see, you work even a tiny muscle, the muscle you want to", "you decide what you want, and you can be very specific, you only move what you have to". This, they reckon, "makes exercise much more effective" and some even claim, "you can see the difference" in a relatively short time. But the difference, as I shall show in the next chapter, has to do with body modification as much as with the positivity of the look, the capacity to gain pleasure from workout, and the satisfaction for one's own improvements. Indeed, the lived culture of fitness training in the gym is intrinsically *paradoxical*. At the structural level, fitness gyms feed on broad cultural ideals of the body which are on the spot in promotional incitements to join in, and yet they must ask training clients to rework and somehow suspend these body ideals to make exercise involvement adamant. At the subjective level, in order to continue exercising, clients may have to put aside the bodily objectives which initially brought them to the gym. Clients must, to a degree, learn to immerse themselves in a world where there should be no competition with others, because everyone is a client with universalised rights to the trainers' attention and highly individualised forms of physical capital which can be improved, each in their own right, via a positive investment in the strenuous display of a self-challenging commitment to the exercise. It is precisely because they are spurred on to "keep doing more and doing better" that clients may learn to put to one side not only their own specific performance, but also the results of their efforts. A focus on surpassing one's own limits in training while looking appreciatively at one's own achievements may help, as it were, in bracketing body ideals and hierarchies, while keeping them available in the background.

5
Discipline and Fun

While gym-goers subject themselves to relatively demanding bodywork, time spent in the gym is typically coded as "leisure". Many sociologists have thus interpreted their role as the de-mystification of the leisure, free-time, cheerful quality attributed to fitness (Glassner, 1992; Le Breton, 1990; Maguire and Mansfield, 1998; O'Neill, 1985, Ewen, 1988). In such views, fitness is the example of an allegedly body loving era which is in fact obsessed with the body to the point that inactivity is not an option and work enters the sphere of leisure by the commercialisation of self-discipline. The ultimate objective of many such diagnoses is to maintain that the commercialisation of discipline is itself a consumption generation device: while mere "resting" costs nothing, exercise and bodywork need a paraphernalia of commodities to be carried out. On similar premises, Jennifer Smith Maguire (2007, p. 193) concludes her book on the US fitness industry considering that "the personal trainer resolution of the tension between work and leisure through a vocational disposition is instructive for field participants more widely: to regard working out as a good use of leisure time fulfils the tenets of responsible self-production". She draws on Baudrillard's (1998) well-known *The Consumer Society* to suggest that fitness is essentially inspired by an "ethic of discipline". Whatever "aesthetic ethic of indulgence" may be articulated in relation to fitness, it is just an ideological move: "exercise manuals and health clubs construct fitness as a leisure activity...However there is a particularly narrow vision of pleasure on offer in the fitness field...Exercise is instrumentally rationalized as a means to other ends: reduced health risks, improved appearance, or both" (Smith Maguire, 2007, p. 196).

In this chapter, I shall show that such reading, which is based largely on the analysis of textual sources or trainers' accounts, does not allow for the experiences of gym-goers. To regular participants, in particular, keep-fit workout indeed offers quite involving experiences of embodiment. It may not be strange that fitness magazines and exercise manuals are weaker on these compared to real gym scenes: official discourse tends to be realised with a normative voice rather than an experiential one. There is an experiential moment in fitness, which is procedural and interactional, that cannot be easily reduced to text. In practice, experience in the gym is organised to provide what participants describe as "real fun". I certainly do not claim that such fun is a spontaneous event. On the contrary, the chapter precisely deals with how subjective experiences of fun are institutionally organised and socially patterned. Nor do I claim that fun comes easy. Far from it, the fitness industry sustains quite a bit of consumers' dissatisfaction and frustration (Frew and McGillivray, 2005). It accommodates under-used subscriptions and copes with high drop-out rates. While expert discourse as well as commercial images are often reconciliatory, actual consumer practices are more commonly disputed – with participants having to work hard indeed to find their way through the fitness world, not always managing to transform the received, official meanings in ways that they may feel satisfactory. Still, we should consider that commercialisation has changed the framing of discipline, stressing the relevance of factors internal to fitness practice and the role of individual experience in it, emphasising subjectively rewarding training. Fitness gyms are, to a degree, entertainment industries: they largely manage involvement as fun. And yet, we must take fun seriously to understand clients' patterns of pleasure. This means, among other things, to consider the situated character of fun: as I shall show, experiences of fun depend on how participants locally articulate the cultural repertoire of fitness training, contributing to its ongoing accomplishment. In the following pages, experiences of fun as narrated by a variety of participants shall thus be placed in the context of the emotional structure of the gym scene as sustained by fitness culture as commercial entertainment. Fun has obvious bearings on participants' successful initiation, which in turn has important effects for the success of the whole fitness industry. The fitness industry runs after clients' pleasures – to the point that clients may be classified by the palette of pleasures provided by fitness and how they manage to respond to it. Estranged and marginal clients, or even gym drop-outs, are as much recalcitrant to discipline as they are to "positive thinking" and institutionally governed "cheerfulness".

1. Routine, cheerfulness and the emotional structure of training

In the previous chapter we have looked at the external and internal trim of the fitness frame, at how fitness is positioned in the broader field of sports and at how gym-goers are supposed to orientate to the activity. Here I start by focusing on how they experience and narrate their orientation as related to their sense of self and achievement. If the experience of those who succeed in entering the fitness frame is considered, it is clear that framing is fully achieved subjectively when participants do not dwell on the meaning of what they are doing, but simply do it. Frames have indeed important affective functions. As Goffman (1974, p. 345) recognises, they organise more than meaning, they also organise "involvement".[1] Indeed, regular participants report that they not only behave *as if* they were involved, but also feel affectively involved. They express such experiences of involvement with words such as "feeling at ease", "natural" and "concentrated", not only fairly sure of the reality they are contributing to create, but also absorbed by it. Using a different language, but essentially in agreement with the ideas proposed by Bateson and Goffman, the social psychologist Mihaly Csikszentmihalyi defines the experiences of affective involvement as a "holistic sensation". They are experiences which, far more than others, imply a "mixing of action and awareness". People in a state of "flow" do not have and, above all, do not seek a "dualistic perspective: they are aware of their own actions, but not of the awareness itself" (Csikszentmihalyi, 1982, p. 38, see also 1997). This does not eliminate the self, or the possibility of reflexivity (Perinbanayagam, 2006), but reflexivity is a function of the activity, which is not addressed from the outside.

In a good training session, involved clients do not ask themselves what they are doing or if this will be good for them. Training thus produces an artificial but very stable world of practice (cognitive, affective, embodied). Regular clients describe the quality of their experiences as a heightened perception of the present and of themselves in it: "you really put yourself into doing the exercises". Being at one with the flow of action may have a dual outcome, depending on the *modality of engagement* with the *routine* element of training. It may alert to routines, make routine monitoring infinitely demanding and involving, such as in postural techniques like pilates. Similar routine engagement techniques place emphasis on awareness of repeated movements, making them less automatic. They entail some reflexive coupling of mind and body in the phenomenological engagement with routine, like in body-soul techniques such as tai-chi or meditation (see Slater, 2009). Alternatively, being at one with the flow of action may help in departing from routine: like in cathartic dancing, the repetitive repetition of movement feels so natural that the mind flows away from it and wanders. Routine disengagement techniques, such as running on a treadmill, place emphasis on release from repeated automatic movements. Depending on their preferred technique, regular clients comment on their flow experiences as liberating by either engaging with routine at a deeper, conscious level, or disengaging from it once it has become so much under the skin that distraction can be sustained for a while without routine disruption. Clients' verbalisations thus suggest that if you "concentrate on what you are doing, you can't think very much", or that "once you are concentrated you can put the automatic pilot on". In both cases, working out is characterised as something which creates an *absolute present*. Even some novices or irregular clients seem to experience this. It is their verbalisations, which describe involvement as a sporadic but remarkable event, which tell us about flow experiences more vibrantly:

I am not a fan. I come every week, but sometimes, frankly, it's really boring. Sometimes, though, I have a good session. Like, today I enjoyed it, got focused. but mostly it's boring, I think I should get a personal trainer... [when a class is good] I can concentrate, and even enjoy what I do, like, I don't think all the time: "what time is it?", but I just do what I need to, and do it well, with a focus on the movement and feeling like I'm up to it.

(Claudio, professional in his mid thirties,
isotonic machines and spinning, Milan)

You may end up being caught up in your routine, I do quite a bit when I am running on the treadmill. It's the most boring thing, you know, but if something clicks in your head then you watch this music channel and keep going, and feel your muscles, perhaps you imagine them or just feel them. You keep going and going... you let things go, have a simple task, do it, and do it... I suppose it's like a prayer, you do it but do not know why, just do it hoping it will work.

(Joanne, student in her mid twenties,
cardio machines and spinning, London)

Feelings of involvement are presented by irregular clients and novices as almost a mystical occurrence, something that simply "happens" on some occasions. Regulars and enthusiasts, on their part, tend to present those feelings as a function of their "commitment" and of their capacity to "embrace the spirit" of the gym. They are much more reflexive in their descriptions, including their agency directly in the picture. For them, involvement experiences are clearly sustained by a greater variety of details of the training scene. Besides, their vocabulary is more obviously leaning towards pleasure. Indeed, among the most salient themes in regular clients' narratives are amusement, fun and even playfulness. Regulars describe the time spent in the fitness centre in ways that are reminiscent of play. Here are some illustrative quotes:

This is a good class, I enjoy it, Paola [the instructor] keeps you going, she's fun, the class goes with a laughter... it is important that there are people around, because one looks around and says "hard, but we all work hard", it's stimulus: the music, the rhythm, you feel you must go on and do as much as you can, but no one really tells you what to do! If you like to do machines, you do them, you choose your class, you decide what you do [for your session] in a way.

(Alessia, postwoman in her early thirties, Florence)

[you are there] for an hour, just thinking about your body; I think it feels like playing: coming in, saying hello, and then doing movements, I concentrate on what I'm doing; it's an incredible effort, you have to concentrate. It's a distraction, a kind of escapism, not to go over and over in your mind all the day-to-day problems...It's a bit like playing here: it's the fact that it's like a game which is enjoyable, which gives you energy...and some people to meet. We don't have that many opportunities to play, apart from in here!

(Bonnie, middle-aged housewife, Florence)

Let's consider the analogy with play from a distance. Although it has some of the typical characteristics of play-type situations – elements of sociability and a relatively limited centre of attention which require the filtering of external considerations, the possibility for subjects to test their limits, to face up to the difficulties involved and to do their utmost to carry out these activities – the physical activities which take place in fitness centres are very far from being structurally like play. Relatively more similar to athletics, play is generally defined as an "autotelic" activity, a practice which is an objective in itself, and which can therefore offer an "experience of flow par excellence", that is, in which flow is "sought above all in itself, and not for the incidental extrinsic benefits which may derive from it" (Csikszentmihalyi, 1982, p. 36; see also Bateson, 1972; Goffman, 1961, 1967).[2] Play, in other words, is presented as a field of action which is "not serious", in which "individuals openly participate for the pleasure of it", and not for the consequences their actions may or should achieve. This is probably most evident in role playing and fantasy games such as those studied by Gary Alan Fine (1983). In these worlds, participants may act quite reflexively in relation to the moves of the game and yet they are rather seriously engrossed, and what is more the instrumental pursuits of external gains are typically stigmatised.

Unlike those who really play, those who carry out physical activity in the gym do not do it so much just to enjoy themselves. While play offers the possibility of "sanctioned exhibition", or the "opportunity to *exhibit* attributes valued in the wider social world" (Goffman, 1961, p. 61, emphasis added; see also Fine, 1983; Perinbanayagam, 2006), fitness gyms are backstage institutions. As suggested in the previous chapter, they allow preparatory activities through which bodies may acquire attributes that are positively valued in other, often decisive, social occasions. Keep-fit exercise is not, in the final analysis, an end in itself: clients' efforts are justified as they produce embodied qualities that appear as external incentives to the activity's progress. However, fitness activities do offer the possibility of temporarily playing down their own seriousness and consequentiality. If games are "mimeses of the interaction life of human agents who live in organized societies" (Perinbanayagam, 2006, p. 25) fitness is a body discipline that, in a way, mimics games. The *emotional structure* of keep-fit workout – the spirit participants are required to embrace while training, irrespective of their own emotions – is characterised by the same "surrealistic clarity" (Bateson, 1972) as that of play, only inverting its poles. Fitness reflects and subverts play by trading on its conventional meanings and turning them upside down. Play is a domain of non-serious seriousness, a reality separate from the wider social world by means of a membrane which makes it relatively non-consequential, important in itself and highly absorbing. Exercise, by contrast, is a domain of *serious playfulness*, a field of serious social action which plays down its own seriousness in order to encourage involvement in the furthering of action.

Fitness activities thus rest on a further paradox: physical exercise is presented as having serious effects on clients' bodies, but is to be carried out as something which, like play, is relevant in itself and allows participants a sanctioned self-centredness. Clients are encouraged to experience workout as a time which has the quality of a meaningful, enjoyable present – in the dual meaning of *heightened perception of the here-and-now* and of *gift*, something special for oneself. As a result, clients may become more seriously involved. I have closed the previous chapter by suggesting that a set of body ideals impinge on training, they become crucial when clients are asked to justify their practices as efficient means to get a better body, but they are largely in the background during training. In the training scene, clients have to concentrate on the furthering of action, to the point of bracketing what they want to achieve by their efforts. In this way an enthusiast such as Amy, who prides herself on having really "entered the spirit of the gym", maintains that she is not looking for "the result", that she does not want to "become like Cindy Crawford in a month": "I don't have any external goal, but in a way I'm testing myself, challenging myself, and I notice that if I go to the gym for a month and take care with my diet, my muscles are firmer and my body is more toned."

As emotional leaders (see Chapter 3), instructors and trainers have an important role in promoting this emotional structure. Their job is primarily to manage the playfulness of exercise as a local experience, balancing this against its consequential seriousness. This is a delicate task. They must promote a relaxed and informal atmosphere, but must not undermine the ultimate value of bodywork, reducing it to a game with no purpose. They encourage clients by inducing concentration on the movements to be carried out, coding such concentration as "fun" while simultaneously claiming that exercise will have tangible body pay-offs for those who work hard. Here are some sample verbalisations from trainers' incitements during workout:

Now really extend your left leg back, and pump, and pump, and enjoy that! We can push a little more now, left leg, reach back, lift and lower, niiiice work! Let's keep moving and keep smiling: this is about you having the best workout for yourself!
(Cardio fit class, London, December 2006)

We all have our own bodies. I've got a large bottom, for example – so what?! I come here and exercise every day, so at least it's not flopping all over the place!...Now concentrate, left side, let's repeat the sequence, and, go, and go, go, extend, now back, back back, and step touch, four, three, two, one, well done! And march, this is great, you're wonderful.

(Step class, Florence, December 1994)

In exercise-to-music classes, rhythmic incitements are used as a way to provide a playful twist to the routine. Reference to fatigue is typically matched by cheerful expressions and appreciative comments. What Nina Loland (2000) found in her study of aerobics in Norway, namely a strong emphasis on "corporeal work ethic" emphasising the instrumentality of aerobic workout, was matched by a variety of playful, cheerful accompanying expressions in most of the training scenes I witnessed across both Italy and Britain. Merely ascetic expressions, such as "I know this isn't fun...it shouldn't be fun...however, it will be good afterward" reported by Loland (ibid., p. 120), as spoken from an aerobics instructor during training, were indeed rather infrequent. Common was instead the qualification of training as a pleasurable duty, and not only because it may respond to deferred gratification. To be sure, a "duty plus treat" logic impinges on the training scene – with exercise being coded as work which allows for relaxed consumption afterwards (of food, for example, see Crossley, 2006; Maguire Smith 2007; Spielvogel 2003; but even more so of "wellness" – saunas, spas, massages – which is increasingly offered in large upmarket premises) (see also Chapter 2). But more frequently, bodywork is itself coded via reference to involvement, energy and fun. *Cheerfulness* strongly qualifies the emotional fashioning of training as strenuous self-challenging commitment.

Considering the Italian and British fitness scene, and a broader set of activities besides classic aerobics, what strikes me is that all fitness participants indeed work hard at supporting cheerfulness, coding the sweat produced by physical exertion as effort *and* enthusiasm, considering the repetitiveness of movements as providing energy and exaltation. In this sense, fitness also inverts the emotional structure of many contemporary sports and leisure activities which have been understood under the rubric of "a quest for excitement" (Elias and Dunning, 1986): rather than "mimetic excitement", fitness training is shaped as excited *mimesis*, the cheerful enactment of a quest. Let's explore this with reference to the emotional structure of boxing. As suggested by Wacquant (2003, pp. 94–5), the boxer's "learning of indifference to physical suffering is inseparable from the acquisition of the form of sang-foid specific to pugilism": the boxer has to develop a gradual resistance to being violently punched at and has to off-set his own "initial reflex of self-preservation that would undo the coordination of movements and give the opponent a decisive advantage". On the contrary, what fitness participants display with strenuousness is not so much an indifference to fatigue, pain or fear – such as in the case of boxers who have to become "resistant to excitement". And not only because in the fitness gym there is very little physical fear, much less and much different pain, and relatively less fatigue. Leaving new combat keep-fit techniques aside, the hazardous excitement of games organised through strategic conversational structures (Perinbanayagam, 2006), the euphoric interaction of eventful plays of uncertain outcome (Goffman, 1961) are not there and somewhat need to be artificially recreated. So fitness clients have rather to become – to paraphrase Wacquant – *excited to resist*. They need to display their will to work dutifully and laboriously, to perform their tasks vigorously (in resistance training) or precisely (in postural gymnastics), as fast as required (in aerobics and spininng) or as slow as required (in pilates). As compared to boxing narratives, fitness fans comments appear sanitised and ceremonial. Exercising bodies in the fitness gym do sweat and get tired, but indifference has to be acquired more to the ceremonial exposure which workout commands than to actual physical effort or danger. Being looked at may be as tough as fatigue, and taking responsibility for one's own body while accepting its defects is indeed a major, if different, challenge to one's own reflex of self-preservation.

To steer emotions in this direction, quite often gym instructors include themselves in the scene as training partners, and they use phrases such as "we are really warm now!", "I'd like to stop, but it's not finished", "you really made me work hard today!" (see Chapter 3). They may even draw attention to imperfections in their own body, and they do so to downplay both body ideals and fatigue, to then stress both by complimenting achievement. In doing so they balance the internal meaningfulness of the exercise with its external effectiveness, fun with consequentiality, local experience with embodied performance. Their role in managing the emotional structure of keep-fit exercise accounts for trainers' centrality in the success of any club. However, to a degree, this emotional structure has become objectified in fitness culture. As the fitness manual *Teach Yourself Fitness* says laconically: "the simple truth is that the quickest way to fitness is the one you enjoy the most" (Archer, 2006, p. ix).

Current fitness marketing, in Italy, Britain and the USA, also insists on experience, involvement and fun. The experience of training, says Giuseppe Ricci, a well-known marketing consultant to the Italian fitness industry, must become "irresistible" (Ricci, 2005). The key issue of gym loyalty is linked up to involvement experiences. Consumption must "produce emotions. And the experience with [a club as] a brand must be holistic: emotionally and sensuously gratifying and involving" (ibid., 18). In the USA, the fitness market is considered mature, and management and marketing experts tend to stress that one of the challenges for fitness facilities over the coming few years will be in maintaining the interest of members by offering entertainment and fun (Brown, 2003). Fitness marketing appears to have absorbed the notion of the "experience economy" (Pine and Gilmore,

1998). Branding is no longer enough: a brand must emphasise experience as dramatic action, and demonstrate how it fits in clients' lives. In her book *Successful Fitness Motivation Strategies*, Professor of Exercise Studies, Barbara Brehm (2004), stresses that the problem for the fitness industry and staff is not to help people get in shape, but to maximise their chance of exercise adherence and of commitment to lifelong physical activity. Towards this end, Brehm recommends positive motivations ("I want to be strong, energetic") as opposed to negative ones ("I need to lose weight") and especially internal rewards related to the exercise experience itself, as opposed to external ones related to exercise goals. These advices have percolated in popular guides to fitness culture and options – as the 2006 *Time Out London Guide to Health and Fitness* suggests: "the motivation to exercise has to come from within, so that we can see merit in the process, rather than merely focusing on the result" (p. 17). Again, fun is considered crucial to exercise adherence: managers and trainers are thus encouraged to put emphasis on the provision of entertainment and clients should learn to take charge of their exercise programmes, including the activities that they enjoy most. Besides, the reframing of training as "fun" further legitimates the fitness gym as a commercial institution.

There is clearly a normative element in "fun". This is well illustrated by the fact that companies producing fitness equipment take great care to make them user-friendly, increasingly mixing workout with entertainment. Nerio Alessandri, the founder of Technogym, the major Italian company producing gym equipment and one of the world leaders in the sector, expresses this clearly. Developing the notion of wellness as a way "to promote human life to its fullest potential" (Alessandri, 2001), this company has been one of the first to use design to improve the pleasure of using machines, to develop electronic interfaces to check training and adjust it to each client, and to boost entertainment via the integration of TV watching, video games and virtual reality. Alessandri (in Bernabè et al., 2007) reckons that Cardio Wave, his new cardio machine which mimics skating, is "getting enormous success, in all age groups, because you can train while listening to music, you can move in different ways, leaving space to the fantasy and creativity of all kinds of people". Developments in interactive technology to further personalised entertainment, with virtual reality applications – such as a simulation of skiing, running through mountains or on the beach – will surely follow.

Keep-fit videos also reveal the normative character of "fun". The keep-fit video market has expanded as part of a shift towards home-based leisure (MacNeill, 1998). The trainers-demonstrators on videos often reproduce a hyper-realist version of a keep-fit scene in a gym. They are all smiles, and use continuous encouraging props and appreciative remarks even though what their imagined audience actually does is fact well beyond their reach. In the most popular fitness videos, we typically see a trainer, alone or with some assistants, who provides the imagined audience with a clear illustration of what they are expected to do and feel, demonstrating a sequence of movements in nice surroundings, with some music. The trainer punctuates the movements by a nearly uninterrupted rhythmic litany: "that's good", "that's fine", "that's lovely", "good job", "well done", "fantastic job!" are some of their recurrent verbalisations. The demonstration of cheerfulness is relentless, and enjoyment or fun are repeatedly invoked.

The obligatory nature of feeling is indeed deeply felt by quitters and irregulars who explicitly mention "the false happiness" of keep-fit training. In one case, a gym-quitter even provided me with a bitter caricature: "you should have fun being regimented inside a crowded, small, indoor place: why?" On the contrary, a coercive tinge is not perceived by fans and regulars in the gym, who code pretty similar scenes just as "full of energy" or "enthusiasm". Along with "benefits" and "results", they stress the importance of cheerfulness. They feel rewarded by the most "attentive" trainers, who "inspire enthusiasm", they appreciate a gym where other participants "don't want to muck about", they are pleased with a "serious" and at the same time "relaxed" atmosphere where one "can make a joke". A real fitness enthusiast like Betty from Florence explains:

> I really enjoy myself. When I do step aerobics every day I can feel that I can give all I can, I am totally involved. It was when I began the step classes that I became really enthusiastic; I enjoy myself because when you've learned the basic steps, you can build up the lesson. People also go to the gym to set their mind free, to feel involved, because you've got to stay there and learn the steps... I want to do step classes as best I can: it's become a part of me, I know the basics and every time I come, there are new things to learn. I can do different things, but using the same style, which I like... Marisa [the step trainer] is fantastic! She really pushes you and makes you want to keep going: it doesn't take much, just a joke or a few words.

2. Informality and social embodiment

To be successful, all the fitness gyms I have studied strive to provide bodywork which is both consequential (body modification) and of immediate significance (involvement, fun). For the provision of fun they cannot rely on the possibility of taking up a strategic, dialogic position through competition – something that in the typical structure of games offers a solid basis for involvement and internal rewards (Perinbanayagam, 2006). A somewhat conversational element is injected in the fitness scene though. This happens through informal, aside exchanges. Moments of reciprocal distraction from training – in the form of glances, gestures, laughter and dialogue – are part of the gym and provide for a sense of "freedom". They are thus particularly important to connote cheerfulness as a genuine feature of fitness. Here is a scene from my field notes:

> Megan [the exercise-to-music instructor] is tough this morning, pace is fast, movements new. I can't follow properly. Simona and Giovanna are close to each other as usual, but they are not doing fine either. Claudia in the front row is perfect as usual, how can she manage? She just looks at Megan and does it. Giovanna is at pain with the routine, she puffs, and sighs, and moves far too much the upper arms. And she chats up with Simona, saying the movements are very difficult. We all look at them, which makes the routine even more difficult. What a pressure: we all look at them. Giovanna says something loudly: "Phew! I can't possibly follow these terrible steps, I'm not a professional ballerina, am I?" Simona plays silly, and giggles. But then she closes the incident "you will impress everyone at home with your stamina!"
>
> (Step, Florence, March 1995)

Such exchanges tend to be allowed, and even approved of by instructors and clients, who smile, look on kindly or play along. In other words, they may be managed co-operatively as expressions of *informality*: an appropriate, limited and circumscribed departure from the rigidity of interaction. The availability of these informal moments is fundamental, precisely because interaction rules during training are relatively rigid, and could therefore distance rather than involve clients. This helps create the impression of keep-fit scenes as rigorous, but neither oppressive nor coercive. A controlled reference to external identities alleviates the emotive cost of continuing to perform exercises which risk being beyond the participants' capacities. It may actually be a strategic move for participants, and as such it is often made tongue-in-cheek. In the scene reported above, for example, when Giovanna says jokingly that the step sequence is too difficult for non-professionals, she shows her ability to recognise that during physical activity the body is a malleable instrument and, at the same time, she distances herself from her own local performance. At the same time, Simona shows that what counts is not so much the perfect execution of the exercises, but perseverance.

If difficulties in perceiving training as fun are partly related to the many body definitions which impinge on the training scene, and in particular to the paramount importance of broad cultural body ideals, some external body definitions also work as internal resources. Gender, age and occupational attributes must not be officially deployed to create hierarchies in the gym; they can only nominally be accounted for by trainers in their individualising and universalising approach. Yet, they may work as references for clients to project a self beyond training. Reference to external embodied identity typically happens when clients feel they may become the object of a surplus of ambiguous attention, for example, when they realise they have made a very visible mistake in performing the moves. At the same time, informal exchanges which build on the supposition of an equivalent motivational position (strenuous, joyous self-challenge) work to transform the universalistic, formal equality of participants as clients into a sort of equivalence between their training bodies. Exercising bodies are not in the first place young or old, rich or poor, male or female; they should be pure instruments of training, trainees have to see and feel the movements and actively respond. Such instrumentality may become a heavy burden in itself as poor exercise capacities are the order of the day. Informality and irony come in to lighten the scene. Irony – that is, juxtaposing the specific demands of the activity being carried out with values or classifications which are different, contrasting or irreducible to those demands – engages with both *local exercise performances* and *broader cultural body ideals*.

It is obvious that the toned, slim and youthful body is the cultural icon which sustains fitness. Proposed by advertising and mass media and associated with fitness gyms, this cultural icon is saturated in conventional notions of beauty and merit linked to gender distinctions, reinforced by racial or sexual connotations, and related to a series of prized social roles and identities (Amir, 1987; Bordo, 1993; Ewen, 1988; Le Breton, 1990; O'Neill, 1985). But actual fitness scenes are different from the scenes staged on glossy images in fitness magazines or aerobics videos, where both instructors and clients are perfectly groomed, dressed and made up (Eskes et al., 1998; Markula, 1995, 2001; Morse, 1987). And most clients express distance from these images: for them, the perfect gym is where "you do not feel ugly if you sweat a lot", where "there is no super-blonde who just looks in the mirror to see if her earring has fallen out", and where there is "not too much showing off little designer outfits". The iconic images cannot be simply superimposed on the body actually engaged in exercise. Such a body is an energy system beyond any specifications other than those necessary for the continuation of the exercise, a pure instrument to which are added layers of meanings in so far as actual training allows room for other social specifications (see Chapter 6).

During keep-fit sessions clients are asked to work on their bodies as if they are instruments. The sense of relative "anonymity" which a few of the regulars report and enjoy can be read as a symptom of such instrumentality. Instrumentality objectifies the body, and creates a space between its attributes (that is, appearances and performances) and the self. Ironic reference to body or performance shortcomings fills in this space, effectively staging the self and suggesting that it is elsewhere. Many regulars say they like gyms where they can relax. But what does this mean? That they can stop thinking of how they look and work on the body at some distance from it? The fitness framing is predicated on "role distance" (Goffman, 1961, pp. 85–152) from external role and identity specifications, and simultaneously allows for distance from local roles, performances and demands.[3] Participants may thus project an image of themselves that goes beyond local identity. This implies a complex gate-keeping trading on roles and selves. In its Janus-like character, a keep-fit workout may appear as "relaxation" from both external roles and from the strenuousness or seriousness of training.

Many episodes from my fieldwork, both during individualised training in the machine area and during exercise-to-music classes, could work as illustrations. Here are some telling excerpts from my field notes on different gyms:

> [Two middle-aged women who often meet when exercising] Vanessa and Daniela, exchange brief comments every so often. Vanessa says very seriously to Daniela: "do you need this machine?... it's excellent for your waistline and your laterals". Daniela replies light-heartedly, pointing at her thighs with a theatrical gesture: "yes, but how much would I have to do, eh?!... oh, it's such hard work". Vanessa is very serious, she does not come often and perhaps she is trying too hard. Daniela, a keen participant, plays informal. She seems to intervene not so much to protect her own appearance, but to show her ability to recognise the physical ideals which culturally support fitness training, while stressing their irrelevance during workout. Daniela takes responsibility as to dedication to training, but not as to her own physical characteristics.
>
> (Isotonic machines area, Florence, October 1994)

> [Late afternoon, the gym is full of people. I am just] in the last rows [of the class], close to the two women I saw chatting in the dressing-room, a man just before them. Smooth and easy exercises. The instructor insists on usual advice (posture, concentration, feeling). She says "don't forget your posture when you're out of here, you may be working at a desk or else, but posture is the key". She plays on self-competition when she asks a bit more from clients "lets continue, push on, push on, you challenge yourself!". Clients may look supportively at each other from time to time, especially when things are too easy or too difficult. One of the two women stops and whispers to her friend "I need a break, you know it's been a hard day." She replies half-jokingly "I've got no excuse I've just come back from holidays."
>
> (Pilates, London, December 2006)

> Amy and Francesco [two regulars, a young shop-assistant and a middle-aged teacher] start a series of humorous comments, that get tacit approval of others – glances, smiles. The instructor asks clients to turn right round until they could see their buttocks, Francesco jokingly comments: "oh yeah, can you imagine me looking at mine, you're all young women here!", Amy whispers "lucky you... I can't help seeing mine!".
>
> (Stretching, Florence, February 1995)

Similar exchanges show us how clients deploy informality ironically to bracket either their own performance or their own physical qualities. Irony thus works to include people who may be left behind, neutralising mistakes or defects, and at showing that what counts is commitment and involvement. Informal exchanges allow clients to slip between the formal demands of the situation, if only for a moment, and to refer to their own irreducible specificity. Informality and light sociability though, however pleasurable they may be felt, are not geared to offer spaces of shared direct confrontation with body ideals. The training scene may thus be defined as an occasion which in the main allows to negotiate body ideals *by diversion*: a switch from bodies to character (strenuousness), from specific body ideals to exercise continuation (self-competition) and even from local performances to light sociability (informality). The latter in particular has the effect of qualifying keep-fit training as a relatively leisured scene, something that allows the individual to shine through prescribed, official norms.

Not everyone seems to be in the position to see the normative character of cheerfulness, just as much as not everyone manages to endorse cheerfulness. In other terms, cheerfulness does not work as a performative of fun for everyone. This is partly because keep-fit remains too serious an activity for some, and too meaningless for others. Cultural pressures are there, but individual motivation is lacking, giving way to one of the most salient feature of commercial gyms, namely the continuous succession of people who try to follow a training programme, but who are unable to do more than a few sessions. More than half of those who take up physical activity give up fairly soon afterwards, and quite a number during their adult life try to take up physical activity time and again (Dishman, 1988; Robinson and Rogers, 1994). The issue of consumer loyalty is present in all expert discourse on fitness, and is paramount in fitness marketing, both in Italy and Britain, as well as the USA (Sassatelli, 2003; Smith Maguire, 2007). Enrolment in gyms peaks at times when people most strongly feel the need to take care of their own body, and when the goals which physical activity is expected to achieve are most urgent, both for cultural reasons (that is, in late spring when many people are expecting to have to show off their bodies) or for personal reasons (that is, after pregnancy or injury). However, clients' drop-out rates cannot just be explained by the fact that the need or duty is no longer there, or that the initial aims are no longer relevant. And indeed, the very stories of the quitters and of the irregular clients all stress the continuous relevance of these aims.

Both sport psychology and leisure studies have suggested that a major difference between the expected benefits from exercise and people's own personal physical characteristics has a negative influence on exercise motivation (Le Unes and Nation, 1996, pp. 527ff.; Markland and Hardy, 1993; Roskies et al., 1986; see also Dittmar, 2008). From fieldwork I have learned that fitness training discourages participants if they envision it as a competitive activity where body comparison is at stake. Indeed, one of the findings from my early ethnography was precisely that constant comparison with others and with an ideal body image hinders people from experiencing exercise as a meaningful activity in itself, and reduces the probability that clients will continue attending (Sassatelli, 1999a and b).

We may now start to consider how social embodiment – as manifested in some externally relevant embodied identities and *habitus* – intersects and couples with fun and commitment in fitness. The resources locally available to participants to concentrate on bodywork make fitness gyms successful institutions especially among some social categories of people. The emotional structure of the fitness gym aims at providing clients who are initially quite focused on body ideals with the possibility of not being trapped by their own idealisations, and to focus on the processes of action instead. Clearly, quite a large proportion of the population might care about the body. But some seem to have more incentive to go to the gym simply because of the particular importance which a well-cared for physique has for him or her from a socio-positional perspective. A disciplined, well-groomed body conforming to cultural norms has relatively greater value for women, youth and people whose professions require strong self-presentational skills.[4] People belonging to these categories are also arguably those who may more easily take up informality, joyful strenuousness and positive self-challenge. They are more prone to engage with the display of fun and cheerfulness, adopting quite a reflexive, self-fashioning attitude stressing positive thinking and willpower over physical capital. They are also more likely to be good at a combination of pleasure seeking and self-discipline in some form of "tamed hedonism" (Sassatelli, 2000a). The keep-fit emotional structure, which is meant to protect clients from a risky self-exposure precisely when they are carrying out activity aimed at their deficiencies, is thus particularly adjusted to these categories, which may more easily develop an internal *habitus*. From their social positioning, they have both plausible external incentives to fitness and feel internal, locally realised affinities with the keep-fit scene. In other terms, these clients may more easily play with the paradox of keep-fit training recognising their own inadequacies and disregarding them as irrelevant for the time being.

Not everyone, however, feels this way. Iconic body ideals may be a particularly obsessive reference for those (the overweight, the aged) whose physical characteristics differ greatly from culturally privileged specifications (Dittmar, 2008; Grogan, 1999). As ideals are typically conveyed through costly body decoration, mainstream fashion and cultured body demeanour, they may appear far too distant for people living on low incomes or in culturally marginal conditions. Even when attracted by the image of the "fit body" people belonging to these categories are arguably less prone to take up the keep-fit emotional structure. Strenuousness may be too much, its joyfulness may not appear credible, informality may give way to quite embarrassing exchanges, self-challenge may be difficult when formal equality with others requires a lot of imaginative abstraction, or a willingness to conform that conflicts with one's own social embodiment. And cheerfulness may be felt as a false expedient that only those who do not make much physical effort in their daily life can be ready to embrace. Body ideals may be incentives for joining a gym, but they may work just as much as deterrents for exercise adherence – a double-bind dynamic intensified by the often aggressive marketing strategies of international fitness chains.

Concentrating on their imperfections, quitters are effectively unable to become engrossed in bodywork. Keep-fit training may appear as an occasion where defects are ultimately and intimately ascribed to the subject, rather than an opportunity to govern defects and take distance from them by either shifting one's own body ideals or stressing one's own powers of pleasure. The quitters I have come across belonged to a broad variety of social categories, but they all shared the same difficulty in "entering into the spirit of the gym". They described themselves during bodywork as feeling "tense", "embarrassed", "alone" and "bored". Regulars, in contrast, tend to portray their encounter with the exercise world as a "learning" process through which they have switched attention away from their body defects, and have come to concentrate on performing bodywork with a cheerful, "positive attitude". To understand these differences, we need to explore in more detail the stories of clients with different participation profiles.

3. Fun in tales and the seriousness of fun

Fun is present in many ways in the gym tales told by regular and enthusiastic clients. There is surely a vocabulary of duty in regular clients' justifications for training, but they invariably also view fitness as "recreation", "entertainment", "fun", "diversion", "play", "leisure", "a hobby". Some of them suggest that they are even "surprised by the pleasure" they may "get from exercising". Successful initiation to training is a situated process of learning which, as suggested, a number of external embodied identities variously impinge on. It is a process of varying length that is normally described as "turning in the right direction". To account for their practice, most regulars stress contingency and evenementiality, referring to things such as "bumping into" a "special" trainer, a "good" gym or an "inspiring" technique, which has made them perceive keep-fit as fun, a genuinely uplifting activity. The eventfulness of the encounter with a spirit of fitness is stressed as a way to emphasise the authenticity of both cheerfulness and one's own successful initiation (see Chapter 7). The fitness frame is thus internalised, no longer seen as an external imposition or an objectified set of prescriptions. Most regulars conclude their description by reckoning that "if you're happy doing it, you do not really feel the effort". Barbara, a university student from Florence, explains:

> during the first few days I was not up to it: I couldn't do it, I couldn't do it for the life of me: I remember finding it impossible to

be co-ordinated ... everyone seemed better and more concentrated than I was ... At the beginning, I was much less involved, I wanted to hide, I felt really embarrassed. Then, thanks to Pamela's [the trainer] encouragement, who explained that "those who are perfect, those who never make mistakes, have been coming for ten years" I threw myself into it. So I said to myself ok, let's give it a try". Now I'll stand in the second row, I want to look at my movements in the mirror to see if I'm doing it properly! I'll follow the teacher carefully, I'll do everything, I'll sweat my guts out but I'll do it! And I have learned that I can enjoy myself, perfection is not so important, what matters is that you try hard and have fun.

Let's consider "fun" more closely. In regulars' accounts fun does not derive from time spent free from all rules; indeed, it is socially organised. In particular it is generated by engaging with well-organised social practices and by learning to embrace their rules. The emotional structure of keep-fit workout not only highlights the procedural, present vividness of exercise movements, it also classifies participants' engrossment as "fun". The successful gym-goers that I have met both in Italy and Britain mention self-challenge, on the one hand, and informality, on the other, as sources of fun. In their words doing fitness is "entertaining" because it provides a "moment of concentration: try to do better every day"; because it furnishes a clear arena for self-evaluation: "to find out how far I can go, and I really like being able to measures my performance". But, to be fun, self-challenge is coded via the relational and emotional structure of the fitness gym. Courtesy, little informal exchanges during the exercises, a cheerful ambiance which allows for a respectful joke from time to time, the staging of a supportive attitude, all these small interaction devices are managed to make strenuous exertion and self-challenge pleasant. Rather than friendship, carnal fraternity or shared membership in "a small guild renowned for toughness and bravery" which are the small pleasures of boxing training (Wacquant, 2003, p. 68), fitness training provides a rather more detached, urban, polished sociability to brighten up the monotony of training with a chance for diversion (see Chapter 3).

Besides, regulars and enthusiasts describe their workout experiences as involving an intense perception of their own body as defined by the exercise. Successful initiation to fitness training is often described as the carnal tuning of body and exercise. However sanitised it may be compared to that of boxing, the very carnality of the process accounts for much of the pleasures of training. Carnality or embodiment is achieved, as in sports activities (Chambliss, 1989; Heikkala, 1993) or indeed ballet (Faure, 2000), via the endless repetition of codified movements. This, however, is not felt as mere subjugation to the rather obvious strictures of keep-fit techniques. On the contrary, as I shall show in the next paragraph, a disciplined body is conceived as a proof of one's own improvement, and linked to satisfaction. Thus, the concentration on one's own body while training may be described as a heightened sense of embodiment, which is conceived as a "liberation" from all external pressure. The idea that training represents a form of liberation will be further explored later (see Chapter 7). Here, I must stress that it concurs to the vocabulary of fun. Just like other sports or amateur practices – especially those which are constructed as "the Other" of ordinary urban life, for example, mushroom collecting (see Fine, 1998) or Nordic walking (see Shove and Pantzar, 2005) – fitness training is perceived as a moment of release from the tension produced by urban living, desk-bound professional demands and family obligations.

Experiences of fun are, in many ways, a function of participation: regulars are more likely to engage and feel comfortable with the physical demands, motivational logic and emotional structure of training, while novices play at the margins. This produces yet again a *double-bind configuration* that perhaps lies beneath what we normally call routine: it is only via participation that we learn to relax in a social scene, and yet a measure of relaxation is quite often fundamental for ongoing, successful participation. There is a recursive relation, participation produces fun, and fun produces participation. Of course this may work up to the point that exercise participation, which is tiring and tiresome, can be justified. As my research extended across quite a long period of time, I could witness an increasing emphasis on fun from the mid 1990s to the present. Today, in Italy and in Britain at least, fun appears to be increasingly drawn upon to provide fitness with legitimation, having become a crucial basis for a public account as to why and to what extent fitness is good for people. As we shall see in later chapters, fitness training rests on a specific combination of asceticism and hedonism, both of which tend to stress the notion of individual autonomy. This is clearly consistent with a more general trend in Western consumer culture, one that stresses the role of (domesticated) individual pleasure in the legitimation of consumer practices (Sassatelli, 2000a, 2007).

"Fun" has important rhetorical uses and practical consequences. As such, it is an extremely serious element in fitness. On the one hand, it is geared towards something more than simple entertainment. On the other, it produces effects on the perception of what exercise is, and what it offers. Involvement experiences are important for their effects of reality (see Goffman, 1961). When coded as "fun", involvement experiences are also crucial for their *effects of subjectivity* (see Foucault, 1983; 1984a and b). They become part of the reflexive narratives about self and participation. So, many regulars describe bodywork in the gym as "not work, but a space which must remain entertaining", something which needs "commitment" and yet "you must feel that you are not forced to do it".[5] The sequence of exercises may thus be described, not just as an external given, but as something alive in the clients' experiences, absorbing the whole of their attention for a brief moment but with quite low risks of failure. Fun is both predicated on, and confirms, the intrinsic relevance of keep-fit exercise. By and large, regular clients are adamant that they have learned to enjoy themselves *and* to use enjoyment in order to continue training. This duality of feeling – which entails both real engrossment and reflexive, even instrumental agency – is not to be understood as evidence of the merely ideological nature of fitness. It is rather a feature of all engrossment or flow experiences in games: as Robert Perinbanayagam (2006) has recently stressed it becomes the basis of the possibility of stabilising and narrating the self through games.

For regular fitness participants pleasure, as a subjective experience that is fun, is reflexively considered crucial for exercise adherence over a long period. They maintain that the possibility of "being involved" and of "having a good time" "helped" them to "train regularly". Again, going back to Betty's story, we see, for example, that she "decided" to go to the gym because she wanted to "lose weight", but the "gym has taught" her something more: "to take care of the body". Still she knows she could not continue if she were not enjoying herself:

> It's important for my body, too, because I've seen it gradually change since I started exercising, but pleasure is also a major part, because you're enjoying yourself – if it weren't for that, you wouldn't just go to lose weight or tone up, after a while you get bored, it's too mechanical.

Among regulars, however, fun is seen as more than an expedient for sustained and increasing participation. Pleasurable experiences are also a *value in themselves*. Coded as fun, engrossment in self-discipline is perceived as personal commitment, realisation and freedom. Anna, a regular from Florence, insists that when she "doesn't like something" she does not continue: "if I don't enjoy myself, I don't go", and she adds emphatically, "it would be stupid to go there and sweat if you weren't enjoying yourself!". John, also a regular participant from London, claims that "you have such a little time for yourself, I would not do it if it were boring for me, I go for the fun". Cleo from Norwich says "having so much on my plate every week, it would be difficult to go if it were not gratifying". Fun thus becomes an experience which positively qualifies one's own efforts. For regular clients, in particular, it is a guarantee that their efforts are indeed voluntary, thus becoming itself a principle of legitimation drawing on hedonistic themes, different from self-discipline and partially in conflict with it. What is more, for these clients, the duality of fun – as experience and expedient – is itself sometimes described with satisfaction, as if a source or pleasure: a truly liberating, cathartic experience whereby one's own pleasure is rational and rationality becomes pleasurable (see Chapter 4).

Of course, there is always a limit to the success of fitness framing. All participants in a workout scene demonstrate public respect for the workout frame, but some of them may feel alienated rather than involved. "Fun" enters potently in fitness culture as a cultural code. Yet, subjective experiences that are fun – or pleasurable – cannot simply be produced or planned structurally or institutionally (unlike timetables, fees, training options and so on). Pleasure is a contingent experiential effect activated through subjects: it is neither a purely psychological nor an accidental element, produced as it is by the particular organisation of fitness workouts, but it can only be renewed or extinguished in each new exercise session according to how participants manage reality. In other words, even the most enthusiastic clients may get a "boring" session or "have an off day". A certain amount of hesitation, and quite a bit of reflexivity for the control of such hesitation is to be found among regulars. In such cases other, more reflexive, forms of internal rewards are deployed.

4. The manifold pleasures of successful initiation

In the same way as other forms of physical and mental involvement in a feasible task (Goffman, 1961), workout scenes in the gym offer participants the possibility of validating both themselves and their own choices by confirming the competences being acquired. Clients may therefore be reassured of their value, allowing for positive thinking to move focus from defects to assets, from shortcomings to improvements (see Csikszentmihalyi, 1997; Perinbanayagam, 2006). "I'm not so clumsy as I was at the beginning", "I can see I'm getting better", "I can get right to the end of the class now", "I can look at myself in the mirror now, I not that bad" – these are some of the feelings that especially successful novices of all ages and genders report about their training. They still remember well a recent time when their competences might have been worse or inadequate and they all agree that it is their newfound experiences of competence which make them "feel more secure", "involved", "satisfied".

"Satisfaction" is described by participants as different from fun. Fun is immediate involvement in the present. Satisfaction is the capacity to reflect upon oneself and feel proud. It comes from sensuous experiences of achievement in doing this or that movement; it derives from looking and feeling good during training, that is, fit and fitting into the scene (see also MacNevin, 1999; Monaghan, 2001). All in all, it is a *second-level pleasure*, a pleasure linked to competence in recognising one's own abilities, a pleasure which directly contributes to constitution of the self through time. Here are some verbalisations from successful novices expressing satisfaction:

It's a more familiar environment now, and I feel I can do it. I am not that funny anymore, I know what I have to do, [and] I can more or less do it. And if I work fine, then I can say to myself: "well done, it was hard work" ... it's really satisfying, [and] you gain confidence and are more self-assured.

(High-school teacher in his late thirties, Florence)

If I am working out fine, I am in good shape and concentrate, then I feel I look good, I do the routine well, and I do like to look at myself in the mirror. Managing by and large to follow these tough step sequences, is really rewarding! Sometimes I'm more tired, so I can't keep up so well and then I don't feel so satisfied, I surely look bad.

(Civil servant in her fifties, Florence)

The first few times I came here I was doing mainly cardio stuff and stretching, and at the beginning I found that difficult too, then little by little I've started doing other things, including spinning. I'm quite pleased to see that I'm managing better, it pushes me to keep going even if I'm tired.

(Female mature student, London)

The stories of regular participants are full of similar expressions of satisfaction. While some techniques, such as pilates, appear less obviously coded in terms of fun, at least compared with other techniques such as spinning, all techniques are described by regulars with a variety of expressions of satisfaction. In their physical specifications, these expressions vary according to the main type of activity carried out, ranging from feelings of "control" of the body to "strength", from "energy" and "power", to "flexibility", "harmony" and "expressiveness". Moreover, most clients also use general expressions such as "I feel strong" or "fit" – expressions which, as I shall show, relate to quite precise meanings as to body-self relation (see Chapters 6 and 7). A more strategic involvement of the embodied self – for example, in the learning of a new sequence in exercise-to-music options, or in the negotiation of variation of one own machine programme with the trainer – is also often mentioned by regulars as very rewarding.

Just like they code the display of strenuousness as fun, instructors and trainers praise improvement and suggest it should help clients to be "confident", "pleased", "satisfied". At the end of a session, in all the fitness centres I have visited, trainers insisted that clients should feel "proud" of themselves and their bodywork. The sharing of applause to mark the end of an exercise-to-music class is just one example of this gratification strategy. Just like fun, "satisfaction" is recognised by fitness discourse as having a positive effect on clients' capacity to continue exercising. The social psychology of sport in its turn stresses that feelings of effectiveness, skill and satisfaction help to persevere with sporting activities.[6] And, not surprisingly, clients themselves concur with such a view. But how does it happen?

Satisfaction helps to translate the here-and-now of bodywork into a long-term training programme. We should remember that, as stated by Licia, a regular from Milan, practising a keep-fit activity may be "nice, it's a way to enjoy myself, but if my shape would be perfect by nature, I would avoid it quite happily. I would go for other leisure activities, less demanding perhaps, more fanciful, such as horse riding." Regulars' stories and verbal exchanges in the gym show that satisfaction may provide the initial, fundamental link between the present of keep-fit training and the body projects which is intended to achieve. Particularly important, though, is how present and projects are related. We may appreciate this by considering what satisfaction is supposed to both reveal and produce. As to the former, most regulars consider that their satisfaction is a *proof of hidden talents* which are finally revealed and appropriated by the self. As to the latter, regulars essentially link satisfaction to the construction of long-term exercise plans characterised by the *embracement of fitness variety* as it proposed in the gym.

In general, feelings of physical achievement experienced during work-out are seen as a reward for commitment which allows for wider and longer projects of bodywork. For regulars, satisfaction mediates between body objectives and training programmes, internalising objectives and link-ing them to the specific exercise options available in their gym rather then simply to broad ideas of body modification. Satisfaction looks back at past keep-fit sessions and helps organise training as a forward-looking sequence of bodywork inspired by self-challenge, novelty and variety. Positive rather than negative motivational narratives become more relevant: responding to fitness discourse as spoken by trainers and gym staff, successful novices emphasise getting toned or gaining energy, and tend to consider losing weight or correcting body defects as secondary to their fitness training. Thus, accounts of novices can clearly be distinguished: enthusiastic novices deploy satisfaction as a way to focus on bodywork options; distant novices are often trapped in their initial body objectives or defects. Here are some verbalisations that illustrate this distinction:

> I'm going to start free-standing exercise lessons in October. I have a very long-term programme: I'm starting to have more stamina now, and to have the stamina I need to do things well, I have to train first, and then bit by bit I can do free-standing exercise classes too . . . in that way, training is more balanced, and it really makes you feel better. I feel satisfied as I do the exercises better, I now come more often, and I want to try out new things.
>
> (Sales representative in his fifties, Florence)

> I relish the break I get from the gym, I have discovered what I want from the gym: what I like, what I do best, which gives me really satisfaction: I can see I'm doing fine, that's really rewarding, it's an immediate result. Then, I guess I have stopped fussing about my look that much. You start with some extreme beauty ideas in your head, silly kind of a thing, I know,

but it takes a while to get real and really appreciate the feel-good-factor of having this regular training.

(Student in her twenties, London)

Feeling that you have worked is very important. Sometimes I'm happy and sometimes, quite often, I'm not. In general, I'm not able to follow the steps they make you do, so I feel like a sack of potatoes and I don't like it. However, if I work with heavier weights than the others I feel good; then I really feel I'm doing something to tone my body and make it more supple.

(Shopkeeper in her forties, Florence)

The last comment comes from a distant novice. It differs markedly from the previous two narrations which were provided by enthusiasts. Satisfaction is present, but for the wrong reasons, such as competition. It therefore does not mediate between external, initial body ideals and internal, gym-specific bodywork possibilities.

By and large, a difficult initiation to the gym world typically means that clients find it hard to cope with either the absence of overt competition, the lack of immediate results or cheerful strenuousness. Gym drop-outs are particularly vocal about keep-fit workout being *senseless*: not competitive enough on performance or too competitive on physiques, too tiring and not immediately rewarding as a leisure occasion. In many ways, while the enthusiasts find ways to negotiate or compromise with the organisation of fitness training, drop-outs and irregular clients share the scepticism which critical theory nurtures for it. Their experiences of satisfaction are marginal, and what is more they often deviate from prescribed rules – such as in the account above. The lack of proper satisfaction validated by meanings-sharing with other participants means that keep-fit exercise remains an exterior and somewhat strange experience for these participants, coded as "duty", rather than "leisure", and "tiresomely tiring" rather than "cheerfully energising".

On the contrary, when initiation to the gym world is successful clients learn to draw satisfaction from their abilities to appropriately respond to the exercise scene. They learn to evaluate their responses, which then become the basis for constructing their gym attendance programme, further consolidating the translation of body objectives into a story on bodywork told by a knowing gym insider. Before dealing with what the negotiation of body objectives and ideals entails (see Chapter 6), let's briefly explore what a successful gym career typically means for exercise practice. Regulars claim that they have tried to "understand" right from the beginning which exercise combinations were most suitable for them, and to have tried, as one of them mentioned with telling words, to "structure myself inside the gym". Regular clients are often determined to exploit the potential of fitness centres to the maximum. This matches the emphasis on personalisation which is a feature of expert discourse (see Chapter 3). Exercise manuals, for example, remind readers that a "good rule of thumb for establishing when to stop exercising is to judge one's own tiredness" (Punzo, 1992, p. 28). What is more, they encourage individuals to choose their own "menu" from the most "suitable" activities for their "fitness level" (Goodsell, 1995, p. 28). Personalisation is an individual selection from pre-packaged options, with gym staff and gym instructors typically advising participants to "do different movements" by following the "different classes" or "techniques" offered by the institution.

The construction of personalised training programmes is very important as it consolidates self-challenge, the motivational logic of fitness, through time and matches the provision of structured variety which is typical of commercial fitness gyms. An ongoing personalised training programme is the main way through which a fitness fan can capitalise on the time spent exercising. As gyms operate on a differentiating pluralism, and there are official limits to internal recognition for those who have acquired a better physique, fitness capital may be displayed more easily via one's own "omnivorousness" in fitness. Just as happens in other spheres of consumption such as music (see Peterson, 1992; Peterson and Kern, 1996), omnivorousness becomes a sign of one's own centrality in fitness culture. Now, this is also expressed through participation as much as through a language of fun. Gym enthusiasts like to socialise around fitness activities, engage in small talk about them, display their insiders' *habitus* relishing the horizon of variety available. Structured variety is described as a source of pleasure, offering an apparently not exclusivist sense of achievement which matches the democratic ideology of fitness. Omnivorousness appears indeed well adjusted to that consumer capitalism which fitness culture is articulated with, enlarging markets and allowing for continuous provision of slightly different novelties. Marginal innovation indeed both diminishes consumers' learning efforts and provides a sense of change and choice, being often coded as pleasurable realisation of one's own well-governed curiosity.

6
The Culture of the Fit Body

> June is looming, and now is the time of year when everyone is
> starting to think of booking their summer holidays, and more
> importantly, getting their body's into shape for the summer, is this
> you?

In spring 2007, the central London branch of an international fitness chain
tried to entice my subscription with a succession of emails, as I had enquired
at their health club in the winter, but did not join. While the glossy
brochures of fitness clubs tend to stress a number of accessory motivations –
such as fun, relaxation, sociability and so on – by and large the marketing
of fitness is managed, at its most external margins, via incitements related
to body shaping, including both appearance and health. "Looking good
for the summer" and "tone up for the beach" are a staple of fitness magazines in late spring, just like "a New Year resolution to lose weight" and
"get healthy" feature prominently in mid-winter issues. Fitness magazines
appear indeed trapped in a bulimic seasonality, swinging between health
and beauty. Just a few examples: the 25th anniversary copy of US magazine
Shape in December 2006 guarantees "the 5 minutes workout blasts anyone
can do: get a body you'll love by new year's"; the 2007 New Year issue of
Health and Fitness proposes a three-month shape-up plans focusing on "get
fit, tone up, shift pounds" that can "change your life"; in the same year
the April issue of the British magazine *Zest* produced a cover with a slender girl in the sea with a bikini supported by the claim "fit & sexy in 5 fast
moves!"; and in May *Women's Fitness* sports a similar cover with the claim
"your beach body starts here! Get a head-turning figure to die for". Back
in 1995, the first Italian fitness magazine, *Vitality*, was launched proposing gymnastics as a panacea which rescues the body from hectic modern
life. During its first year of publication, with a similar seasonal dynamic,
keep-fit training figured as providing health by "strengthening the heart
and lowering cholesterol" in the October issue, and allowing readers to "get
ready for the beach: firm breasts, flat stomach, toned buttocks, slender waist

and legs!" in the June issue (see Sassatelli, 2003). While Hollywood stars and media personalities routinely appear on the covers of these magazines thanking their personal trainers for their toned appearances, medical discourse has been attributing an ever increasing value, both therapeutic and preventive, to physical activity (Oja and Tuxworth, 1995; Shepard, 1995). Indeed, the vacillation between health and beauty is a function of fitness magazines location between health and sports discourse, on the one hand, and celebrities glamorised lifestyle reporting, on the other.

Still, these objectified symbolic dynamics do not exhaust fitness culture as lived culture. In this chapter, listening to fitness participants – clients, instructors and trainers – I ask which kind of symbolic work happens in the gym around the body. Fitness gyms are productive environments, not only because they produce "material" effects on the body, but also because they allow participants to negotiate and (re)produce body ideals. As I shall show, consuming fitness means working on the meanings of the "fit body". This involves a dialectical play between objectified fitness ideals as responding to broad cultural ideals and lived body objectives as negotiated through training. Such dialectical play matches the dialectic that I have shown operates between the external trim of the fitness frame (the embodied performance of normative body ideals) and the internal one (self-competition and involvement) (see Chapters 4 and 5). Broad cultural incitements and body ideals may have prompted clients to get into a fitness centre in the first instance. However, these ideals are not simply taken up by gym-goers. Indeed, while fitness culture is so obviously part of contemporary consumer culture, enticing a vast public of consumers to engage, via commercial transactions, with goods and services that are produced to be sold, my journey into the world of the fitness gym demonstrates the productive force of consumer practices and the permeability of the division between production and consumption in consumer spaces such as commercial gyms. By taking part in gym activities, regular participants contribute to the production of the notion of fitness upon which the whole industry is predicated.

1. The naturalisation of fitness knowledge

In backstage conversations, in casual encounters in the gym and in structured interviews at their homes, the regular gym-goers that have contributed to this study, from both Italy and Britain, have referred to keep-fit practice as an entry into a new form of knowledge. Clearly, training does not imply the mere obedience to the precepts of whatever exercise technique may be the order of the day, as it does not simply imply physical efforts or effects. It is precisely because it ultimately influences people's understanding that training succeeds in modifying the clients' bodies without being experienced as an imposition. By quitting the gym, individuals reject, and sometimes question, the soundness of what is on offer; by continuing to go, clients inevitably *negotiate* the rendering of the body and self within fitness culture.

Regulars describe the knowledge they maintain they have acquired not only as "new", but also as "deep", "better" and "true". Such knowledge is often identified as an objective and complete *knowledge of the body*. And yet, from an observational point of view, it also very clearly amounts to *practical body control* in response to *specific exercise requirements*. Leo, for example, refers to muscles, repetitions, breathing, synchrony, co-ordination and so on – all items which are standard features of the kind of keen stepper he is. For this 30 something architect from Florence:

> [knowing one's own body] means understanding when your heartbeat is above a certain level, and deciding whether to stop or continue, or understanding that breathing is important: with breathing, you can syn-chronise heartbeat with muscle exertion, and the blood goes to the areas you are using at the same time, not before or after … it means that you are in control, and it becomes automatic.

In this and other regulars' verbalisations, knowledge is indexed to keep-fit training, but is felt as usable beyond the training scene, precisely because it concerns *the* body as such. Cleo, a secretary in her late thirties from Norwich stresses that "if you stick to a [exercise] routine, it becomes a way to keep an eye on yourself, to check your body regularly … just to know what you need, what is bad for you". The oracular power of routines is stressed also by a Florentine fitness fan like Marica, also a secretary in her late twenties:

> the gym is very important because you are controlling your body every day. It's a way of controlling yourself: you've got problems you're not aware of, you could weigh yourself, but if you can't see yourself and you don't do anything about it, it isn't of much use. I never weigh myself on a scale, scales mean nothing. What's important is that, when you look at yourself in the mirror, every day doing your routine, you say: "this is fine, this isn't".

A similar line runs through official expert discourse on fitness. It can be repeatedly found in fitness manuals. Typically written by famous instructors and/or personal trainers, each of these manuals provides its own special recipe for fitness. But these recipes are variations on the same theme: what counts is to learn to exercise appropriately, that is, according to the proposed technique. Self-surveillance during training helps in this, but also important is to "feel" how one's own body responds to the solicitation of training. They agree with what Callan Pinckney (1995, p. 49) wrote in her popular manual: those who want to keep fit must "throw away the scale": "the important thing is how your body reacts to the care and attention it receives from training". Typically designed for DIY fitness, all manuals indeed exploit similar rhetorical strategies. For example, *Escape Your Shape* by Edward Jackowski (2001) suggests that following his advice will allow the "true body shape" to emerge. The founder of one of the largest one-to-one fitness companies in the USA, Jackowski reckons that all bodies can be placed into four body shapes, each of which defines the truth of the body, which can be known through exercise and demands different exercises. Here is a telling quote:

> In truth, you're only temporarily caught between [body] types. Deep down you are a pure Hourglass, Spoon, Ruler or Cone... You may have problems in determining your body type, but it is only because you are carrying extra weight. Fear not, simply follow Hourglass workout [...]. As you become slimmer and your natural shape begins to emerge, you can start adding some resistance and weights to your exercises.
> (Jackowski, 2001, p. 31)

Gym instructors and personal trainers also insist on the idea that fitness provides for body knowledge whose worth goes far beyond the exercise performance, even though it is grounded in it. In their words, fitness training must become something which can help all of us to "feel our own body" not only "inside", but also "outside" the gym. While working out with a personal trainer in Bologna, I have also been given similar advice, with the personal trainer suggesting that "the work" we were "doing together" and the "knowledge" which I was "gaining" as a result were "meant to be a resource in life". During classes, gym instructors stress the cognitive value of training, qualifying the capacity to respond to keep-fit techniques as knowledge. While working out with a group, they may provide little incidental lessons on body knowledge mixed up with training encouragements. Here are a couple of such lessons from trainers during group activities:

> [trainer:] you have to think of your body, get to know it, understand which positions you're adopting and try to correct them. We get backache because we don't walk properly, or we don't sit properly, or some of our muscles are too short or squashed, now you can feel yourselves, so learn to adopt the correct posture.
> (Stretching class, Florence, November 1995)

> [trainer:] the technique is very important. Put your hands on your tummy, you can really feel you muscles and your spine. Now roll on your spine, slowly, slowly, one by one your vertebras are set free – and bend, bend, bend gently. Remember once you know these stretching movements, that's for life. You can do them everywhere, you can just take

5 minutes off wherever you are, to keep in contact with your body and avoid back pain.

(Relaxation after step aerobics, London, February 2007)

As is apparent, fitness practices are predicated on the idea that fitness knowledge is somehow *absolute*: knowledge of exercise movements is presented as thoroughly useful on a daily basis, competing with other forms of physical awareness, and providing a nearly objective measurement of one's own body (health, capacities and appearance). This amounts to a "claim to truth" (see Foucault, 1983; see also Chapter 7) on the body, which indexes the truth of the body to keep-fit training.[1] Gyms draw people into a specific consumption or participation-based set of institutionally sustained body classifications. In tales of successful initiation such classifications come to coincide with what one knows and one believes to qualify as knowledge, being thus both "subjective" and "objective". Fitness knowledge becomes naturalised in the sense that what is a *conditioned* and *conditional* knowledge becomes *unconditional*. Thus, for example, in the process which brings regulars to construct a personalised training programme (see Chapter 5), knowledge of the training *alternatives available* in a gym is turned into knowledge of the *most suitable techniques* for one's own body. This is predicated on fitness gyms structured variety and on trainers' encouragement towards a pluralistic, but gym-bound, vision of the training alternatives.

2. Coping with body ideals

Fitness knowledge has dramatic consequences for regulars. Instructors and trainers insist that their clients must learn to aspire to body characteristics that are within their reach and are actually produced by fitness activities. Indeed, in patterns of successful initiation, fitness knowledge helps change original individual body objectives. Motives for continuing training in a fitness gym are typically different from motives for joining – not only, as suggested, because internal or intrinsic aspects of training become more important (see Chapters 3 and 5), but also because external aspirations change. As self-challenge, fun and sociability acquire relevance, body objectives shift in their specifications. In the gym, clients' body objectives are formed and transformed. Many regulars echo trainers in suggesting that fitness training helps people "get real" about their bodies. Let's explore this by reconsidering patterns of successful initiation.

As participants manage to organise their efforts into a training project, somebody characteristics acquire a fresh, prominent and foundational importance. These characteristics, in turn, form the basis for an awareness of the body as being something "useful" and "real", an embodied awareness which can be used to negotiate initial subjective aspirations as related to broad cultural ideals objectified in commercial images and the like. In their verbalisations, the "feeling" component acquires relevance for many regulars, suggesting that cognition is far from purely mental, but practical and embodied, a reflexive experience of bodily presence (see Crossley, 2001, 2004). But there is more. The paradoxical emotional structure of the exercise appears to induce participants to play with their motivations by organising their experience in a similarly paradoxical manner. Clients may learn to say to themselves and to others the opposite of what they mean in order to understand the opposite of what they say (see Bateson, 1972). That is, they can learn to say that initial body characteristics or acquired body capital do not matter, which allows them to keep (certain) body images in the background as ideals, and to work on their own bodies without too much self-exposure.

This configuration may generate a variety of responses, which are more mixed and articulated than the simple "aesthetic masochism" diagnosed by Frew and McGillivray (2005) as endemic among Scottish gym-goers. In this study, the fitness industry is reported as largely dissatisfying its consumers' desires for an ideal healthy and attractive body. Yet, in my explorations I found a much more nuanced, and in fact different, picture. A sense of frustration maybe there, and it is very clearly so among quitters, novices and irregular clients. But it is alleviated by a shift in body objectives among those who stick to a club and become regulars: regular clients typically learn to suspend their initial aspirations, concentrate on performing the exercises, and then reconsider their aspirations in the light of what may be provided by locally organised fitness options. The process which leads to a successful gym career is described as having a *circular structure*. But rather than having the "vicious" quality of a contradiction, it is portrayed by gym staff and enthusiastic clients alike as a "virtuous circle", a spiral in fact, that in cognitive terms may be seen as reducing dissonance and organising preferences (Elster, 1979), thus offering a way forward. In different, more embodied terms, bodily presence as experienced during the routine offers appreciation angles which are very practical and feel very real as compared to ideals. Thus, we may say that when initiation to training is successful, clients return to the *purposive* moment of their practice having lived through its *procedural* moment, learning what they consider "new things" about themselves and about exercise, learning to feel rewarded by their bodywork and choosing exercise options on the basis of such satisfaction. In successful gym careers, the gym becomes important not only because participants get accustomed to going and acquire insider *habitus*, but also because they acquire insider agency, they begin to set objectives which the gym can meet. The very variety of keep-fit exercise is taken as a palette of possibilities which circumscribes the body objectives one may aspire to, rendering such objectives more "realistic" indeed – namely both "within reach" and "truthful" to the body as practically known through keep-fit techniques.

Regular participation in gym activities tends to produce the endorsement of the body characteristics which are promoted by keep-fit workout (typically tone, stamina, energy, co-ordination, strength and so on). It is partly through this that the initial body objectives – those which clients enter the gym with and which are typically formed whilst fantasising about one's own physical appearance, health and condition against the backdrop of broader body ideals – are worked upon and reappraised. Let's consider regulars' verbalisations, both in Italy and Britain. As suggested by Jo, a middle-aged woman from Norwich, "I see a lot of people who are just more real, or perhaps modest [than the stereotypical image of the gym queen]. They hold down a job and still find the time [to work out], and this is definitely nothing to do with their image. It's about something real, about feeling good." Many acknowledge initial goals as "dreams of perfection" which often insist on appearance and refer to celebrities, models, singers and the like. Thus, Loretta, a young shop assistant from Florence, says she started going to the gym to "look like an artist's model", defines her original objectives as "false", and is adamant that "anyway, I am happy with the gym, because I have improved my body [as] best as I can".

A recurrent theme to describe one's own initial objectives among regulars is "weight", or better the fear of being "overweight". Emphasis on weight control is increasingly present in fitness official discourse, especially in Britain and the USA (see Frew and McGillivray, 2005; Maguire, 2007, see also Chapter 7). Exercise manuals often incorporate nutritional tips, as much as manuals about dieting incorporate exercise sections, which, as in the case of *Body Business* by Donna Ashton (2001, p. 21ff.), treat exercise as the "flip side of the equation": the one that allows us to burn calories. This is reflected in provision developments with, for example, joint ventures such as "Together", a British campaign for joint membership with a major fitness chain and slimming organisation.[2] Not surprisingly, therefore, many people of all ages, both men and women, maintain that they began exercising because they had "put on weight" which they wanted to "lose". However, when asked to consider the specific benefits of training, many of them end up providing a far more articulate, and positive, image. In regular clients' verbalisations there is a marked shift towards affirmative, constructive language: "keep slim enough" generally replaces "losing weight". This positive attitude is reflected in that "tone" becomes paramount, and effectively replaces slenderness: crude versions of weight reduction are rare among regulars, weight reduction being mostly coded via functional elements. For example, among regulars I have met quite a few women who had begun to go to the gym after giving birth because they wanted to be "slim" again: the gym ultimately "made a lot of difference" to them because they have learned that what they "really wanted" was "to be toned". Men also mention weight control and reduction as amongst the major initial aims, even though muscular growth is also very prominent. Still, they also shift objectives, and talk of getting "energy", keeping "fit" or "releasing tension". By and large, regulars usually observe that weight control may be facilitated by keep-fit training, but "exercise as such doesn't help you to lose weight", "you put on weight when you exercise regularly": exercise "helps" in that "you tone your body", you "increase your muscles, don't lose them".

As seen, this is facilitated by trainers' attitudes (see Chapter 3). A negotiation of body objectives is also a feature of the institutionally sustained equivalence between keep-fit activities in the fitness centre. In many of the premises I have visited this is expressed via pluralism, with the diversity of individual desires being encouraged and, at the same time, kept in check. Here are some telling quotes from instructors:

> Of course fitness is not only about what you do in the gym, [it is] also about what you do outside it, trying to live a more regular life, checking your food, eating well, sleeping well, we give them information for healthy living, not false hopes about getting Angelina Jolie or Brad Pitt's bodies, which is what some people initially seem to want.
>
> (John, gym instructor, London)

> The initial objective becomes the last objective, they [the clients] have other smaller objectives along the way which are more sensible which they can see, and they learn to stick to it...When a woman wants to give up? Mostly it's because she is not able to recognise the changes, she is fixated on the original objectives and can't see how she has improved. Then you [the trainer] must be very good, you must change the way you train her, give her more advice, push her to do other things in the gym, so that she will feel more attached to the gym as a whole, as a place, not only to you as a trainer, suggesting that she can have a sauna if she is tired, but she must come, never stay at home...we must keep a variety so that she will not get bored and she will think that if she comes she will find something, anything, to do.
>
> (Valentina, gym instructor, Bologna)

Regular clients appeared to respond to similar incitements. As suggested, the most dedicated clients often end up trying and enjoying forms of physical exercise which they had not initially considered. Very common, in their verbalisations, is reference to what are described as "discoveries" (see also Chapter 7). Paola, a Florentine secretary in her late fifties, explains

> It took me nearly a year and a half before I wanted to use the machines. The fact that there was this nice girl in the machine area has helped. I do not feel that weird now, or at least I do not care...I only do exercises for my legs and arms, and I've built up my repetitions...My arms and legs are much stronger now, and I've really noticed something...It would be

foolish on my part to claim I really do weights, and I would not even dream of becoming seriously big, but a bit [big] is good, it works with my strong personality... I will never have the body I dream of, but I have learned to work on what I have, also what I didn't think I had.

By trying out new techniques, regulars ultimately perceive their bodies from a different angle, placing less emphasis on some of their original objectives, and more emphasis on others. Francesco, also a middle-aged Florentine, was quite dubious as he initially thought of the gym as a place where you "build up your muscles". Yet, "as a man" it was easier for him to "start off with weights and machines". However, after a year, he has built up a different programme: he has added a lot of stretching, soft exercise and tai-chi, and says that he was "wrong to have done exercises for the arms which were a bit too exaggerated in some ways":

I was overdoing it with my shoulders, and I would have ended up less physically healthy, less mobile, with less physical tone in general, and slower at performing the movements. Here you learn other things, other possibilities, and understand that there are stereotypes for men to be big, but not agile, which is totally wrong... Each is an individual and I really needed more flexibility and relaxation... In the gym there are so many things to do, aerobics, weights, step, soft exercise, dance-fitness combinations, and so on... a variety of things which all have one aim: providing exercise for people who live in cities to get a better body.

For some, buying a fitness pass is like buying a dream of perfection and plasticity. As we know (McCracken, 1988; see also Sassatelli, 2007), consumption may allow the cultivation of utopias that may not be realisable in ordinary life. Goods represent bridges suspended not only towards others, but also towards broad cultural ideals of a deep mythical force that on average escape us, and which we do not want to give up. The consumption of what may be called utopian goods, or the participation into utopian practices, may not so much change the nature of the utopia, but it can change how we relate to it.

Working on media representation of the fit and slender body, some authors, such as Susan Bordo (1993), have identified in a similar mechanism a sort of *disempowerment machinery* for the reproduction of the gender-laden normative ideal of the slender body. Bordo (1993, p. 191) sees "an important continuity of meaning in our culture between compulsive dieting and body building" and, by extension, fitness bodywork, which are "united in a battle against a common enemy: the soft, the loose, unsolid excess flesh... simply to be slim is not enough – the flesh must not wiggle". This is ultimately linked to the possibility of demonstrating a disciplined self – which, given that self-control is decisively coded as male and middle class, becomes more demanding for women and the working class. Empirical work in fitness gyms may also reach similar results. For example, Frew and McGillivray (2005) carried out their study of Scottish fitness mainly amongst personal trainers, with whom they conducted personal interviews, and supplemented these with focus groups of clients solicited to comment on a six-minute video clip representing an array of body shapes. With such objectifying methodology, it is no surprise that the study comes up with the result that "desires for the attainment of physical capital is constantly open to objectification in the health and fitness club", that "mediatized celebrity bodies become a sough after accessory", and that consumers' desires are "caught in a theoretical and practical vacuum" being unable to "practice the stoicism required to achieve their dreamscape desires" (ibid., p. 166). Rather than listening to the voices of fitness participants, such a study brings them to focus quite narrowly on official body ideals, allowing for very little attention to the many, different mechanisms that different clients put to work to negotiate or appropriate such ideals.

In her study of Norwegian aerobics classes, Nina Loland (2000, p. 118) reports the verbalisations of Ann, an aerobiciser in her early thirties, who thus justifies her participation: "I started with aerobics to do something about this [body] dissatisfaction...At that time, it must be ten years ago, I didn't know that it was that difficult to attain the thin, well shaped model body...however, even if I now see it as impossible, I still dream about that body and it is still the reason for taking classes." Loland does not explore how a regular, loyal participant such as Ann manages with what appears as a contradiction, nor does she tell us to what extent such a contradiction comes to be felt as painful or irrelevant, central or secondary to other rewards in fitness. However, it is precisely such dynamics which need exploring. They have been addressed by Debra Gimlin (2002) who has maintained that aerobics in many ways helps in steering the contradiction. Working out with aerobics fans and collecting their narrations, Gimlin has considered bodywork as something of an *empowerment opportunity*. "Women" – so she writes (ibid., p. 52) – "are capable of using aerobics classes to fuel a reconstruction of the self that releases identity from the physical, denies individual responsibility for socially constructed bodily 'imperfections', and provides new resources for identity formation".

From my fieldwork I have emerged with a clear sense that neither disempowerment nor empowerment offers a precise picture. My journey through fitness has helped me to consider fitness training very much as a *coping mechanism* – a device through which one's own inadequacies with respect to body ideals are negotiated, without necessarily implying a shift in those ideals.[3] A fitness pass represents in many ways a bridge to ideals of beauty, health and fitness, but – to follow the metaphor through – consumers may be able to walk on such a bridge only if they actually use the gym. And by using the gym, they modify their initial body objectives, the ones the bridge was directed to in the first place. At the very least, they emotionally qualify these objectives differently. At a subjective level, it is thus certainly true that we see a shift in body objectives, with "realistic" aspirations becoming more important for the self, and with ideals becoming less pressing as faults commanding strong dissatisfaction. This, as I shall show in the next chapter, is also accompanied by a shift from body to character, with emphasis on one's own determination and authenticity. We should not underestimate such shifts especially since they are grounded in lived bodily experiences which are described as deeply involving, and which allow fitness fans to devise often quite imaginative patterns of use. But use, involvement and exercise adherence itself become important as stabilisers of a positive attitude, a "realistic" attitude which may not be sustainable if we stop training (see also Burgess et al., 2009). As a coping mechanism, fitness training may need to be continuously activated.

Patterns of successful initiation shed doubts on the apocalyptic conclusion that fitness is an "unsuitable field" for the pursuit of health, at least a genuine version of it "untainted by consumer culture" (Smith Maguire, 2007, pp. 197ff; see also Frew and McGillivray, 2005). Sure, like most individualised coping mechanism, even when successful, keep-fit workout might simply provide consolation for our defects, offering some emotional relief. This, rather than dramatic bodily or life changes, may be the most significant outcome of fitness training. Moreover, a shift in body objectives or their subjective emotional requalification does not automatically mean that we actually renounce, once and for all, broader body ideals, and even less that we manage to contribute to their overall change in objectified commercial images. As a coping mechanism, fitness may indeed remain quite ambiguous, because it offers individual satisfaction and enjoyment in culturally prescribed and highly localised forms.

We shall at least analytically identify two political issues here, which I shall expand upon in the Conclusion. The first one has to do with what is the social role of the fitness gym in current health and stratification issues. Fitness training in the gym may provide some real individual relief for problems – of health and fitness – which are larger and social, sustaining the impression that they may indeed be simply solved by individual resolution. The universalistic and individualistic profile of commercial gyms may exacerbate this, contributing to foreclose the possibility that fitness be addressed also by other, probably more collectivised, informal or public means. This opens the way for a discussion on fitness promotion and policies tailored to reconsider body care as part of citizenship. The second issue has to do with how fitness training is organised in a gym environment and how this facilitates successful coping that provides for more than emotional relief. A commercial context, so it seems, has the potential to widen the gap between the internal and the external trim of the fitness frame: large, international, sales-oriented fitness chains often advertise by using all the mythic powers of accepted, dominant body ideals, only to orient training clients to internal rewards via the provision of rather standardised elements of joyful strenuousness. But commercial contexts may also provide for quite different routes. For example, the study of Leslea Collins (2002) on a group of US self-proclaimed feminist exercisers and their use of aerobics offers an example. Deeply critical of the gendered nature of fitness, the women in her study used strategies for participation that both downplayed oppressive aspects of training (the focus on the look, non-functional or embarrassing movements) and enhanced their personal empowerment in aerobics classes (sociability, criticism, refusal to participate). She concludes that constant adaptation of practice testifies to both the normative gendered views incarnated by keep-fit training and the capacity of fitness participants to take (some) distance from them while training.

Examples such as this do not represent the bulk of the phenomenon and feminist notions of "empowerment" have often been cosmetically incorporated in fitness discourse (Eskes et al., 1998; Markula, 2001). Yet, we should not undervalue clients' capacity to resist particular aspects of fitness while carrying out their routines. Actual training and the performing of physical exercise changes both how exercise gets done and how people perceive themselves and their objectives. In many ways, gym participation initiates cultural dynamics that entail a shift in the subjective rendering of body ideals. It is through such dynamics that not only broad, objectified body ideals may remain in the background as powerful utopias, but also the position of fitness in such a landscape is negotiated.

All fitness insiders – trainers and regular clients – contribute to the negotiation of what is fitness as against broader body ideals and images. Their narratives illustrate very well the kind of "boundary work" (Lamont and Molnar, 2002) they are engaged in. Boundary work occurs mainly with respect to four entities: *general media images, fitness commercial images, inactive people* who dream of fitness and gym *novices* – including their past selves as novices. Before going to a fitness centre, so goes the typical script, a lot of people tend to have a "fairly unrealistic idea" of the effects of keep-fit exercise, they hope to achieve "astounding results in the space of two weeks", they dream of "crash fitness programmes", something which is promoted by "media images", "consumerism", "advertising" and the like. But in actual fitness training "there are no crash programmes", no "quick fix". Clients thus learn, sometimes at their obvious distress, that fitness takes time. Regulars and fans come to prioritise the idea that "we need to know our body" through routine, which distances them from standardised commercial images by stressing individual appropriation: "everyone follows their own path", "we all have different bodies", "each is unique, and must learn what is good for him". In the gym also, "you realise that it's important to *feel* well", and this means "accepting yourself and improve what you have": "you may not have an exceptional physique, but a more harmonious, proportioned physique". Just as clients are asked to learn that "no-one has the so-called 'ideal body'" (Pinckney, 1992, p. 26), they are asked to disengage from the standards of beauty prevalent in mainstream advertising and dramatised by the last Hollywood beauty. The fitness gym, for regulars, does not make the body "beautiful as such". Not conventionally at least. Not if one thinks in terms of "an image based on fashion". Not if one just thinks in terms of objectified body parts, as many indeed do when they buy a gym membership and fitness magazines. In contrast, keep-fit training may institutionalise an active version of the "sour grape" logic. Thus, if fitness magazines' discourse often surreptitiously reproduce oppressive body ideals through visual images that may even contradict written text (see Markula, 2001), regular clients distance themselves from most fitness magazines in so far as the latter offer a "crude image" of keep-fit workout and the gym. At the objectified, commercialised pole of fitness culture, in magazines and adverts, "it's all about losing weight", while the "reality" of the insider is that training is actually "far more varied". Again reference to variety, personalisation and acceptance are prevalent among fitness fans to determine what appropriately lies within fitness as lived through the fitness gym.

We should be wary of providing a reconciliatory vision of fitness gym culture though. Indeed, one of the features that may strike the observer quite sharply is that in the fitness gym the ongoing surveillance of the body demanded by training adumbrates a likewise *constant negotiation of body objectives*. This is indeed the mark of the fitness fan, and may have ambivalent results. Marica and Carmelo, for example, both with ten years' experience as clients in the Florentine fitness scene, say they have continued to learn new techniques and movements and to set new physical goals. They both tend to provide triumphant narratives of participation. Carmelo, a middle-aged medical doctor who began doing weight training as an adolescent, maintains that his way of going to the gym matured along with the gym itself. "These days," he explains, "the issue of diet is much more precise and refined" and training is done on machines which are "very selective, there's a machine for one group of muscles, and one for another" and the new machines "don't have a violent impact on the joints". Carmelo's aims developed along parallel lines: he still wants to "have a presentable physique from an aesthetic point of view", but rather than "becoming broader", he is aiming at "reactive muscles", which "respond correctly no matter what you do", and which "burn off fat" so that you can always allow yourself to "go out for dinner with friends". Even though he presents his participation pattern in a low-key tone, he would "feel lost without the gym", he "hate[s] to skip sessions, especially due to injuries", as the gym provides him with a "place where I can concentrate on myself", working precisely on his embodied identity. Marica, who loves aerobics classes and circuit training, says:

> I choose what to do also according to what I see in magazines: they have loads here in the gym. I always try to keep up to date, and then you

look at other people, [I] don't know, maybe I'd like to have shoulders like the one over there, or buttocks like hers, so I say: "I've got to work harder!" ... You change your training here and there, someone may even think you are obsessive, and in a way you are, like every day in the gym a couple of hours, you know, it's quite something... But on the whole you learn what is good for you, and you get a bit more patient with your shape.

While these clients clearly negotiate with their received body ideals, below their superficial serenity, their narratives also appear to accommodate a measure of stress. As repeatedly suggested, fitness gyms contain quite a bit of variety in terms of patterns of participation. We not only have quitters and irregular clients who clearly never manage to get into an insider perspective. We also get a few fitness fans that dangerously linger on the contradictions of fitness culture, with a continuous negotiation of body objectives becoming itself a goal. And if in other pursuits collectivised through official competition such as body building and boxing (Klein, 1993; Wacquant, 2003), looking at other participant's bodies, being keen on locally specific performance and focused on body hierarchies are, as it were, sub-culturally sustained practices, in fitness training clients who become obsessed with the negotiation of their physique are left much more alone. There may be an element of fun in this, as body negotiation is largely predicated on self-competition and satisfaction. But fun is not always good, and in some cases, as I shall show in the next chapter, it may evoke the spectre of addictive behaviour.

3. Health, beauty and fitness

In general, clients agree that the fitness gym may respond to a multitude of different, specific and personal body objectives. Insiders in particular emphasise the plurality of these environments: "everyone – I have heard over and over again – has their own goal". Novices reiterate a number of stereotypical descriptions: there are "the body builders who just want to develop their muscles", the "older women who want to relax" and "the gym beauty who wants to look perfect". Regulars tend to have more nuanced pictures, mentioning those who "want to get rid of their stomach" as well as those who "just want to move", to "feel more energetic" or to "be more supple". As clients' careers in the gym advance, there seems to be a degree of convergence. While even quite different participants to specific keep-fit techniques (such as aerobics, spinning, stretching or circuit training) may converge on certain body objectives, what seems to unite regulars is their capacity to negotiate body objectives, and through such a process to cope with broad body ideals. Broad body ideals themselves are partly reworked by fitness culture. Let's focus on fitness culture and its body ideals (see Sassatelli, 2003).[4]

Beauty is often referred to within fitness discourse. It comprises features within a semantic area that refer to the body as an exterior instrument of self-presentation in everyday life, and in erotic relations in particular. Working towards the surface may be an aim in itself, and indeed, quite a few of the incitements from fitness periodicals deal with such a dimension. In general, they suggest that the gym is to be expected to help clients "look good" and "have a presentable physique from an aesthetic point of view". Slimming down is in this case often quoted together with "problem areas" as a primary target for bodywork. Problem areas are quite obviously heavily gendered: attention is drawn to the lower part of the body for women, to the upper part of the body for men. The ideal is a small, round bum and slim, long legs for women; a muscled, flat stomach and broad shoulders for men. These differentiated shapes, which evidently stress the complementary relation among gendered bodies sustaining heterosexuality, are paramount in fitness magazines. Sexual attraction, sexual problems and tips for a better sexual life often feature in dedicated articles in these periodicals, where the beauty and the prowess of a gendered fit body is correlated with the capacity to boost the "magic" of sexual intercourse.

Still, in many ways, notions of beauty are weighted against the idea of being in "good physical form" or "being fit". Energy, together with other factors such as strength, resistance, agility, elasticity, vascular capacity, breathing and so on, charts the territory of the "fit body". *Fitness*, as good physical form, covers a number of broad aspirations which relate to the body as an instrument to be used in sports as in ordinary life. Providing a list of benefits which combines mental and physical health with improved self-esteem and appearance, standard exercise manuals often stress this. A classic, matter-of-fact Italian exercise manual *Sentirsi in forma* (Feeling in good shape) (Cella, 1989, p. 7) thus suggests:

> accurate research has shown that a person who is physically fit resists fatigue far longer than a person who is not; that a person who is fit is better prepared to cope with physical effort and has a stronger, more efficient heart; and finally that there is a direct relationship between physical fitness on the one hand and intellectual alertness and absence of nervous tension on the other.

But also a more fanciful manual, written by the world-famous American belly dancer Tamalyn Dallal, *Belly Dancing for Fitness* (Dallal and Harris, 2005, p. 15) considers fitness as offering essentially "cardiovascular and muscular benefits", "relaxation and stress reduction" and "weight control and self-image". The book illustrates that even sexual attraction passes though a vision of beauty informed by the (gendered) functionality of the body, its movements and its activity as reflected in "skin tone". The book recalls that belly dancing "originated as preparation for childbirth ... helping women by massaging the internal organs", and that it "has evolved over thousands of years to tone a woman's body from the inside out":

> The exercise of belly dance stretches us, makes us sweat and smile at the same time and so improves muscle and skin tone. Belly dance also inspires women to acknowledge, express and celebrate their femininity, which makes them want to dress with little more sizzle, or even show a little bit of belly that they finally realise is beautiful and natural.

As a deep bodily feature, good physical form is opposed to beauty as a "superficial" feature. So for many regulars both in Italy and Britain "the gym doesn't relate to appearance as such, but it's something more physical"; it is about "feeling physically good with yourself. It doesn't mean looking in the mirror and saying 'Oh, I look great!'; it "means feeling at ease with your own body." This does not mean that beauty, or the pursuit of attractiveness, is not an issue. Rather, as I shall show in the next paragraph, beauty ideals are shaped by the notion of the "fit body", and the ideas such as vitality, energy and functionality.

The emphasis placed on functionality has obvious implications for the third semantic area which is paramount in keep-fit discourse, namely *health*. The particular notion of health promoted by fitness is evident in manuals. A popular Italian gymnastic handbook appropriately entitled *Sempre giovani* (Forever young) maintains that "feeling good" is above all to "be healthy and efficient": "one can be strong, healthy, active and in love at any age"; thus the objective of fitness training is "not only that of adding years to the lifespan, but rather that of adding some life to one's years" (Cianti, 1994, p. 5). Such a notion of health goes well beyond the absence of illness and may be placed alongside what is now defined, by the World Health Organization among others, as positive health. It may be conceived as a healthy physical form, or a "general functional adequacy to withstand physical challenges without overstrain" (Oja and Tuxworth, 1995, p. 7). Rather than an environment of function to preserve, the body which can reach such a healthy form is an instrument whose internal functioning is to be stimulated in order for its utility to grow and work submissively for the subject in the world. A healthy body may work as a sign of a deep internal environment in which organic functions are carried out and either facilitated or threatened by external factors, rather than a body-instrument to be used or presented in an external environment.[5] Even as a deep set of functions, the body demands an active use of energy and fitness training is presented as fundamental to the preservation of the physiology of the internal organs. Health may therefore be seen as a specific goal of fitness, and it is indeed presented as such in expert discourse, especially in so far as exercise is seen as a means to counter the current increase in obesity.

It is evident that the three semantic areas that gym-goers engage with are not equivalent. Being healthy and beautiful are important aims in themselves. Some clients contrast these aims with, and prefer them to, fitness. However, the "fit body" is clearly hegemonic, and it is this ideal that – independently of initial aims, age, social standing or gender – the vast majority of regular clients refer to as "normal". Fitness takes central position in the symbolic work that regulars perform to account for training and keep motivated. Indeed, even amongst those who prefer to concentrate on beauty, there is a widely held perception that this goes beyond the purpose of fitness. They tend to stage some self-distance, suggesting, for example, that their desires for beauty are "not normal" or "a bit exaggerated" (see Chapter 7). Self-monitoring is paramount: many indicate that they would indeed pursue extreme aesthetic ideals if only these were sensible. Not surprising, given the conspicuous association between beauty and workout in commercial images and commercial fitness magazine, references to health are often deployed to keep fitness central. Contrasting what they perceive as a "frivolous image" of the gym, many clients refer to health and distance themselves from purely aesthetic objectives. A number of clients single health out as a discreet body objective, and clients prefer bodywork which they consider "health related". This is especially so with mature clients that may look at more strenuous techniques, such as aerobics or body building, with suspicion, reckoning that "at the end of the day it's actually not good for your health". Even in these cases though, fitness produces a particular kind of health attuned to functionality; health that is, above all, vitality and energy. Even clients of mature years, those who felt the need to exercise for "health reasons", associate increased levels of health with the capacity to be "active" and "independent", both to socialise (as many retired men said) and to continue helping their families (more characteristic of older women). Body maintenance thus becomes central. This may be discovered occasionally in the verbalisations of very young, female participants such as Elisa or Federica, who we have already encountered. Federica reckons she needs to "move", to "tone up" her body, because "with sitting down all the time, I'm beginning to be a bit flabby". Elisa states that "if you're not healthy, you can't plan for the future: it's not as if by exercising you will end up beautiful, but you keep doing it because of the hard times ahead, you should start thinking about your blood circulation now".

Clients are called upon to recognise that a good physical appearance cannot be obtained without being fit, and that fitness is the best and most obvious sign of good health. As an arena of cross-referencing body ideals, the fitness centre stresses the centrality of fitness. Such centrality is then variously nuanced by different clients:

> I want to be fit, just supple and full of energy...if I have to run to get the bus tomorrow I know I can do it. [I want a body that] doesn't age so

much and so quickly, which is in good shape, firm muscles, oxygenated skin, a body which is obviously healthy.

(Middle-aged clerk, stepper and stretcher, Florence)

[the gym] helps to keep you fit. I do resistance training, I don't want to increase muscle mass but to be lean, and to benefit from it outside the gym... my girlfriend, for example, started smoking like I did, but it makes her wheeze, and it doesn't affect me at all.

(University student, light weights and cardio machines, Florence)

Balance is of the essence. You know, this is to keep me fit, I may dream of a fantastic body, but I know I want a normal body, which is quite something... I want to function and look healthy, and just to feel healthy and strong.

(Clerk in her early thirties, pilates, cardio and weights, London)

Such claims illustrate that for regular clients the rationalised movement of muscles produces muscular efficiency as much as muscular efficiency produces greater physical fitness. As much as this is the route to fitness as "muscular tone", fitness semantic reach appears to broaden to include health and beauty, thereby remaining fluid enough to accommodate different subjective aspirations.

To explore this further, let's take a brief look at the genealogy of the notion of fitness and at its rendering in an ever evolving expert discourse. The historian Roberta Park (1994, p. 61) has shown that "the Victorians thought of fitness in terms of biological adaptability, and from this idea are derived a number of racial, sexual and other differences" to the extent that "athletes were often portrayed as biologically superior males". Adaptability and the capacity to withstand the world and its demands are still central and so is muscularity. Yet, what once might have been a measuring instrument, exercise is now co-extensive with the notion of fitness: "[t]oday fitness is often linked to muscularity, the shape of the body, and/or the ability to perform an exercise session of 30 minutes" (ibid., p. 62). Fitness fuses bodies and exercise together. An *instrumental vision of the body* lies at the heart of fitness. In keep-fit culture, instrumentality becomes a value in itself, and as such it is signified by external marks that may be used to adorn the self. Taking a broader look at the history of exercise, the "fit body" may be considered the contemporary incarnation of instrumental or functional notions of the body which were already juxtaposed to morpho-structural notions by the beginning of the twentieth century. Morpho-structural notions informed body building and entailed a "semiotics of physical appearance that looked for an indication of strength in the body", whilst functional concepts were typical of long-distance running and concerned "the invisibility" of a "peculiar, intangible and 'profound' quality of physical movement", similar to "the unique ability for running races" (Louveau, 1981, p. 305). Functionality today has come to the surface: fitness is predicated on the notion that the body must be kept active, yet energy emanates from the body's shape and becomes a crucial indicator of the subject's worth. A fit body is appreciated as a *sign* of the subject's energy, vitality and strength. If, as Foucault (1991, p. 137, see also 1975, 1976) claims, "the only truly important ceremony is that of exercise", a body which has visibly incorporated exercise acquires ceremonial properties, it becomes important at the level of signs as well as function, and tells us something about the subject and its worth.

Instrumentality and its display via external bodily signs such as tone and stamina are at the core of the fit body in today's fitness manuals. Here are some examples from manuals circulating in Italian and English for more than a decade:

> the muscles direct each and every thing, and the more they are toned...the more easily one moves, and every activity becomes less tiring. Exercise is a muscle tonic, it is the most effective medicine, and the best restorative.
>
> (Punzo, 1992, p. 10)

> [fitness training] will make you a more resistant sportsperson, if that is what you want, but at the same time, it will turn your body fat into muscle...and will tone your body and improve your appearance. You will also derive strength and energy, and this will help you relax and sleep better.
>
> (Goodsell, 1995, p. 10)

Clearly, the ideal of fitness here legitimates the training which produces it, just like the capacity to work out is both an instrument and a feature of the ideal figure. This has broad implications for individual identity which will be dealt with in the next chapter. Here I want to stress that, with the development, specialisation and differentiation of fitness manuals, we are witnessing not so much a marked switch in this broad underlying characterisation, but a layering of repertoires (both in terms of body techniques and vocabularies). This is well illustrated by a recent, internationally successful manual, *The Energy Booster Workout*, written by trainer and fitness manager Dan Brown (2003). This text reflects the entrance of Eastern body-soul techniques in the fitness domain, increasingly emphasising feeling, relaxation and body awareness and de-emphasising concerns for "the look". Presented as "unpretentious, funny and easy to follow", featuring "appealing cartoon illustrations" rather than "super-slim models", "a quick and easy way to energize your day", this pocket-size book mixes stretching techniques with self-massage exercises derived from an ancient Japanese technique known as "Do In", to "provide an all-round workout that will make you feel energized and relaxed at the same time" (ibid., pp.7–8). We know that Eastern body-soul techniques, and yoga in particular (Strauss, 2002), have been locally adjusted in various ways through their global penetration. While proper consideration of how these techniques become Westernised in keep-fit training would require a dedicated study, the impression I received from both discourse analysis and participant observation is that hybridised forms of gymnastics – such as Combat Yoga, Yoga Fitness, Power Yoga, to mention some of the more popular definitions – emphasise relaxation, feeling and wellbeing, but ultimately remain framed through the dominant cheerful, self-challenging instrumentality of fitness training.

4. The fit body and gendered modulations

Let's consider the notion of the "fit body" more directly, focusing on one particular, very salient, aspect of its negotiation, namely its different gender modulations. The available literature has stressed the gendered nature of fitness, and more broadly of exercise as related to body modification (see, among others, Leeds Craig and Liberti, 2007; Maguire and Mansfield, 1998; Markula, 2001; Wacquant, 1995). Loland (2000, p. 119) summarises this quite bluntly: "[w]hereas many women are concerned about appearing to be too large, men are dissatisfied with areas of the their bodies that are considered too small". Such findings need to be qualified though. For example, a strong cultural preference among Japanese women for tiny, slim bodies and a strong aversion for building muscles was precisely found by Spielvogel (2003) as a deterrent to the diffusion of fitness gyms in Japan. Size and muscles matter in quite subtle ways.

Clearly there are differences between men and women. They have emerged constantly from my empirical enquiries both in Italy and Britain – from observation, participation, interviews and discourse analysis. Gender differences, articulated via the normative male/female dichotomy, are often expressed in terms of size, but are best qualified considering "fears", "worries" or "problem areas". The number one enemy of the feminine ideal figure is "cellulite", the change in body tissue which primarily affects the hips and the buttocks, making them flabby and poorly defined. Cellulite is often portrayed in expert discourse as a real "pathology, both aesthetically and physiologically" which can be combated through "organised movement" (Mangano, 1995, p. 17). The "tummy", "a distended stomach, a waist that is too fat, a protruding abdomen" is presented in expert discourse as "a threat" on the masculine side, "a problem which no man wants to have" (Selby, 1994, p. 9).

Male and female fitness fans often comment along these lines. Here are a couple of quotes, which stress the awareness of broadly shared gendered bodily desires and the importance of achieving a properly gendered body shape:

> You may want to tone your legs, and your bum, mainly. I know very few women who really like their bum, it's always too big, even if you're slim: so the only way is to tone it up!
>
> (Woman in her early thirties, Milan)

> You could be the same weight but a poor shape: a man with a slim waist, or at least without a big stomach, with wide shoulders and a good posture is more pleasing to look at than one with rolls of fat.
>
> (Man in his late forties, Florence)

Even though men and women often identify different critical areas, for both the real problems are where they believe they have accumulated too much "fat" and where they feel "flabby". Gym-goers seem to have declared war on chubbiness: although it is possible to work in order to increase or reduce volume and to correct asymmetry, the ideal figure is above all defined by "sculptured", "solid", "firm" contours. All clients seem to view fat as "dead weight", a useless and, at the same time, disobedient part of their own body weighed down with "toxins", a sign of "old age", a bearer of "illness". Fat is ugly because it is of no use, and unlike muscle, it is not manageable and functional. In other terms, it is the clearest indication of the body's lack of discipline. This has been observed in women who do aerobics, but it is also typical of men who go to a fitness gym. The majority of men and women that I have met in the course of many years in Italy and Britain stress that they are working towards a dual purpose: reduce fat and increase muscles. Sure women express this by words such as "tone" which reveal a concern for bulky muscles. Of course men may verbalise their desire for "muscles" much more, and much more culturally legitimately than women (see Wacquant, 1995). But legitimate muscles in fitness culture are in general toned rather than bulky. By and large, all the clients of commercial keep-fit gyms are discouraged from developing extreme muscularity.[6] In the rejection of large, visible muscles there is, therefore, something more than the "patriarchal domination of women" based on the assumption that men are, and must remain, biologically superior, in other words, stronger and bigger (Bordo, 1993; Dinnerstein and Weitz, 1998; Lloyd, 1996; Maguire and Mansfield, 1998). Likewise, in the masculine attention for bodily fat there is more than the cult of healthy living, or the femininisation of male body ideals (see Segal, 2007). In the ideal of a toned, lean and visibly reactive body there is something characteristic of fitness. Let's explore the gendered modulations of the fit body more closely, considering that they do appear to exist on the backdrop of an apparently gender-neutral notion of functionality.

As early as the 1980s, feminist Margaret Morse (1987) wrote that aerobics promotes a "new muscular femininity". Based on "cardio-vascular resistance which, perhaps wrongly, is linked to health", aerobics works out "an ethics of activity" and it is "linked to beauty", so that "the world of exercise, once exclusively masculine, has become part of a commercial beauty culture" (ibid., p. 23; see also Bordo, 1993; Kenen, 1987; Markula, 1995). Whatever its emancipation potential, it is clear that this image of the body has gradually replaced in Western culture both the cult of slimness of the 1970s and the soft voluptuousness of the 1960s. A new composite ideal of the female body – strong and attractive, muscular and long-limbed, toned and blooming – ultimately contradicts the traditional association of femininity with inactivity and passivity, and is closer to the athletic image of an energetic, resolute subject. Rather than the absence of an aesthetic dimension, clients learn a different aesthetics. It may well be true, as Markula (1995, p. 348) claims, referring to her female aerobicisers, that you can aspire to "the toned look of the ideal body, but for functionality, not only for the look". Yet it seems even more correct to state that the majority of women who go to gyms tend to develop a particular aesthetic taste, inspired by functionality. Some of the more assiduous clients, even among the youngest enthusiasts from diverse backgrounds, explain that fit people perform even minor gestures of everyday life such as "picking something up" or "bending" in a "physically" and "aesthetically more correct way", with "agility", without "squatting" and "springing up nicely". The regular gym-goer "glows", she leaves the gym "with a certain way of walking", "standing straighter", being "more oxygenated" and "more energetic". In many ways, to be fit is to look positively functional.

While women appear to linger towards a *muscular femininity*, men seem to orientate themselves towards an *agile masculinity*. Many regular male gym-goers are indeed wary of what they consider excessive muscular growth, and include energy, flexibility and stamina in the picture, placing emphasis on lean and elongated muscles rather than on bulgy ones. Fitness, therefore, is also aesthetically expressed in a model of toned, compact body mass and well-defined curves indicating muscular energy. This is what I call the *aesthetics of active functionality*. It demands that the body be not big, but strong. Rather than swollen, muscles must be strengthened, firmed and elongated. It also means that strength and energy are signified by tone and firmness.[7] In its turn, tone signals reactivity and visualises vitality and the capacity to feel and live to the full.

Most men and women, amongst the regular clients that I met in Florence, Bologna, Milan, Norwich and London, elaborated on such aesthetics. Paola explains that those who practise fitness manage to perform simple everyday activities such as "picking up something on the floor" in a "physically" and "more aesthetically correct manner in terms of the muscles", without "hunching", "springing back up" in "the correct manner", or as Glenda, who works as a physiotherapist, suggests, obtaining an "agility" which helps to avoid "bending over a patient badly, who is already bent badly". In general, as Bonnie says, fitness training encourages "a different way of standing from others" since, as she explains, "you leave the gym and walk in a certain way", a certain "attitude of movement", "you stand more straight", you feel "more full of oxygen and more energetic". The aesthetics of functionality means that the body should not be fat, but strong, springy and agile. The more the muscles develop, the more powerful, firm and stretched they become. Despite their different ages and professions, most male participants state that in no way do they want to "increase their body mass" and even less "resemble Schwartzenegger". They want a "well-balanced body" and "reactive muscles". Together with "resistance", they also want more traditionally feminine characteristics such as "co-ordination" and the ability to "move well". The musculature of a fit body seems in some ways to challenge the traditional associations between strength, bulk and visibility: muscles which are too large and visible are "ostentatious", but are not necessarily "strong", or "active", "resistant", "agile" or "flexible". Regulars may get to demand from gym instructors movements which they consider in line with this view. Several gym fans told me they appreciated when "less emphasis" was placed "on aesthetics" by gym instructors, and this both in their body presentation and their proposed routines. This goes well with an emphasis on "feeling" the body that indeed characterises some of the new combinations with body-soul techniques (see Chapter 7). Even among men who only train with machines, there appears to be an increasing distance from body building, justified precisely by the notion that they are working not only on aesthetics, but on functionality, mentioning qualities such as "energy", "breathing", "resistance" and "suppleness" as a way to reiterate their point.

The aesthetics of active functionality may appear to promote androgynous or unisex ideals precisely because they relate firstly to a toned, flexible and energetic body. In the early 1980s Catherine Louveau identified the promotion of unisex ideas of beauty as a fundamental characteristic of fitness. Louveau (1981, p. 318) provided a feminist interpretation of the phenomenon: "the unisex body, like unisex clothes, constitutes at the same time a demonstration of a reality and a demand, acceding – or aspiring to accede – to the same professions, women of the new bourgeoisie clearly aspire to model their bodies in order to avoid a figure which recalls their belonging to the weaker sex". Other feminist readings have interpreted similar trends as the assimilation of feminist values into commercialism, with the consequential veneering of masculine domination (Bordo, 1993; Maguire and Mansfield, 1998). What I have observed in my journey into fitness culture as lived in the gym, is both less triumphant and less apocalyptic. The widespread emphasis on functionality is both intertwined with established gender differences and gendered ideal figures, and allows for their negotiation.

In many ways, the emphasis on functionality seems to enable several clients to at least keep possible anxieties concerning their own femininity or masculinity under control, and to encourage them to try out new activities which do not conform to very strict, traditional views of gender. What we have here is an important propellant for the gym's emphasis on variety (see Chapter 2). Instructors and personal trainers, both in Italy and Britain, also appear to have an incentive to promote an aesthetics of active functionality, as it appears compatible with a great variety of activities, body shapes and publics. Gym instructors' incitements to work towards more "complete" and "balanced" forms of training may entail that masculinity and femininity be somehow de-constructed and reconstructed in the development of fitness training options. What is presented as ideal indeed is a combination of exercises that burn calories and build vascular resistance with ones that aim at strength and muscular resistance and others that provide for co-ordination, flexibility and agility. New forms of training often appear to work upon and reappraise, if not transcend, gender dichotomies. The once masculine province of isotonic machines has been changing with the introduction of circuit training – a form of group training that involves a class of people led by an instructor moving rapidly from one machine to another, lifting light weights and working more on muscular resistance and variety of movement (Crossley, 2006). Likewise, spinning has become popular, which is a type of aerobic training on stationary bicycles in which a class of students pedals to music, together with a trainer, on an imaginary uphill and downhill track, varying pedalling speed and the position of the body on the saddle, also using the arms and the back. These developments stand side-by-side with the endurance of gender segregation – as demonstrated in the growth and success of women-only gyms (see Craig and Liberti, 2007). They are also rendered via the enduring relevance of both a gendered division of keep-fit workout in the unisex fitness centre and traditionally gendered body ideals as manifested in the different problem areas reported by men and women. Thus, while subtler and subtler gender differences are continuously inscribed into it, the fit body is constructed as a gender-neutral terrain of individual emancipation. And in some ways, for its tendency to abstraction and instrumentality, it does create a space which accommodates continuous ever changing gender play.

7
Fit Bodies, Strong Selves

The notion of "fitness" implies what Michel Foucault (1983) has called "a claim to truth". Such a claim concerns not only physical activity and the body, but also, and more fundamentally, the subject. For all their emphasis on instrumentality, the cultural legitimacy of fitness gyms rests on strong and specific notions indeed: views about the correct way of transforming the body and views about the (valuable) self as the transforming agent. Fitness culture works on a particular articulation of the body/self dualism. Fitness fans are adamant that the gym allows them "to do something *just* for the body". Yet, what is at stake is not just the body. If actual bodywork demands emotional and cognitive involvement, fitness becomes visible at the discursive level as a tale of subjectivity. A "well-disciplined body" is paramount in contemporary rationalised Western cultures, not only because, as maintained by Foucault (1991, p. 135ff.), its ceremonial functions are downplayed in favour of its docility-utility, but also because discipline acquires symbolic value: fitness culture shows the centrality of exercise as *discipline* and *display*, as well as that a body which has *visibly incorporated exercise* may yet again have important *ceremonial properties*. Although body language is not the direct object of bodywork in the gym, a fit body speaks of the subject in certain ways. In their classic *The English YMCA Exercise to Music*, Rodney Cullum and Lesley Mowbray (2005, p. 10) consider fitness or better "total fitness" as "the ability to meet the demands of the environment, plus a little in reserve for emergencies ... you will have to develop an independence of attitude that makes you self-reliant". Fitness makes the subject active, ready for everything. "Be active!" is the slogan of Joanna Hall, a popular British fitness icon. And activity in fitness takes on clearly moral connotations. A body with toned contours and erect posture, with more muscles and less fat is appreciated as a sign of "energy", a "vitality" and a "strength" which the subject can put to use in everyday life. Still, this energy is visible in the shape of the body, and becomes not only an instrument but also a precious indicator of the self and its value. All in all, through concentrated bodywork, gym-goers *perform character*, alluding to a self which is both stronger and more authentic.

As noted at the outset of this study, that the self is ultimately in question in gym culture, is a widespread cultural perception. However, the precise contours of fitness subjectivity remain largely unexplored. Just as happens with sports or games (Perinbanayagam, 2006, pp. 69–158), fitness participants may indeed narrate themselves through fitness. In this chapter, I will deal precisely with this, looking both at experiential narratives from gym participants and expert discourse. Fitness training, thus goes the hegemonic narrative deployed to account for gym practices, brings out the body's "natural" plasticity. Yet, it does so somewhat contradictorily. Naturalness is predicated on the backdrop of a vision of "artificiality" which is exemplified by the urban, desk-bound patterns of work with which the fitness gym lives in a relationship of symbiosis and opposition. Fitness culture thus is not only predicated on "body projects" (Featherstone, 1991; Giddens, 1991), but also on natural ones; projects that bring out one's own true "nature". As a significant corollary of this, fitness is presented as a temperate body modification technique, enhancing the self without compromising his or her "authenticity". Narratives of self through fitness appear to work on a contradictory space, of symbiosis and opposition, at three different levels: with the kind of urban living and desk-bound jobs along which the fitness gyms have developed, with the broader area of commercially sustained body maintenance and modification techniques, and with the very dualistic notion that we need to be doing something just for our otherwise neglected bodies.

1. Predicating nature

In the last 15 years the fitness centre has been the home of a shifting constellation of training techniques and accessory body practices (from sun-bathing to saunas). However, what has remained remarkably stable is the *benchmarking function* that consumers and producers attribute to regular fitness training. Following a popular trainer such as Lory in her many classes at BodyMove in my early Florentine ethnography, I got a very good taste of such function. On a busy morning, Lory reminded her soft-gym class that exercises learned in the gym can accompany us everywhere ("an elastic band is like a mini-gym that we can take with us anywhere, thus enabling us to do our exercises on holiday or wherever we are"). She told her body-conditioning class that keep-fit exercise can help us convert idle moments into useful time ("no one can see you're doing this exercise [a light squeeze for the buttocks] so you can do it anywhere, while you're waiting for the bus or queuing at the post office"). She admonished her step-aerobics class that training may alert us to good practices ("we have to learn to drink more, because it's good for us and it replenishes fluids that are lost during training"). Lory then spent some time with the clients pedalling on the static bikes and casually dropped the line that exercise is "fundamental for a healthier life". In the intervals between her classes, in small chats with individuals or little groupings, she had often variously repeated that keep-fit training can help us counteract the effects of bad daily habits. What emerged from these scenes, and from countless others which I have witnessed since, is that its benchmarking function places keep-fit workout at the centre of body management.

Let's explore this, starting from fitness publications (see also Smith Maguire, 2007, pp. 106ff; Markula, 2001). Fitness periodicals across the world, from *Ultrafit* to *Health and Fitness*, from *Zest* to *Shape*, from *Men's Health* to *Self*, from *Salve* to *Vitality*, to mention only some of the magazines which I have considered, regularly associate keep-fit exercise with food management. More broadly, exercise is said to have a "balancing effect", it is something through which one may "care for the body as a whole", helping each individual to "choose a healthier and more balanced diet", to appreciate "when and how much one needs to rest", and even counteracting bad habits, thus being "mentally better prepared to give up smoking". Fitness manuals also regularly stress the centrality of keep-fit training with respect to one's own body conduct. A pocket-size manual such as *The Anytime, Anywhere Exercise Book* (Price, 2003) lists a number of exercises that can be done while doing something else, provides a number of tricks for active life which incorporate training in people's daily round, and suggests how to choose a gym if finally one does find time and acquires a taste for the gym. Even in this case, the author is adamant that "simply changing from inactive to moderately active yields dramatic health, fitness and weight-loss benefits", and to start every morning with some exercise helps "mental productivity... The stress of the day won't get to you as much. Exercise is like taking an energy-plus calming pill with no side effects" (ibid., pp. 15, 27).

Fitness fans collude with such public rendering of fitness training. Keep-fit exercise is presented as an opportunity to reorganise body conduct as a whole. The body knowledge acquired in the gym (see Chapter 6) helps define body priorities, and bodywork becomes a benchmark for managing other body practices. Jenny from London says that "by going to the gym, I eat the right amount and don't put on weight. I just get full faster... Maybe it's a nervous thing. I have more energy, but need less fuel"; Alessia from Milan says "you are more careful about eating healthily because if you don't then going to the gym is pointless". Some of the fitness fans I have spent more time with in Florence were even more vocal, articulating similar claims independently of their preferred gym activity:

> I have learnt to listen to what my body is saying when exercising, and this now functions as a yardstick. The gym acts as a double check that

tells me if I've put on weight because I haven't walked all day, or because I ate too much the previous evening. So then I say to myself that I really shouldn't have done that because it's bad for my inner balance, and it's the gym that makes me realise that.

(Amy, university student in her twenties, regular participant of soft aerobics classes and stretching)

[going to the gym] means following a few little rules, like not going to the gym when you've just eaten a lot, and then if you have eaten, you have to absorb everything you've consumed, or not eating too much fat and eating fruit and vegetables that fill you up without excessively increasing your calorie intake.

(Carmelo, middle-aged medical doctor, ex body builder, weights and machine area fan)

a new relationship has developed between body and mind. Perhaps it is because I exercise and use my muscles, but I have been struck by the fact that my body will make itself felt... sometimes I feel lazy but I'm used to concentrating on my body, to feeling it and looking at it... and this habit sort of takes over. Instead of sitting at the computer using only my mind, I now think about how I'm sitting and I'll sometimes worry that I'll get scoliosis every time I'm tense. In short, I take my body more seriously and I'm more attentive about how I physically perform certain activities.

(Francesco, university lecturer in his forties, stretching and tai-chi fan)

By and large, fitness producers and consumers stress that the practical role of fitness training is "restructuring routines", restoring a "natural balance" by countering, limiting or modifying potentially damaging conducts. Reference to "nature" has striking importance in fitness culture. While contemporary fitness workout in the gym is clearly man-made, often requires the use of machines, and takes place indoor in quite artificial environments, it is invariably presented as "natural": it is described as a "natural solution" to re-establish the "natural balance".

In the first place, the notions of nature and balance are articulated on a *macro cultural level*, as part of a broad discourse against the ills of modern, urban life. The gym is portrayed by participants, both in large cities such as London and Milan and in smaller ones such as Florence and Norwich, as counteracting the increasing levels of stress and inactivity which accompany urban living, "with its cars and pollution", where "you don't even have to walk up the stairs" and where "everything is done at breakneck speed". Urban life, I have been repeatedly reminded by fitness fans, leads individuals to "forget about the body" and the gym is the "antidote". Instead of displacement – looking for a space or moment of reimmersion in nature, such as mushrooming (Fine, 1998) or windsurfing (Dant, 1998) – fitness gyms provide *emplacement*: they supply an interstice, integral to urban living and environment, where "the body" may be woken up to its nature.[1] Reference to the "inactivity" of the body during the day as constrained by demanding "desk-bound" jobs and to "sedentary lifestyles" far removed from the "healthy lifestyle" of the "countryside" or of "our ancestors" often provides the lead into the whole argument. "We could give up going to the gym only if we pursued a more natural way of life" – says Jenny – "otherwise you need to spend time [in the gym] to get balanced again." Expert discourse thrives on similar premises: "get your body back into balance" declares *Bodydoctor*, a fitness and nutrition manual that promises to help readers to "lose a stone, double your fitness" (Marshall, 2004, p. 5). Exercise may be presented as a form of "natural" treatment, no longer "repressive and aimed to eliminate the symptoms of illness", but inspired by "the detailed search for the real causes of illness and, therefore, to long-lasting cures" (Ruffier, 1991, p. 11). The spectre of urban malaise is evoked in one form or another in many fitness manuals. The importance of the gym is associated, firstly, with the fact that "in this day and age, our legs have been substituted by wheels as the main form of transport" (Cella, 1989, p. 7) and, secondly, with the constant build-up of "tension" and "stress" accumulated daily "at work and in the home, without taking into account the body's ability to withstand the pressure to which it is subjected" (Caplin, 1992, p. 309).

Reference to urban life as inescapably nervy and physically draining is particularly evident in the local renderings of fitness discourse in a metropolis like London. The *2007 London Time Out Guide to Health & Fitness* (p. 19) suggests that:

> It's an inescapable fact that we Londoners operate in the fast lane … such speed is leading us into a life of ever-greater extremes … forces us into ever-longer and more stressful working patterns and dramatically tilts our work-life balance. We may be cash rich, but we're also increasingly time poor … There is however a way forward … it is important to make exercise an integral part of our day … and think about why we are going to the gym.

This is however a culturally overarching and historically deep script. A number of historical studies have indeed documented that the spread from the big cities of Europe and the USA of individualistic physical and recreational activities, including gymnastics, was coupled with a crusade against sedentary lifestyle and urban stress (Green, 1986; Grover, 1989; Jackson Lears, 1981; Rabinbach, 1990; Ulmann, 1971; Vigarello, 1978). Keep-fit activities may be discreetly proposed as the natural helping hand to nature: "for most of us, nature needs a bit of encouragement, and it is at this point that exercise comes into play", as suggested by Callan Pinckney (1992, p. 42). Alternatively, reminiscent of the original evolutionist connotation of the notion of fitness (see Chapter 6), the gym may even be proposed, somewhat pompously, as the necessary "final destination in the development of the human race", as suggested by one Italian manual (Castiglione and Arcelli, 1996, p .viii):

> scientific research has demonstrated that we have been programmed to do at least a certain amount of physical activity, and if this does not happen, then problems begin to appear. For many thousands of years, up until the beginning of the 20th century, we were always required to exceed that limit because our lifestyles demanded it. However, within the space of a few years – too few to allow us to adapt genetically – everything changed and man was freed from the obligation of having to rely on his own strength. There were, however, negative consequences. Nowadays, we should spend some time every week exercising in a gym in order to complement the (little) physical activity required by modern life.

Gym instructors and trainers all deploy slight variations on the same script: movement is natural, but only organised, disciplined movement done regularly in a gym works when our daily life has become unnatural. Here are a couple of their verbalisations, spoken both during training and interviews, in different places and times:

> we have arms that were made to grasp things and legs designed to bend but we don't use them anymore. People don't move like they used to, but the gym helps them to achieve a balance with their own bodies.
> (Informal interview with gym instructor, Florence, 1995)

> Feel your centre, slowly, slowly. This is the most natural thing, only we do not realise it because of the rushed life we now live.
> (Pilates class, London, 2006)

In this rendering, fitness corresponds to the notion of diet in its original, etymological meaning. Diet as derived from the Greek work *diaita* means "regulation, regime of life". It concerns the careful balancing and management of the activities which are important for our body to live, rather than the therapeutic cure for symptoms of an illness that we have to eradicate. A dietary element is a typical feature of today's health promotion campaigns. Considering the spread of fitness awareness in the USA, Michael Goldstein, for example, has suggested that this was inspired by the "Hygeian model" in which good health is seen as something that each person can obtain by living in harmony with nature. Debates on health differ from official medical thinking, which is dominated by the "Aesculapian model" that views health as the result of specific therapeutic treatments designed to cure diseases (Goldstein, 1992; see also Whorton, 1982). Fitness fans and instructors claim that training encourages us to organise (at least some of) the daily activities that are related to the body – that is, food and drink consumption, various forms of body care as well as rest, illness or malaise prevention, sex and so on – in more balanced, natural ways.

The concept of "regime of life" may be useful here. The gym acquires meaning according to a visualisation of action as "close examination of behaviour" on the backdrop of "a nature to which one should conform" (Foucault, 1984a, see also Foucault, 1984b). Unlike "lifestyle" – defined as a way of organising individual choices to express identity and personal preference (Giddens, 1990)[2] – the notion of "regime of life" grasps those forms of choice organisation or agency that are predicated on a "nature" to be recognised and accomplished. While organised as consumer culture and addressing participants as clients, customers or consumers, fitness gyms do not ask participants to rely solely on their freedom of choice to account for their participation. To be sure, consumer choice is evoked in the selection of the particular gym (see Chapter 2) or preferred type of bodywork (see Chapter 5), but keep-fit exercise is presented as *more* than choice. Fitness fans vibrantly distance themselves from the idea that fitness culture might respond to snob or bandwagon effects: doing fitness is not, they reckon, a way to express status (distinction or identification), nor is it a fashion statement. Not for them, at least.

The vehemence with which many clients criticise commercial images of the fitness gym, describing them as "false" and "superficial", quite often relates to this. Fitness fans, just like fans of popular TV series such as 'Dallas' (see Ang, 1985), are aware of the critiques that are addressed at fitness culture as consumer culture. They feel it necessary to justify themselves and use a vocabulary wherein "nature" and "necessity" feature prominently. Fitness, I have repeatedly been told, is "more than just a fad or fashion" and it "is not a luxury" either. In contrast, "it is something necessary" that "should be a part of our everyday lives, because we are naturally designed to be active". Regular gym-goers in my initial ethnographic study in Florence were very keen on this. For instance, in Leo's opinion, "the gym, as portrayed by the media, is a fashion statement, but this just isn't true", because "going to the gym is not a formal choice. You do it for your body and for your inner self." Betty is aware that the gym "these days has become a status symbol"; but for those "who train seriously, nothing could be further from the truth". Of course, she continues, there are people who "try" and go to the gym thinking solely "about their appearance" or to "fit in with a certain type of lifestyle", but the latter has nothing to do with those "who have a real passion for it, that is people like me who have real motives and a real awareness". The fitness gym, says Alessia, provides for experiences which are "far more profound than that superficial representation which is actually to do with consumerism and the desire to make everyone the same". Training, she continues, "has allowed me to use my own mind" and "to be aware of who I really am". This kind of rhetoric incorporates counter-consumerism into fitness culture as lived culture, and is often directed against elitarian, snobbish or narcissistic images of the gym. Here are some telling verbalisations from later interviews:

> [the gym has become] popular among people from all social classes. Perhaps initially, it was a purely female thing, for upper-class women, but now it's really widespread and for all; there are gyms in working-class areas and sessions for pensioners organised by the city council everywhere... There's an element of imitation and fashion, like in most things, but [the gym] is about a general sense of wellbeing, something that everyone needs.
>
> (Antonia, manager in a cultural organisation in her
late thirties, pilates fan, Milan)

> [in magazines] fitness clubs are represented in a mistaken, over-the-top manner... people have the impression that gym users are full of themselves, narcissists or a bunch of fashion-victims, people that go to the gym in designer clothes to lose weight and look beautiful... and of course this is untrue, it's too tiring to be just "cool".
>
> (Polly, university student in her late twenties,
regular step-aerobics, Norwich)

To reinforce the distance of fitness culture from the superficiality of consumerism, fitness fans typically choose either an experiential or an empowerment rhetoric: they thus justify their practices based either on experiences of involvement and fun or on their capacity to negotiate body ideals via bodywork (see Chapter 5). In the latter case, they may deploy irony to reframe the fit body and its limits, displaying a "knowing" attitude and affirming that they are aware of both the advantages and the dangers of keep-fit training. As suggested in the previous chapter, the illusion that whatever body can be obtained fast is stigmatised by fitness insiders and this often spills out into a critique of crude consumerism. Similar forms of reflexivity are generated in the gym largely via the lived interaction between clients and gym staff.

This does not prevent fitness gyms from living through predicament. The fitness gym is as much opposed to, as it is symbiotic with, hectic urban living. It shares, and in many ways intensifies, the latter's fast pace, instrumentality and emphasis on visuality as well as its finely guarded, detached social mixing. It allows people to address their body, but does not allow much strategic self-investment in the highly prescriptive, non-dialogic moves characterising keep-fit training. It does so in a fashion which resembles the bureaucratic slant of many urban low-middle to middle-class jobs peppered with the buzz of personal, creative investment defining what has been called the "new spirit of capitalism" (Boltanski and Chiappello,

1999) and incidentally deriving from the incorporation of counter-cultural critiques (see Willis, 1979). It goes well with the home-work-home pattern that characterises the urban, self-contained bourgeois family while providing individualistic refuge from it. It offers space to move, but an indoor space, sanitised and courteous. It provides for sociability, but one made of casual chats, without the risks of hazardous encounters in the park or sidewalk, rather than one made of more deep emotional attachments. Finally, it is predicated on the notion of balance, something that requires more than a quick therapeutic fix. And yet even the promotional language of fitness does recur to similar plots. Quite often sold as a handy balancing trick, the gym may much less frequently work as such. The gym is, thus, a natural solution which needs to be naturalised: it does not come easy and must be fitted in the midst of what is described as an overwhelmingly contradictory, wearing and stressful urban condition.

Still, fitness discourse itself is growing in reflexivity, especially at its expert core, as opposed to its commercial edge.[3] Fitness discourse increasingly acknowledges the contradictions of contemporary urban living, and the fact that the gym may just add to it. Thus the *London 2007 Time Out* guide to fitness suggests (2007, p. 19):

> Feeling guilty after yet another snatched junk food lunch, we resolve to get fit and suddenly launch into a concerted bout of gym-going... after only a couple of weeks of intensive treadmill trudging, dragging ourselves even deeper into a spiral of tiredness and anxiety, we feel wore than we did before. And instead of trying to find a more moderate approach, more often than not, our reaction is to give up.

The gym becomes a balancing tool, I have often heard, only if it is itself taken with a sense of balance: allowing time, reconsidering priorities, enjoying and making it into something beneficial to ordinary life. If the only "way forward" is, as mentioned, to "make exercise an integral part of our day", this suggests that a sense of balance has to be applied to one's own life as a whole. A balanced approach to life clearly goes beyond the gym and may be incompatible with other basic commitments. Also, it is differently accessible to different people in different times and place, something that the individualistic and universalistic slant of fitness culture tends to obfuscate. Finally, a balanced approach to the gym may require the capacity to enjoy not only keep-fit activities themselves, but the associated local relationships – with gym mates, trainers, staff – however purpose based they might otherwise be.

2. Plasticity and its limits

The notions of nature and balance are also articulated on what may be called the *meso level*, referring to the field of body modification techniques. Reference to naturalness potently enters the qualification of the kind of body modification provided by fitness. In fitness culture the body is characterised as plastic. Plasticity in turn is not conceived of as absolute, but it is tied to the ability to work out and limited to what may be achieved with workout. Fitness workout not only delivers body transformations, it also sets the limits to body plasticity. Gym instructors' constant mantra is that it is *only* through keep-fit exercise that real changes can be achieved. During training or in gym chats, they stress that there are "limits to how much the body can change", or that it is "pointless going on unrealistic diets: if you're born with a large behind, the most the gym can do is ensure that you don't have cellulite as well". Even more than this, personal trainers stress that a lot of their work has to do with keeping clients motivated while helping them switch to more achievable goals (see Chapter 3).

As suggested previously, regular clients learn to aspire to body characteristics that they appreciate they may achieve with their keep-fit routines. Clients, too, insist on the limits to body malleability. Francesco, a Florentine university lecturer in his forties is blunt: "if you're ugly, you're ugly, even if you go to the gym; it's not magic! You think that you can completely change your body but in reality, that just isn't true. It's better to consider it as something that can improve the body and help you to keep healthy." Here are some other telling quotes from regulars:

I'd like to have Anna Falchi's [an Italian TV starlet] body, and you think that if you go to the gym, go on a diet and put on a bit of cream, that that's what you'll end up with. The problem is that if you don't have the right shape in the first place, it's almost impossible. For me, it's going to be very difficult to achieve my aims because of my bone structure, and my large hips and ankles... Still I got to terms with it, because I can concentrate on myself and my energies in improving what I've already got.

(Loretta, shop assistant in his twenties, Florence)

In the gym I sometimes find these magazines, they are full of wonderful women, and you think "yes! That's gorgeous, I wish I could get a bit like that", and you may still have the dream, and perhaps you do a series of push ups more, while you fantasise about a smooth, round belly that looks like perfect... They [the dreams of perfection] are there but they are just a dream, and you are here: you do what you sensibly can after all.

(Petra, professional in her late thirties, Milan)

Angelina Jolie's arms and legs, that's what brings a lot of people in here, you know. But that's just a dream. You can improve your shape, not turn it upside down... bring out the best of you.

(Chris, mature student, London)

How plastic then is the plasticity promoted by fitness? The notion of the fit body is predicated on bounded body modification. Body modification is bounded to *direct, active bodywork*. Most gym-goers I have met with were keen to stress the importance of using one's own body to transform it: keep-fit training is effective because "you work on the body directly", it changes the body because it "works on its inherent capacities", and it is nat-ural because it "works on the body through the use of the body". Keep-fit training is also "a form of responsibility-taking", allowing for "improve-ments" and "changes" which are "earned really with your sweat". Compared with the kind of epic which is articulated in the narration of the boxing *habitus*, these claims adumbrate a different emotional structure and a differ-ent carnality (see Chapter 5).What is more, at a difference with the boxing narrative, reference to endurance is not used against visions of an undisci-plined underclass masculinity, against uncontrolled violence and grotesque idleness, in a word against the image of the black Ghetto (Wacquant, 2003). The boxing gym is inextricably articulated with and against the Ghetto as an "antidote to the street", a "dream machine" and a sub-culture of "controlled violence" (ibid., pp. 239–40, 83ff.). The fitness gym is instead inextricably articulated with and against commercial body modification techniques avail-able in the clients' horizon of possibilities as commanded by promotional culture and the intense presentational needs of fashionable urban living. These are indeed the rather more blurred mainstream cultural formations and bourgeois sites with and against which the fitness gym is articulated.

While most regular clients are very careful in stressing the limits to body transformation inherent in fitness, and likewise willing to embrace them as natural, they also recognise the potency of an ideal of perfection and of a utopia of total plasticity. These are made flesh by media icons, film stars or sport idols and by the commercial diffusion of a variety of body modi-fication techniques that are presented as safe and accessible. Many regulars candidly admit that "Hollywood stars all have a personal trainers, and it's easy to think 'oh well, if I get PT I may get that body too!'." They also admit to looking eagerly at images of well-toned, well-proportioned and genuinely "exceptional bodies" in magazines, including health and fitness magazines addressed to the broad public. Quite often these images appear to func-tion not so much as a source of inspiration, but as a form of day-dreaming or vicarious consumption. In a relation of responsiveness and opposition, most regulars somehow accept as culturally given an ideal image of the body which is different from theirs, relying on fitness as their way to "get real", and at the same time "think positive" about their bodies (see Chapter 6).

I shall come back to the limits of similar divestment rejoinders as to broad cultural body ideals, visions of perfection and body malleability. Before that, I would like to focus on how differently defined are a variety of body tech-niques. In her interesting book *Bodywork: Beauty and Self-image in American Culture*, Debra Gimlin (2002, p. 10) looks not only at aerobics classes, but also at plastic surgery and the hair salon. She develops the category of "bodywork" to explore "how health and beauty organizations provide both resources and limitations on women's negotiations of identity" (see also

Brace-Govan, 2002). While Gimlin clearly understands that hairdos, keep-fit activities and plastic surgery provide different examples of bodywork, she tends to undervalue their differences to argue her thesis, derived from symbolic interactionist theories of stigmatisation, that "arenas of bodywork provide women with the 'socially approved vocabularies' that explain their failure to accomplish ideal beauty and thus serve to neutralize the flawed identity that an imperfect body implies in Western society" (ibid., p. 15). However, studying keep-fit activities, I could not but notice that some techniques came more readily to mind to gym-goers, while others were mentioned with greater difficulty commanding much more moral investment. The vocabulary to justify fitness is very specific and is predicated on boundary making with respect to other forms of bodywork. Not every technique is felt as equally legitimate. This partly reflects the fact that the notion of direct active bodywork cannot be applied to all techniques equally, at least because *who* does the work and *how* it gets done matter greatly. Intrigued by the subtle differences that clients individuated among body modification/maintenance practices and by the strong emotional reactions that some of them elicited, I was interested in capturing what qualified fitness in their eyes as a superior form.

Participants in the study mentioned different techniques, but they were adamant that going to a gym has to do with "being active", its alternatives and possible substitutes being practices such as brisk walking, swimming, cycling, jogging and tennis. Other options – creams and cosmetics as well as massage and hydromassage which are present in fitness centres increasingly inclined to "pampering" – were mentioned as "nice but different". Francesco, whose stern attitude we have already encountered, warns that:

> [having a massage done] works wonders and is relaxing, but it is not enough. If you need to have a massage, it means that your way of life is wrong. If you have a massage you feel great, but if you can't have one you're going to feel even worse ... It's better to change your lifestyle! In the gym, you're using your own body; but when you have a massage, you're using someone else's surplus energy. It puts you back on track but if you can't have one for a few days, you feel rough. In the gym, it's you producing this surplus energy.

This account contains many elements that are used by clients to structure the cultural space of body modification techniques, positioning fitness training within it. Such space is defined by the degree of invasiveness or superficiality, risk or passivity of any technique. Whilst beauty treatments (creams, depilation and so on), make-up, hairdos and clothes are clearly recognised as valuable, they are generally considered to be comparatively "superficial" and "external". Clothes and make-up may "cover you up", and "may help you look better but your real body is not changed, it's just a masquerade, not your real self". They are thus fairly ceremonially risky: they "make you seem as though you are different", "they make you fit the situation, but you are not more fit". Massages may actually be a safe, truly relaxing practice, but they are also "passive", they do not change the body from within. It was only with some prompting that my interviewees discussed more drastic, and likewise increasingly popular, techniques such as plastic surgery. Plastic surgery commanded, if not outright rejection, quite a bit of emotional and moral distance in most clients: many described it as "scary" or "unnatural", others joked about resisting the social pressure to "avoid looking like a Barbie" and only a few declared their "interest", suggesting that plastic surgery is "becoming less invasive". Invasiveness was typically charged against plastic surgery: it works deeply and may be quite consequential, effective in changing the body, but precisely because it cannot be controlled by the individual on a routine basis, it is a "risky", "external tampering" with the body that may not be conducive to real balance and harmony. Most techniques were discussed as not belonging to the individual, or to their embodied selves. They rather appeared as referring to personal appearance or instant gratification. Fitness training instead was deemed active, deep and embodied, conducive to harmony and safe. Reference to direct, active bodywork was, indeed, prevalent when gym-going was discussed in interviews compared with other options of body modification, maintenance and care. Expressed succinctly, what characterises keep-fit activities as a superior form is the use of the body's own energy for body modification via direct self-discipline.

Let's focus on the narratives around plastic surgery, as they commanded indeed quite a bit of emotional investment. I have investigated them only in relation to fitness, as I was interested in comprehending the legitimating grounds for fitness training and to see how it stands when the possibility of plastic surgery is factored in. Fitness fans were all aware of plastic surgery and clearly agreed that it may produce quite dramatic changes. But the majority were also quite sceptical and felt plastic surgery was neither for them, nor morally undisputable. It may change the body, many reckoned, but does so in an "unnatural way", without making it work and without using its own built-in capabilities. Because of this, many of the fitness fans I have talked to conceive of plastic surgery as diametrically opposed to keep-fit activities. Even a young woman like Loretta, very preoccupied with her own appearance which she deploys as a fashion shop assistant, says that she "do[es] not trust" the plastic surgeon's "knife":

> I don't like this method of change . . . tightening the skin and having face lifts goes against the nature of old age. Old age is something that comes to us all sooner or later and anyway, you are the way you are. I can't imagine it, it's unnatural. Going on a diet and working out are natural. Make-up

has its uses too but, it's just a temporary measure, whereas with plastic surgery there's no going back and you have no control over it.

Plastic surgery is often deemed as "false", the aesthetic improvements it may afford risk rendering the individual a fake. The fear of losing one's own legitimate claim to one's body, its naturalness and one's own authenticity is often mentioned by clients who declare they would never undergo plastic surgery. Here are some of the strong reactions I got about plastic surgery: "[I] would never do it: this is what my nose is like and there is no natural thing that will change that, I should accept it"; "if you change that way you are no longer a real person", "it means that you can't really be happy with yourself"; "we should take pride in our wrinkles and accept aging, but be active though". Against this, fitness means "improving oneself and accepting yourself", and "doing something…with your own body and your own capabilities: I'm still myself, and I've brought about a change through my own actions". These clients thus articulate what I like to call a *modernist critical narrative*, one that develops the notion that a natural body can be improved only through the hard work which the self manages to do on it, that only improvements which are earned by the subject through some form of self-discipline are authentic.

Over the 15 years timescale of my research I have seen acceptance of plastic surgery growing, to a degree. While this was not my focus, again the narrative terms of such a shift related to keep-fit activities are telling. As time passed, I did witness less hostility towards plastic surgery, but I did not find that a post-modernist narrative, one predicated on absolute body plasticity and on the embracement of artificiality, was gaining much ground among fitness fans. Also, very few clients maintained that "no one is really natural" and that we are all "artificial to a degree" – as a mature student from London indeed said. There seems to be scope for including (some) plastic surgery as part of the body maintenance/modification repertoire of the fitness client: some of the more recent interviewees displayed relatively less distance from plastic surgery, and often deployed a therapeutic script. "I am not against plastic surgery" – "says Licia, a 30 year old clerk from Milan that does aquagym regularly – even just for aesthetic reasons, because it may help people to feel better inside. Personally I would have breast enlargement, one size at least, and liposuction in the tights, but I do not do it because of money and fear." In general, many suggested that "small, not invasive interventions may be good if they make you feel better". Here we get closer to what may be termed a *neo-modernist psychologistic narrative*, one which prioritises feeling and feel-good factors together with self-control and autonomy. In these accounts, clients tended to discriminate between different types of intervention – suggesting that "soft treatments" – such as the use of fillers or liposuction – were not like a facelift or breast enlargement.

The use of "the knife", the expensive recourse to the surgeon in a heavily medicalised setting, and the idea that one was not in control of what others were doing, were often presented as deterrents. In contrast, soft treatments appeared closer to everyday body care practices, such as the use of hydromassage or of creams, which act more slowly and require some direct involvement on the part of the subject.

Clearly, the boundaries cut out by fitness culture are never stable. This partly reflects the fact that keep-fit activities are positioned within a shifting arena of body transformation/maintenance techniques which may be synergic as much as they are in competition. Ever new and more extreme techniques solicit clients' fantasy, while established sub-cultures such as body building are long present. The world of professional body builders is fascinating for some. For example, Roberto, a Florentine university student who spends almost every morning in the gym doing mostly resistance training, says:

> I've bought a few magazines that had guys with good bodies on the cover, I'm doing the same thing, so I always ask myself "if I carry on, will I really be like this?" So I start thinking that it's impossible and that I'd have to use drugs and anabolic steroids. I think it's ridiculous but at the same time, I'm still curious.

Steroids are also typically deemed unnatural, but their appeal may lie precisely in the fact that they may be self-administered and require some routine, long-term, direct involvement of the self, which offers the illusion of control. On the whole, techniques which may be accommodated within narratives predicated on active, direct bodywork or body control appear to have greater chances of endorsement by fitness fans. Thus, the paramount association between keep-fit and dieting. As suggested in Chapter 6, the fitness industry itself is moving in the direction of such a synergy, while it remains wary of partnerships with even soft surgery companies. Whereas the most external, commercial edge of fitness culture realised by fashion-oriented fitness and health magazines is typically organised as to avoid direct challenges against the plastic surgery industry and even to wink to it, trainers tend to be much more vocal in their judgement.

The personal trainers interviewed both in Italy and Britain in particular positioned fitness against plastic surgery and close to dieting. They suggested that with the new millennium they have to face a duality: on the one hand, "more awareness of the importance of fitness activities for health and wellbeing", on the other "more negative pressures towards aesthetic perfection". Adam – founder of his own personal training company which has operated in London since 1998 – illustrated this prettily. The following interview exchange shows also the kind of boundary work done by trainers to limit fitness plasticity:

Q. Is there a predominant "type" or "model" of body today?

A. Cosmetic companies are pushing this. It's unrealistic, but the media push Angelina Jolie, David Beckham, but that's not good. It's putting too much pressure on women, particularly girls...they are saying you have to look a certain way regardless of spirituality, psychologically. Nothing about the inside...Cosmetic surgery has become as popular, that's not good...The whole concept of plastic surgery and people looking for the perfect body is damaging. But overall with the emphasis on nutrition people are realising the health implications and the real importance of training, they realise that they are not doing it just for their image, but they are actually doing it for their life. People realise that the lifestyle they live is unhealthy, and sedentary, and very stressful and they need to set it in balance by looking after themselves.

Q. What motivations do you encourage or discourage?

A. I am going to be honest with them so if people come to me with unrealistic expectations I will tell them the truth. I say that we can work with what you have but that's the best we can do. Otherwise they can go for plastic surgery which doesn't work anyway. Some people do look at plastic surgery but when they see what it really is about and what you have to go through, they give the idea up.

Reference to nature has a double, both cognitive and normative, slant. It is used to account for why fitness works and why it is moral. As suggested, expert discourse on fitness claims that the transformations gained via keep-fit bodywork respond to the true nature of the body. Fitness is said to be valid as it is the only method that really works, allowing for a continuous self-monitoring of one's own body (see Chapter 4). Keep-fit exercise uses the body's "true" capacities and therefore brings about a "true" transformation. Techniques that work differently may be more or less acceptable, but they are doomed to fail or at least be ancillary to exercise. Thus, make-up "improves your appearance" but "it starves the skin of oxygen"; and with plastic surgery "you can tighten the skin all you want, but it will always sag again, and then you'll look worse than before!". These other techniques cannot give individuals what they desire because the body will react against them. Naturalness also validates fitness from a moral, normative viewpoint. As I will demonstrate in the next few pages, fitness training is not only sensible and effective, it is also virtuous and proper. Fitness fans are indeed quite concerned to distance themselves from vanity and narcissism. They also claim that whatever body transformation they may have achieved via bodywork is morally justified: they have earned it and it is just the result of a natural process which the subject has carefully managed, demonstrating his or her "will". They therefore get to claim that looking good "isn't vain if it is the result of training", if it is obtained "through natural means, and being careful about what you do with your own body". It is this kind of slow, regular, controlled work on oneself which is seen as providing naturalness (to the body) and authenticity (to the self). And, as I shall argue, the possibility of convincingly articulating these two notions appears to grant fitness its moral centrality.

3. A productive dualism and bourgeois embodiment

The notions of nature and balance are finally articulated on what may be called the *subjective level*, referring to keep-fit training as a balancing act between the body and the mind-self that re-establishes nature. Acting directly and exclusively on the body, keep-fit exercise is seen by most regulars as a way of providing some "relief" to the overexcited mind. During a work day, so goes the typical script, the body is neglected and the mind overused, keep-fit activities come in to re-establish some harmony:

> [during the whole week] I must get my mind into gear, and do things with my brain ... it's as though my muscles don't exist because there is no link to the rest of my body, so this is just my way to strike a balance.
>
> (Antonia, manager in a cultural organisation in her late thirties, Milan)

> it's as though only a part of you [the mind] is functioning and you're definitely missing something, still if you do an hour of exercise, you're missing slightly less, you feel more whole.
>
> (Anna, natural food shopkeeper, Florence)

In clients' accounts the mind-self, on the one hand, and the body, on the other, are presented as two interconnected, yet distinct and diametrically opposed entities, the equilibrium of which is threatened by the modern way of life.[4] The body is not transformed into an end in itself, one of the core values of fitness being instrumentality (see Chapter 4). As regulars explain: "looking after the body a little more carefully helps to have a more efficient body", not losing "contact with its capabilities" helps in "making the most out of it". To balance out mind and body, we are asked to work exclusively on the body. The mental effort which accompanies training is often described as the capacity to "think about the body and nothing else", and, therefore, to "not think about anything or about matters that are worrying you"; and also to "eliminate the effects of tension" and to "relax your mind". Even clients who refer to the notion of "harmony", tend to conceive fitness as a balancing act between the body and the mind visualised in separation: "finding a balance between these two aspects, the body and the mind, is fundamental ... because if you betray one of these two aspects, you betray yourself!".

All in all, the emphasis placed on balancing body and mind must not lead us to believe that fitness culture as predicated in the West overcomes dualistic thinking about embodiment and selfhood. The space given to the body in the gym is more to do with finding new forms of body management that can increase its energy and capabilities than overcoming the body/self dichotomy. This may be better appreciated if we look at fitness historically, considering the slow transformation in body care recreational activities. Still at the beginning of the twentieth century, the idea of body care, typically reserved for the haut-bourgeoisie elite, found expression in physical activities, such as visiting thermal baths, aimed to preserve energy. These recreational practices were inspired by what may be defined as *negative* body management, centred on preservation and rest. During the same period, however, other more *positive* forms of body care were making headway. They were linked to the bourgeois appropriation of physical education (Chambat, 1987; Defrance, 1976, 1981; Haley, 1979; Hargreaves, 1986; Pociello, 1981, Vigarello, 1978, 1988; see also Chapter 1). They involved stimulating the body rather than inhibiting it, thereby producing energy instead of containing it. As George Vigarello (1978) has demonstrated in his *Le corps redressé*, together with the concept of the body as a meeting point for the unconscious where it found expression and external demands which repressed it, techniques developed which aimed to rediscover the body in all its aspects (see also Elias and Dunning, 1986; Lears, 1981; Thirion, 1987; Vigarello and Mongin, 1987). The body thereby became an arena that can and must be explored, visualised and appropriated to new profit, something that gradually took hold of bourgeois strata. The body/self dichotomy was not therefore altered in terms of structure, but in the way these two terms constituting a structural opposition related to each other. The self and the body remain separate; the self is still the intangible, sacred part. Yet, the body is no longer seen as the source of error and wickedness. Instead it is viewed as a forgotten, precious territory waiting to be rediscovered, a territory of unexplored possibilities whose proper development may lead to a better, stronger, more complete self (Shilling, 1993; Turner, 1984).

Current philosophy largely reflects these developments in its attempt to draw the body back in. In particular, criticism of the body/self dichotomy is widespread: numerous authors, from Richard Rorty (1980) to Judith Butler (1990), have rightly criticised the dualistic philosophical stance on the basis that our identity is characterised by practice and performance; that is, subjectivity is a doing, a creative praxis which involves both the body and the self in ways which challenge dualism. This resonates with contemporary sociological theories of practice and embodiment which try to fully appreciate the creative properties of social activities and their ongoing, situated, embodied character (Crossley, 2001). Following from this, in my journey into fitness culture I've been trying to appreciate the experiential moment in training, and the role played by immediate involvement in the execution of exercise. The experience of involvement is the fundamental subjective ground on which keep-fit exercise is validated – and clearly it is not about the self becoming distinct from the body, by simply governing it. In contrast, involvement precisely erases the line of demarcation between the cognitive and affective, between the mind and the body and, indeed, between ends and means of action as the notion of flow suggests (see Chapter 5). Still, once we emerge from the experiential moment and consider the narratives generated by gym participation as to fitness objectives, validity and general significance, a dualistic code remains fundamental. While involvement is rooted in the immediate persuasiveness of the scene for the participating subject as a whole of body *and* mind, the value and validity of fitness are confirmed by projecting the self beyond the body as an intelligible object to be managed. The value of fitness rests on the pursuit of a better body, more efficient, more useful. And from the ensuing achievement of a stronger mind, one where self resides, and one which is more "in control". The opposition between the body and the self-mind thus remains a productive discursive device within fitness culture, effectively used by gym enthusiasts to represent themselves as moral individuals. Given this configuration, a sociological approach should critically examine the rendering and workings of dualistic thinking (rather than rejecting it, as philosophy may legitimately do in spite of its admittedly inadequate linguistic means).

On these premises, we should also be wary of echoing expert discourse on fitness. In an early contribution to the sociology of the body, for example, the French sociologist David Le Breton (1990, p. 133) suggested that in contemporary society the "ontological alliance" between man and his body has been broken: the gym is nothing more than a compensating "parenthesis" of "real life", "a privileged place where the usual hindrances are removed, and where the ritualised displacement of the body is partially suspended" without resolving the ordinary "atrophy" of the body's "functions", but in a "voluntary and temporary" way. Such arguments are somewhat ingenuous. Firstly, physical exercise can never be sociologically equated with the freedom of the body *tout court*. Yet, this is because *the* body is a theoretical abstraction, one which does not exist beyond the set of situated social practices that both mould it and are moulded by it in countless but precise ways. I am here siding not so much with disincarnated constructivist perspectives, but with practical theories of embodiment, which may be found in both Goffman (1963b, 1967, 1974) and Bourdieu (1977). The very notion of embodiment as situated, symbolically rich practice does not accommodate the possibility of going back to an original and pure body. To stigmatise gym activities on the grounds that they are incapable of overcoming the body/self dualism and consider the latter as a merely repressive ideological form may unwillingly draw us back to biologism. As if the body were a natural and given object and not, more correctly, an ongoing, often taken-for-granted, practical accomplishment linked to definitions of nature and naturalness.

Secondly, the desire to reclaim the body may prevent us from appreciating that dualism and transcendence ambitions are co-extensive. In other words, we should recognise more fully that keep-fit bodywork develops in a relation of symbiosis and opposition with body/self dualism. Just like naturalness, transcendence is predicated on the backdrop of a vision of "the neglected body" in disciplined desk-bound professions and formal urbanity. Le Breton somehow endorses fitness discourse and its idea of natural balance, only to criticise it on the grounds that the balancing activities offered are partial and vain. We should instead consider that the very development of special institutions such as the fitness gym, dedicated to physical activity and predicated on the desire for health and wellbeing, has contributed to promoting the idea that there exists a natural body which has been lost and must be rediscovered.

A critical sociological analysis of the dualism found in fitness should neither accept nor transcend it. It rather should look at its effects, especially those which appear quite paradoxical. In other words, it should take seriously the fact that a dualistic language is not just an unfortunate trait of Western thinking and an aberration to be rejected. It is also, and above all, a *productive mechanism* for discourses and practices of transcendence whose value is predicated on the persistence of dualistic forms. It is the idea of a (harmful, unnatural) separation and opposition between the self as mind and the body which allows to attribute special value to places such as the fitness centre which are targeted for their (healthy, natural) recomposition and harmonisation. In turn, the creation of specialised spaces defined by the possibility of "taking care of the body" strengthens the impression that modern urban living otherwise is – *and can only be* – unhealthy, unnatural and harmful to the body. The fitness centre may be confined at the margins of urban daily rounds, but as a marginal, highly specialised and separated institution it reinforces the functional structure of urban living. Its diffusion may have rendered less urgent the provision of parks, outdoor exercise tracks, cycling paths and other urban fitness solutions, which may incidentally be less prone to commercialisation, more universally available and more incisive in changing urban living. Its diffusion may also make us accept more readily that other daily practices, such as work, for example, may be harmful to the body.

All in all, fitness culture is predicated on the "natural" body, its deterioration and its possible rescue. And we must then go back to the questions: how is the natural body portrayed by fitness culture? How universalistic is the rescue? Such questions may now be answered by looking at the particular *economy of energy* which is presupposed by fitness. The notion of the fit body impinging on a particular vision of bodily energy, and its generation. Anson Rabinbach (1990) has shown that, especially from the nineteenth century onwards, the idea of the body as a "machine" was essential to calculate and rationalise individuals' energy as productive potential.

The metaphor of "the human machine" was tied to the rationalised use of the body for work-related purposes, while generating worries about its de-humanising potential. This metaphor has had an impact on the debate about physical education. It was to "combat the loss of physical energy" produced by the "rational use" of the body during work that at the beginning of the twentieth century "hygiene experts, moralists, and physiologists" were already thinking about equally rational forms of gymnastics, maintaining that "exercise should no longer be a disorganised and diffuse distribution of exhaustion and pain, but a rigorous and standardised collection of activities based upon the repeated application of energy" (Rabinbach, 1990, p. 224; see also Bonetta, 1990; Vigarello, 1978).

On several occasions during my journey into the world of fitness, I have met with the thought that the body is indeed a "machine", even though a "strange" one, one that defies the laws of thermodynamics. The body needs movement: by burning and consuming its own energy through keep-fit exercise, the body acquires more energy. Fitness trainers often use similar arguments both to define their role, and to encourage clients. They proclaim themselves proud of the fact that they can "give a burst of energy" to those who train with them. In their classes they encourage clients with incitements such as this: "Come on girls, one more time! Just wait until this evening and you'll see how much those stomach muscles hurt. They'll feel really good, really firm and relaxed, and anyway, how else are you going to get rid of all that energy?!" They stress that whatever energy is "spent in the gym, it will be gained in life", and that the latter will be a "positive energy" as opposed to the negative one which accumulates during the day, especially at work. Reference to the interplay between *negative* and *positive* energy is paramount in expert discourse. It links up with the notion that modern urban life and work patterns are unhealthy for the body: they produce negativity. Echoing this, regular clients insist urban life harms the body, not only directly by reducing its capabilities because of sedentary life patterns, but also indirectly because of wrong movements and psychological stress in bureaucratised jobs. The lack of movement, or movement constrained by job requirements, makes the body and indeed the mind into a recipient of negative energy, stress and tension that can exhaust the individual. Only movements that are purposely designed to cultivate the body may do so and provide positive energy. The rationalisation of the exercise thus ensures that the energy acquired is positive. In many ways, rationalisation is presented as both the disease *and* the cure.

Just like strenuousness is brightened up by cheerfulness (see Chapter 5), rationalisation is rendered in triumphant accents. Emphasis is placed on the development and growth of one's own energy potential rather than on mere maintenance. Within the domain of fitness, conservative views predicated on avoidance of illness, on physical fragility and inertia, are put to one side. By and large, all fitness fans I have met with spoke of "energy gains" and "growth", rather than mere "retrieval". In their verbalisations: "you can do things you thought were impossible and most of it's down to training"; "I really did not expect to get to feel so well, like I feel relaxed and strong at the same time!" Even with mature clients, the body is first and foremost something that can recharge itself with ever increasing energy: "my energy has increased enormously, I can now do things that I doubt I could have done as a boy". Physical degeneration is for fitness fans an acknowledged horizon that may be turned upside down thanks to fitness transmutation of negative energy into positive energy. If properly exercised, the body reveals its potentiality and power.

Rationalisation of keep-fit activities also helps present fitness in univer-salising tones (see Chapter 4). "Everyone can go to the gym and get fit" is a recurrent theme in fitness expert discourse, vented through a plural-istic vision of exercise (it is "not important which exercise you do, only that you do some") and body shapes ("no matter what size or shape you are, the thing is to get toned"). This is matched by an equally uni-versalising portrayal of the negative external influences which come to bear on the body as a energy system. External menaces come, it appears, from urban living and rationalised, sedentary patterns of work. Although it is presented as a universal feature of urbanisation, the particular econ-omy of energy adumbrated by fitness training is in many ways spoken in the voice of the bourgeoisie, the urban dweller engaged with rational-isation and bureaucracy. In expert discourse, this is often expressed in a tone which glosses over distinction. Fitness workout "allows the body to make use of the huge reserve of energy" that helps to "make a positive change to the way it meets the challenges of life" and "face everyday life activities with ease", proposes an Italian manual (Punzo, 1992, pp. 5, 83). Fitness may provide "everyday readiness [as] defined by the demands of our lives...we all share the demands of daily life", suggests a British manual (Mills, 2006, p. 18). As the clients of fitness centres come from a mix of social backgrounds and a variety of jobs, it would be sensible to imagine that actual specifications as to the ills of urban life and job require-ments would vary accordingly. However, narratives about the economy of energy are, in many ways, surprisingly similar, if differently accented, across all fitness participants. They typically reiterate the very same economy of energy, with rationalised, specific bodywork providing positive energy. In particular, reference to the "de-stressing" or "anti-stress" qualities of fit-ness is paramount. It clearly appears to effect a shift from the body to the mind-self, sanitising bodywork and emphasising its civilised and civilising capacity.

Let's get closer to clients' narratives. The emphasis on releasing negative energy and regaining positive energy via organised bodywork is prevalent among both clerical and manual workers, males and females. Here are some verbalisations from my interviews which reflect general views:

> [the gym means] an hour of physical exertion. I'm exhausted from work, but the hour I spend there is energy and nothing else... it de-stresses me and keeps my body efficient.
>
> (Sandro, a decorator in his mid thirties, Florence)

> I don't really use my body at work, I like to be well groomed and all that, but I spend my working day at a desk... the energy I use when I'm moving around or doing housework isn't at all like the energy I use when I'm training... [fitness workout] is precise... I like pilates it's natural, and feels good for your overall balance.
>
> (Stella, administrative secretary in her early forties, Norwich)

> I accumulate much nervousness at work, people are often rude, and I must always repress my feelings... by doing some physical work, it's a mechanism probably, I take out all my nerves, all that negativity, which then becomes positivity with people, I really do not like to be nervous.
>
> (Alessia, postwoman in her early thirties, Florence)

> work is work, it's either sitting down or lifting up boxes, [it] soaks up your energy, and I need to be cool when all the clients are in a rush... coming here charges you up, it's the other way round... with machines you more or less follow your rhythm, it's relaxing.
>
> (Carlo, mid thirties cash desk worker in a supermarket, Bologna)

Exploring these claims in some detail we may exemplify different accentuations which appeared recurrently. Stella, like many women I met, especially in secretarial jobs, and even more so in managerial or professional ones as well as in those related to fashion sales, is surely particularly alert to self-presentational needs. Carlo and Alessia, in different, working-class and low-middle class jobs that require contacts with clients also feel strongly about the emotional burden of their jobs. They do mention these as stressful demands on the body. Stella, as many clients with good cultural capital, refers to balance and feeling, while Carlo and Sandro, as quite common among clients in jobs of a manual sort, use markedly more instrumental vocabulary. Indeed, a differential accentuation may be noticed in the gym-goers' accounts I have collected, bearing precisely on the qualification of rationalisation. Reference to "harmony" is more often articulated with an opening to body-soul techniques such as yoga, tai-chi and even meditation among participants from advantaged, culture-rich backgrounds. Thus, looking back into the interview excerpts reported in this chapter, we may notice that an intellectual worker like Francesco has moved away from machines, and likes tai-chi based exercises, stretching and soft-gym techniques which appear to prioritise reflexive engagement with routine and "feeling". Indeed, as commercial fitness centres have become increasingly mainstream, I have gradually witnessed a certain rebound against heavily rationalised bodywork. As we know, class attachments to specific sports and body modification practices change across time (Bourdieu, 1978). And looking at distinction from within the field and its internal evolution may help to account for such ongoing change. Indeed, participants from working-class backgrounds in my study appeared to adhere to the lesson on utility and rationalisation even more than upper-middle class ones. As Bourdieu maintained (1984, 1978), the working classes display a remarkably functional ethos towards their body, as the body is for them, after all, a quasi-mechanical tool of work and they live in closer proximity to "necessity". On their part, the middle classes, and cultural intermediaries in particular, may be the first to endorse an experimental ethos, having access to a broader variety of therapeutic, cultural and sporting discourses which centre not only on more finely tuned details of appearance, but incorporate elements the of the holistic health movement and Eastern body-soul disciplines (Baer, 2001; Bennett et al., 2009).

As much as they speak with different accents, fitness participants converge in their portrait of the natural body which needs to be rescued and the fit body which is to be pursued. For gym-goers, the body which is to be rescued from the pressure of urban living is far from the grotesque proletarian body, it is the too disciplined, bureaucratised body of the urban dweller. This may allow for glossing over the specific physicalities associated with working-class job requirements, and may push for the generalised embracement of the release mechanisms of a more properly bourgeois embodiment, whereby rationalisation may be countered by further rationalisation. In a way, in the qualification of fitness and its value by fitness fans, internal fitness *habitus* takes precedence over social embodiment. The local dominance of the fitness *habitus* illustrates that worlds of practices based on consumption offer participants narratives of self which are only loosely coupled with their positioning in the external social structure. This may work as ideology (covering up differences), but it may also offer spaces for integration (offering access to more culturally favoured forms of embodiment) or extrication (in the different accentuations of practice and embodiment).

If we move to the characterisation of the fit body, we see a likewise convergence. The fit body, so I heard over and over again, is essentially a body that is "more ready for everything". The long-standing dominance of such a script in fitness culture has probably induced Barry Glassner (1992) to maintain that the greatest force that pushes men towards keep-fit exercise is "insecurity". But while he sees male exercisers as engaged in "a battle with their own sense of vulnerability",[5] he sees females as concerned with "accomplishment, beauty, affiliation with others"(ibid., p. 123). In my journey into the world of fitness, I have come across a different scenario: the genders differ in their relative body ideals, but a sense of vulnerability is there for both. And what is more, among male and female fitness fans training provides feelings of command, self-government, accomplishment that assuage one's own perceived vulnerability. For all fitness fans, reference to the "hectic pace" of contemporary urban living underlines the need for a docile and powerful body: "these days you're always in such a rush", "you never know what's just round the corner" and only a "fit body will never let you down".

Fitness gym insiders associate the energy produced by training with the possibility of living a fuller life and using the body to the fullest: fitness provides the body with energy that helps to "do everything better", with "less effort", to "organise the day", to have "more drive", to "get more done". The energy produced in the gym is "good" because "it charges you up", and "enhances your life and your environment". Asceticism is thus coupled with hedonism. This is the polite, efficient and tamed hedonism which contributed to the diffusion of mass leisure in the twentieth century (see Chapter 1). It is a script which resonates with the cult of individual autonomy and self-control which are both crucial to Western consumer culture as intertwined with bourgeois embodiment (Sassatelli, 2007). As rendered through commercialisation, fitness training not only displays the capacity to "suffer a little" to fulfil one's own "obligation towards oneself", the will "to improve yourself instead of complaining". It also stresses "accomplishment" and "positive thinking", articulating an ethic of self-control with one of self-realisation (Lears, 1983; see also Green, 1986; Grover, 1989). The energy acquired by training is thus positive because it is docile and expansive, making life grow. "Ready for everything", the fit body is a powerful, docile universal utility. Its instrumentality matches the individualistic universalism of the fitness gym. What is more, it illuminates an allegedly infinite horizon of potentiality, adumbrating the existence of a self that is not confined to different social roles. A self which is able to master and govern roles and contingency by self-control operated, quite dualistically, via body control.

4. Authenticity and addiction

I shall conclude this chapter by looking at the kind of subjectivity that goes hand in hand with such an empowered, fit body. As articulated in fitness, body/self dualism produces a particular normative subjectivity and is rendered through a particular narrative of self. Of course, people do not go to the gym to discuss philosophy. By training they, so to speak, elaborate the body as materiality. The ultimate significance of the gym, however, shifts from the body to the self. Many clients indicate what gym attendance has given them as a "greater mastery" over their bodies, and the notion of the body as a docile instrument accentuates the idea of the self. More control over their bodies is often translated as more selfhood: working out at a gym enables the individual to "acquire energy and strength and, consequently, confidence and trust in themselves"; and with this comes the "awareness" of having transformed themselves into their own "masterpiece" (Brusati, 1992, p. 9; Rizzi, 1992, p. 7). Individuals are no longer at the mercy of unhealthy urban environments. Instead, they become confident, rational managers of their resources: keep-fit exercise trains them to "control their own emotions and feel more balanced" (Caplin, 1992, p. 298). Training in a gym is thus often described by clients as "a twofold phenomenon" which not only "serves to separate" the individual from everyday life, but also helps to "rediscover oneself". These words allude to the centrality of the notion of *authenticity*.

Being acutely aware of the danger of discrediting oneself in the search for the perfect body, fitness fans refer to "authenticity" as a moral guarantee of the transformations they seek and may obtain. Gym insiders (instructors, trainers and fitness fans) articulate an overarching script stressing that fitness participants can claim physical improvements to be legitimately theirs. Let's explore this more analytically. Clients often insist that a fit body is a "fair reward". It truly belongs to the subject because they have learned, through sustained dedication, to put body to work, rather than pursuing fast, external, ephemeral transformations. Reference to asceticism, stressing active, direct, constant work on the body through the body is paramount. According to an Italian fitness manual for women (Brusati, 1992, p. 7), the gym conforms with the idea that

> [a better physique] is not a free gift that accompanies us at birth, but rather the result of self-study and an informed choice that can turn every woman not only into a better person, but can give them real individual beauty, which is both fascinating and above all shows a strong personality.

Indeed, going to the gym is presented on moral and moralistic grounds as the "right thing to do": everyone has to "to look after themselves", "we are the first responsible for ourselves". All clients I have come across both in Italy and Britain seem convinced of the moral stance of fitness training, on the grounds that it allows for a legitimate appropriation of body transformation. An irregular novice from Florence like Raffaele, for example, suggests that he does not even want to "have abilities" that are not his own: "I don't want to be Tomba [an Italian world skiing champion], he trains ten hours a day". For Raffaele the gym is something "healthy" that "doesn't make you look silly" because it allows you to "be in full possession of your own abilities!". The transformation brought about in the gym is *not* a sign that the fitness fan aspires to be something or someone else. It does not "betray" the subject as much as it does not betray the others. Marica, an enthusiast, thus states that she does not want to "hide behind appearances, I want to be me! I want my own muscles!... When people look at me, I want them to know that I am the way I am and this helps my self-confidence." The naturalness of fitness is reflected in a certain subjective quality: fit people are more authentic than before because they have worked on their potential and are aware of how to use it. Clearly keep-fit bodywork has a moral value which transpires in interpersonal relationships: it may provide for better social relations because authentic body improvements make people "feel good about themselves". Fitness fans thus suggest that training helps you "to be at ease with yourself" and "therefore with others too"; or that "I try to have a good relation with my own body and feel at ease with myself; and this improves my relations with others."[6]

Reference to authenticity is supported by engagement with both routine and rupture. On the one hand, authenticity is predicated on the natural plasticity of the body which is demonstrated by the gradual character of the improvements. Gradualism is the result of "long-standing", "regular commitment" to the routine of keep-fit workout. Some fitness fans suggested that they may "perceive the changes and be aware that they are natural", that "you only become aware of them very gradually" because "there is no overnight change". Gradualism is both the cause and the result of clients' engagement with the routine of training, and of their emerging as reflexive trainees that continuously control their training programmes. This allows clients to claim that some of their body defects are just a temporary condition that will be redressed with work and exercise and to feel they own whatever body amelioration they may obtain. This also allows them to reject and take distance from crude versions of consumerism which propose quick-fix solutions to body defects and dissatisfaction. On the other hand, while many clients stress choice and commitment, they also feel as though they have acquired something that they "did not expect", which was "almost accidental" and "spontaneous" and therefore all the more authentic. Amy, for example, concludes her account with the assertion that her efforts have opened up a new, unexpected self-awareness: "I now have a relationship with myself that is different, confident and self-assured. It has been an enlightening change." Claire, too, claims to have "discovered something" she was "previously unaware" of. Such comments from fitness fans echo fitness discourse as expressed in manuals. As a trainer wrote in her gymnastics manual, engagement with fitness routine helps people "to meet their aims and discover their hidden qualities" (Goodsell, 1995, p. 9).

In the context of fitness culture, commitment to both routine and rupture or discovery is particularly interesting. It helps us explore embodiment as ongoing emergent practice. We may do this by looking at how routine and discovery are articulated in experiential narratives. Reference to "discovery" is used at least twice in fitness narratives. The initial discovery of something wrong is described by clients as having prompted them to go to the gym. In success stories, this is matched by the discovery of something good and unexpected. Those who join a gym often tell stories about having become more conscious of their bodies as a result of an embodied misfit experience in everyday life which derived quite often from some breaching experience, a rupture in ordinary routines. A salient misfit experience mediates commercial images or medical discourse on the body. In the interviews I have gathered, misfit is not derived from facing normative discourse or idealised commercial body images. It is an utterly practical experience through which we may read such norms and ideals. Misfit experiences often have to do with a comment from a friend or a lover, with facing one's one aging body when carrying out everyday ordinary activities, or with finding out that one has gained weight when trying on an old favourite item of clothing. Some, even the youngest, had not even been aware that they were, in fact, "becoming weaker" up to when their bodies "did not respond" as expected in one or more instances in ordinary life – to the point that "simple activities like going up stairs were an effort" or one "got out of breath just running after a bus". The fitness gym is thus described as a response to a (mostly sudden) realisation that ordinary routines and taken-for-granted requirements of daily life cannot be easily sustained, a response which provides names for discomforting experiences, and solutions to named problems. A response that requires one to come to terms with routine again, to engage with the repetitive nature of workout, investing time and effort to bring out, discover, the fit body – something that, as previously suggested, is normatively measured against one's own embodied capacities in ordinary life. Thus, while fitness culture identifies problems and offers remedies this happens through lived culture. Embodiment, as a dialectic of routine and rupture, should not be underestimated: in many ways people feel neither fit nor unfit because they see a magazine; they feel fit or otherwise because they experience their bodies in certain ways. Clearly expert discourse on fitness contributes in shaping the language of fitness, but it does so articulating people's ordinary experiences, of failure and success. In a likewise fashion, attending a gym is less a rational choice than it is a creative learning process.

Turning to the normative side, commitment to routine and discovery also helps us explore the particular rendering of the work ethic within fitness culture, considering how asceticism and hedonism are intermeshed. Gym insiders deploy slight variations on the same script, which elaborates a rather Puritan work ethic (Weber, 1904).[7] Reference to the notion of "discovery" is often used by gym insiders to complement the idea that fair rewards are the result of sustained bodywork. As in the classic version of the work ethic, mundane asceticism is working towards something which is *already* inside us. Discovery, rather than invention, furthers the claim to authenticity: the subject of fitness has found the strength to work on their body to realise their nature. In other words, discovery is something which cannot be simply factored in as part of a rational project, and brings authenticity back to normalising reference to nature. Keep-fit workout is certainly described as a moral imperative, a secular form of salvation (see Pronger, 2002; White et al., 1995). Rather than the demonstration of a desire to be aesthetically pleasing, fitness fans often claim that training is just like "taking responsibility for oneself". This may well be a strategy to gain control over the sense of self which derives from the mastery of physical activity. Yet, self-mastery may be jeopardised by presenting oneself as primarily an object of gaze, something which is implicit in bodywork as beautification or aesthetic technique (see Brace-Govan, 2002). The aesthetics of positive functionality discussed in the previous chapter may indeed translate, in contemporary terms, the "austerity of appearances" (Perrot, 1987) through which the modern bourgeoisie controlled the meanings of their bodies and ultimately legitimated their moral claims to superiority and power. Thus it may be true, as Christopher Lasch (1979) suggested, that self-realisation is now explored in leisure and consumer culture rather than in work, but commercialised leisure, such as keep-fit activities, is often organised in ways that both draw upon and subvert work. An economising rationalisation, made of effectiveness and efficiency clearly places fitness workout close to the bureaucratic sphere of work. But trainees have to make sure that all benefits are theirs. Routine acquires a liberating potential for the individual, if it is taken both seriously and lightly. Engagement with routine is officially geared to the discovery of one's own hidden qualities, to the realisation of one's own potentiality. And, what is more, the process of routine engagement itself has to become pleasurable, involving, relaxing – to the point that neither routine or rupture, duty or pleasure may take over the autonomy of the self.

Visions of normality, as a balancing of duty and pleasure, were ultimately implicated in fitness narratives. They were evident in the often-repeated notion that fitness fans are just "normal", "natural" people, quite "distant from Mr Perfect", more real than the "cheer-leader image" that was associated with aerobics (see Chapter 6). Normality means habit and habitual practice. Something which is both taken for granted and essential. As one fitness manual says, once people have settled into the routine of going to the gym "very few are willing to give it up, for the simple reason that if you returned to the inactive life you led before, you would no longer feel at ease with yourself" (Jackson, 1992, p. 8). With regular participation in fitness activities comes, so it is suggested by fitness insiders, a new, deeper awareness. Because of this, breaking one's own fitness routine may be risky: those who give up may put (their) nature in jeopardy. Here are some telling quotes from fitness fans and trainers:

> I would no longer feel myself if I'd stop training... When you start working out, you learn to see yourself from a different perspective, and then you can never turn back, you feel different, you feel better... you develop an awareness that you don't want to lose.
>
> (Amy, university student, Florence)

> everyone goes to the gym for a thousand different reasons, each one with their own aim in mind, or even if they go just for the sake of it, those who continue will end up feeling they can't easily give it up... They have

to come in order to feel good, and also because it provides structure to their day.

(Omar, gym instructor, Florence)

the objective is to get to the point that training is a way of life, a natural, normal way of keeping contact with one's own body.

(John, personal trainer, London)

Normality, though, also means that such habitual practices, which are deemed to help control the body, are themselves somehow controlled. Normality means regularity, stability, order. In some ways, something that we habitually do, but is neither eccentric nor deviant. That offers sound pleasures, rather than obsessive cravings. And here we do get to a final set of issues indeed. The more enthusiastic fitness participants I have come across, those who train almost every day, those who go to the gym despite injuries, are clearly aware of long-standing medical findings referring to "The Runner's High" (Wagemaker and Goldstein, 1980). As early as the late 1970s, these findings suggested that exercise is a stimulant which leads to physiological arousal in the brain. Fitness enthusiasts often mentioned "endorphins" and the internal physical arousal mechanisms which would be activated by training. Some of them reported to have had such physical experiences, and a few even considered themselves "a bit extreme" in that they felt it "difficult to do without" training (see Chapter 6). This kind of self-awareness has been recognised as one of the diagnostic features for addiction in the literature on exercise dependence in psychology and psychiatry, and may or may not be associated with eating disorders (Adams and Kirby, 2002; Bamber et al., 2000; De Coverley Veale, 1987; Griffiths, 1999).[8] Such literature not only provides definitions of addiction that stress withdrawal symptoms and increasing priority of exercise over other activities. It also suggests that addiction is often accompanied by the narrowing of training repertoire leading to a stereotyped pattern of exercise. It furthermore suggests that the gym is used in a rather obsessive, individualistic fashion, with the continuation of exercise, the repetition of the exact sequence becoming an absolute, unstoppable focus of attention. Of course the issue here is not to draw a clear line between committed exercisers and addicts, something that even psychologists recognise to be quite difficult. It is rather to show that fitness consumption, like other forms of consumption, is normalised (Sassatelli, 2007). That is, fitness participation is not only predicated on unconditional increases, on uncontrollable desires, on untamed pleasures. It is rather conditional to self-governed appropriation.

Only a consumer who is sovereign of themselves can surely be trusted to be sovereign of the market, thus legitimating commercial culture as rooted in (bourgeois) freedom (Sassatelli, 2000a). Broadly speaking, our anxieties about addiction reveal the centrality of the cult of individual autonomy as self-government in Western consumer culture (Eccles, 2002). In many ways addiction and "normal" consumption are co-constitutive. More to the point, inherent in the fitness instrumental vision of the body, in its individualistic slant and rationalised character, in its demonstrated, joyful strenuousness, we may find the very root of addictive behaviour. Yet it is also in fitness culture and organisation that we find the means of normalisation. The picture portrayed of exercise addiction in recent diagnostic literature suggests which positively evaluated elements of fitness organisation may indeed have a strongly normative value: structured variety is not just a selling technique, omnivorous patterns of training being witness to clients' capacity of both involvement and detachment from each specific routine; gym sociability is not just a cunning side benefit, the development of gym interaction requiring an alertness to irony, informality and courtesy which may not be compatible with obsessive training. Participants in fitness not only contribute to fitness culture, but also to its normalisation: boundaries of normality have to be drawn and participation in fitness needs to be kept within these, stressing individual desires, but keeping them geared to culturally approved visions of subjectivity and projects of wellbeing.

Conclusion: Embodiment, Subjectivity and Consumer Culture

Fitness gyms occupy a strategic position for the study of embodiment and embodied subjectivity in contemporary, Western consumer culture. Largely organised via commercial relations of some sort, they intersect body discipline and consumership. The promotion of physical efficiency and health is surely still very much part of a governmental logic for the nation state, in particular as it faces aging populations. But efficiency, health and beauty – as summoned up in the notion of fitness – are more and more pursued via market relations and the consumption of commoditised services and goods. While the list of dietary products which claim to be both pleasant and healthy is longer and longer, fitness gyms promote themselves as places where, with a bit of effort and some fun, clients may gain long-lasting results to their otherwise forgotten bodies. Gym-goers are typically addressed as individuals who may take control of both the market and themselves, and act as consumers. To critically consider fitness culture as part of today's consumer culture, we thereby need to explore the social persona of the fitness consumer and the notion of choice associated with it.

The ethnographic approach adopted in this study has been ultimately geared to this broad problematic. Sustained participation and observation in a variety of fitness gyms in different urban contexts has helped in considering the actual space cut out by what, initially, was merely a rather elusive theoretical triangle, defined by the notions of consumer choice, body discipline and fun experience. Ethnography is widely credited with the merit of depth. It allows to get close to people, share their experiences, learn their ways of interacting (including non-verbal ones), understand their meanings as realised through practice. This quality was crucial to appreciate how people become fitness participants, and how their participation in keep-fit activities acquires meaning. Seen from the ethnographic close-up, choice is revealed as a process, rather than a cost-benefit decision. A transformative, ongoing practice rather than an accomplished, rational calculation. Instead of revealed preferences, we get a rather hybrid mix of decisions, constraints, habits, contingencies, aspirations, interactions, relations – each of which may be more or less satisfying, and may or may not lead to further consumption. The notion of rational choice – operationalised in mainstream economics through the cunning conflation of "revealed preferences" – obliges us to either imagine a sovereign consumer, or to reject it altogether opting for notions such as "induced needs" and "false consciousness". Ethnography has offered a third, less dramatic, but more daring picture. In such a picture, the boundaries between production and consumption seem to be shifting and, to an extent, blurred. Consumption is revealed as ambivalent practice, with consumers increasingly asked to be active producers of cultural forms that are nevertheless largely circulated and managed by producers who need to consume much of the very same sort they produce.

Let's consider this a little more. As demonstrated throughout the book, gym-goers' reasons for taking up fitness training, developing a gym routine and sticking to it do not easily fit a rational choice model. This finding is all the more relevant as rational decision models have dominated exercise research and health promotion. Normative reference to widely accepted body ideals including health may easily become a deterrent rather than an incentive to exercise participation, and once inside a gym, the local organisation of practice is of the essence in providing internal rewards. Rationally choosing a gym would be based on a series of cost-benefit, instrumental decisions, narrowing down possible alternatives, moving from the recognition of an abstract need to exercise, to an objective assessment of all the activities which may satisfy this need, an evaluation that keep-fit in a gym respond to one's own aims, a choice of the best-suited fitness centre among those available and finally the purchase of a season ticket. Any subsequent action, except sustained participation, would count as weakness of the will. Clearly such characterisation stand miles apart from what gym-goers experience, and it provides little insight into what gym drop-outs may go through. The inadequacy of a rational choice model is briefly summarised as its incapacity to take seriously consumer choices as cultural processes and transformative practices. As lived consumer culture, gyms are transformative environments, they change subjects as much as, and indeed more than, they change bodies. For example, using up gym facilities, interacting with trainers and other clients, gym-goers not so much achieve, but certainly identify body objectives in the light of what is relevant within fitness culture as realised in each gym. Instead of a clear means-end logic, we find that gym participation is a mix of habit, self-challenge, emotional release, light sociability and, broadly speaking, a culturally approved way of coping with one's own shortcomings. Nevertheless, as typically articulated through market relations, fitness cannot dispense with the idea of choice altogether. Indeed, fitness culture has flagged out choice conceived as the capacity of the individual to choose what is best for themselves. The services of a fitness gym as well as the efforts of a personal trainer are truly legitimate and successful, so goes the dominant script in fitness expert discourse, only when clients "really want" to train, when they "have made a true choice for themselves".

In many ways, thus, a fitness participant is a good consumer. The point is not just a nominalistic one, even though gym-goers are often referred to as clients, customers and consumers by gym staff. Neither is it a purely economic one, even though regular gym-goers often buy a variety of commodities associated with keeping fit. Fitness fans are good consumers primarily because they tend to portray themselves as such: subjects capable of making their own individual choices, deriving pleasures from choice and making pleasure coincide with long-term wellbeing. In this sense, studying fitness allows us to consider the broad cultural politics of consumer culture, exploring the ambivalence of the emphasis on individual responsibility and self-control.

To be true, the regular use of a fitness gym lies in the province of voluntary action, it is predicated on clients' possibility to exit and the development of loyalty to a gym (Hirschman, 1979). Fitness managers themselves place emphasis on the client as someone who pays and who makes the final decision on the quality of service. As with the majority of other consumer practices, use of the gym cannot simply be explained away by the manipulation of clients by cynical, self-interested managers and trainers, partly because experts themselves believe in the advice they give and the goods they provide. In social sciences, on account of the authority of neo-classical economic models of action, the voluntary nature of consumption is often traced back to the notion of rational choice, that is, it is associated with the idea that each individual acts according to clear, well-defined needs, and that to satisfy these needs, individuals are capable of identifying and evaluating various alternatives and remain faithful to their own preferences (see Sassatelli, 2007). Approaches which are influenced by rational choice are therefore not concerned with the process of needs formation, neither are they concerned with the way in which some products or services are identified as substitutable alternatives, nor with the ideas of subjectivity and morality which these alternatives imply. Attendance at a gym, however, takes place in far less instrumental and linear ways than those suggested by the idea of rational choice: its processual, situated and open-ended character seems to require a different model of action. Quite interestingly, marketing experts also seem to lean in this direction. In proposing a taxonomy of decisions for the purchase of leisure services, Ian Reid and John Crompton (1993, p. 198) maintain that the "the choice to buy a service is normally the outcome of a process which may start much before actual purchase, but last much longer than its initial use" and that services like fitness or swimming courses require "a long period of training and experience" on the part of participants "before their attributes can be fully appreciated".[1] As we have seen, independently of the level of interest or identification shown at the beginning, it is only when clients enter a gym and learn to use what is on offer there that they seem to become attached to the gym and to keep-fit exercise, attributing meaning to it. For this reason, it cannot be said that the majority of clients rationally choose to go to the gym, and that they *then* put this decision into practice. Rational discernment can only suggest the choice of one gym over another when fitness activities taking place in the gym have become a non-substitutable alternative. As suggested in the first part of the book, this identification of the activities carried out in the fitness gym as a non-substitutable, superior alternative for keeping in good form happens via a situated and open-ended process of which clients are only partly aware, and which they may come to partially govern only with sustained participation.

My journey into the lived culture of the fitness gym has clearly shown that quite often gym-goers learn to recognise what they define as their "need for exercise" through actual practice. Not prior to, but after, choice. They often mentioned the desire to "do something", for their body, themselves, their weight and so on, but the precise need for exercise, and for keep-fit exercise, is recognised only via participation in fitness activities. In other words, the identification and specification of what is otherwise a rather abstract longing takes place through concrete practices. These practices may be more or less satisfying as such, but they act as a pivot, giving access to answers that then allow questions to be asked in the pursuit of further answers. If we go back briefly to the comments made by gym enthusiasts, we see that some consider that they "started off just by coincidence", to "try it out", being "dragged there" by friends or relatives; others describe much more conscious decisions often mentioning the desire to overcome experiences of inadequacy and explore new sources of positive self-evaluation. For both these groupings, the gym is recognised as having produced "something new", an "unexpected relationship with the body" to the point of "finding you are different almost without wanting to". They "found out after" a number of lessons "what" it was that they "really wanted", and even scorned at their initial body desires. They might have reached this stage after a period of dullness and habituation, up to when they felt relaxed and at home in the gym. These stories illustrate that fitness is rarely a well-defined project from the start: participation is often the main initial project, while detailed body projects typically come with participation and need to be continuously fuelled. A corollary of this is that many clients "discover" their own "essential" need for fitness in *one* particular gym. Generality is thus construed through particularity. In this process, the very idea of *the* fitness gym, as a precise alternative to other forms of bodywork, is stabilised. The mainstream economics notion of consumption as revealed preferences is reversed: needs only exist in contexts where subjects try, more or less successfully, to satisfy them (Sassatelli, 2000a, 2001).

We may certainly read clients' stories as normative narratives or *ex post* rationalisations, but we cannot avoid considering a great deal of clients' knowledge, including the ability to evaluate and choose different clubs, as deriving from their experience of training. Most clients considered that the gym is a highly visible institution, a familiar part of their own urban environment well before it became important to them. Many of them remembered having "always seen" gyms in their neighbourhood, having heard the music from aerobics lessons or glanced through large widows into the machine area. From the outside, however, the fitness gym is opaque. This is partly because what the media presents us does not fully correspond to what takes place in a health club. But it is also because a fitness gym must constitute itself as a meaningful world of meanings by (partially) cutting itself out of ordinary life. Access to this world requires more than the purchase of a membership or the payment of a fee. The increase in the number of gyms, and their consequent increasing accessibility, does of course have an influence on fitness popularity.[2] But supply driven explanations for the fitness boom do not hold. As we know, most people do not exercise, even though they have the means to do so and display vaguely positive attitudes towards physical activity.[3] This crucial fact can probably be understood only if we appreciate the gap between the external, abstract visualisation of keep-fit activities and local, specific scenes and practices. Clients really learn to want to train only by continuing to attend. To a certain extent, the importance of the gym is always a result of its use. For example, although they do not act in an irrational or casual manner, in general, most people do not know if they will enjoy a new type of leisure activity unless they try it out, and they learn to enjoy activities with time and practice.

Given this configuration, fitness gyms cannot be fully understood by referring to shared, abstract cultural values which encourage people to work on their bodies (Bordo, 1993), or to an equally abstract social function responding to a psycho-physical need to give vent to emotions (Le Breton, 1990). Nor can we consider that gym attendance can largely be grasped as a mere function of the fitness industry (Ewen, 1988) or the realisation of identity and tastes constructed according to external determinants such as economic and social position (Smith Maguire, 2007). In much of the available literature fitness tends to be described as a uniform training culture throughout the globe, with multinational corporations being seen as driving forces behind its expansion (Maguire, 2002; Maguire and Mansfield, 1998). While not the focus of my research, the picture that emerges from it is different. The local/global relation cannot be reduced to diffusionist visions whereby US-dominated forms spread out in other countries. This is so, not only because fitness culture is variously translated across the globe as a function of different systems of provision, professional organisations, sports histories, and consumers' expectations (Sassatelli, 2000c; Spielvogel, 2003; Steen-Johnsen, 2004) but also because locally realized resources are crucial in developing the need for fitness, and its actual realization, into practices. Consumers in particular play an important role in variously translating hegemonic fitness discourses and trends coming from the USA. Consumers are effectively co-producers of the training scene in the gym. A focus on the co-production of the actual scene of consumption, and on the ensuing creation of locally specific body dispositions may indeed be very helpful. Spaces of consumption, such as the fitness gyms, create taste as much as they attract people endowed with certain dispositions. The productive role of local, lived cultures of consumption must be factored in as it largely organises fun as a consequential experience. In other words, the way in which the correspondence between goods and services and tastes is established is of uttermost importance, as it is in the social organisation of such correspondence via consumer practices (spaces, interactions and relations) that these services and goods are finished and acquire meanings. As such, goods and people within a particular domain of consumption may form a relatively separated order of reality which may (partially) filter external determinants (gender, class and ethnicity) and reorganise them in its own peculiar way, contributing to new hierarchies of taste, and new paths for the stabilisation of individual, broader and long-lasting dispositions.

This of course does not mean that we need to take what consumers say at face value. Rather, while I listened to gym-goers carefully, I needed to go beyond their often-repeated phrase "I'm going to the gym to keep fit". I needed to explore how they came to think and feel this way, what this actually meant for them, and how it resonated with fitness expert discourse. This exploration brought to light that the cultural strength of the fitness gym lies in its promise of external, culturally prized, gains (that is, body improvement) in both a rapid, controlled manner, and in a morally acceptable manner. What is fitness culture's cultural strength is also, however, its experiential limit. As a rationalised, rational and moral form of recreation, keep-fit activities in the gym may look too much like work. As suggested, they are indeed perceived as boring, tedious and tiring by many irregular clients, and even embarrassing by gym-drop-outs. Not surprisingly, gym instructors and trainers consider "motivation" as their major concern, as they are utterly aware that keep-fit exercise may be perceived as a sterile activity, directed entirely towards the future, producing no meaning for the present, and consequently alienating clients. The emotional codes and qualifiers of actual keep-fit training, and in particular the promotion of joyfulness and positive thinking, were crucial elements in the definition of what keeping fit means to gym participants.

The physical abilities, emotional codes and cultural scripts which clients appropriate as they participate have been the centre of attention during my journey. Implicit in my focus was the idea that in fitness gyms, as indeed in many other consumption spaces, consumption is best understood as a learning practice. Not always do we learn good things, of course, but let's put aside this normative question for the time being, and concentrate on the model of action. To be true, consumption comes in many guises, and processual, learning-like elements may be more significant for services, leisure services in particular. Yet, consumption is the use, and not simply the acquisition, of commodities. We may come to fully appreciate consumption as social action only if we put aside the idea of purchase (which resonates with choice) and consider instead its situated character. This allows us to appreciate use as realised through social relations and see how participants – both producers and consumers – continuously stabilise and accomplish both their identities and materiality. This provides quite an active image of the fitness participant, but activity is what allows gym-goers to be transformed by practice as much as they appropriate it – showing that the space to criticize the ideal of the autonomous, strong consumer is inherent in consumption as a social practice.

The evidence gathered though fieldwork may now be placed in a much wider perspective. Ethnography is often accused of not being able to grasp macro-reality and structural dimensions. Yet, in many ways, it is up to the ethnographer to step back and inject breadth into the depth of fieldwork. To help me towards this, and to consider keep-fit gyms as institutions which organise the much broader cultural principles of fitness culture, I have looked into fitness discourse through the experiential lenses of clients and trainers. Manuals and fitness periodicals provide normative injunctions in a clear, condensed form. It is such injunctions which are variously articulated in the lived culture of the gym, chiefly by producers (instructors, trainers) but also by consumers. Having shown that, as a form of consumption, fitness participation cannot be equated with rational choice, I had thus to come back on the notion of choice, which is indeed very much central to fitness culture as a symbolic formation. Bodywork is presented by gym-goers as testimony to their capacity to choose to realise themselves. While it is essential not to launch into an intellectualised interpretation of fitness culture, it is true that clients account for keep-fit practices using legitimating scripts that dwell on choice as a *normative model*: they recognise chance and contingency, they allow for relational elements, yet ultimately they stress that what is needed for participation is to "make a choice and stick to it". Gym going is described as reasoned commitment, a form of self-government that responds to one's own true, natural needs. This allows fitness fans to define themselves as moral subjects, the best judges of their own "nature", and the wise managers of their own lives and bodies.

Choice is thus seen less as a rational cost-benefit calculus and more as self-government towards culturally sanctioned projects of wellbeing. As such, individual choice is ambiguous: inadequate as a description of actual practice, it functions as a normative claim sanctioning a view of subjectivity and wellbeing centred on self-government and its pleasurable pay-offs. Informing clients' legitimating scripts, choice becomes a practical method of linking micro and macro, allowing fitness to exist, not only in particular local scenes, but also as a symbolic cultural formation that, as it were, sits in a pantheon of positive activities all contributing to the consolidation of a valuable image of the self. Fitness fans therefore help to legitimise fitness culture by realising a particularly normative view of subjectivity. Fitness gyms acquire value by referring to individuals as subjects who choose responsibly. As a normative category of consumer action, choice is based on culturally specific anthropological assumptions which in turn are associated with the development of commercial culture. Consumership refers to subjects who are masters of their will. As a study of the fitness consumer, and of the lived culture of fitness as consumer culture, this book has hopefully allowed explore a bit more the nature of such mastery, how self-government and involvement may be subjectively intertwined and socially organised, how desires and objectives get defined and normalised while being felt as genuine expressions of the self.

The very active, powerful image of the consumer sustained by fitness culture can be problematised. While engagement with routine may indeed become pleasurable, cheerfulness in training has clearly a normative slant. Thus, not surprisingly, cultural parodies of fitness often deal with the quasi-compulsive character of "fun" – such as in the case of Japanese director Nagi Noda's short film "Doggy Fitness" which has been used for the cover of this book.[4] Moreover, positive thinking, fun and self-discipline all point to the joyous pursuit of self-sufficiency on the part of a rather strong self. As suggested, the fit body corresponds to an ideal of absolute utility. The very idea of health, increasingly defined as a set of abilities rather than the absence of illness, has become something that the subject can acquire and for which they are personally responsible (Crawford, 1985). This tends to attribute responsibility for body care and bodywork solely to the individual and discounts everything that may be in the way of effective self-government. Thus, while only such strong selves can be left alone to decide how to care for their bodies, positioned on a different and differentiated social map, they may also be quite lonely in bearing the whole weight of their lives, physical defects and misfortunes.

Sure, fitness consumers are no cultural dupes or market slaves. Yet, the emphasis on their capacity to be active and responsible, and their duty to do so, may have structural effects on the social provision of physical recreation and may legitimate certain ways of organising commercial relations. The fact that physical exercise is no longer part of an explicitly political sphere has ambivalent outcomes. Unlike the physical education rigidly organised by states in order to control their populations, fitness training largely responds to a heterogeneity of consumers who also wish to enjoy themselves, seek variety and novelty, and can be persuaded but not coerced. This does, however, reinforce the erroneous impression that care of the body is an extremely personal act, which is beyond distinction and free.

Like other leisure pursuits, both organised via for-profit organisations or provided by city councils and public authorities, fitness culture quite poignantly demonstrates the ambiguity of the notion of free time. Training in the gym is essentially a limited fraction of time spent free of ordinary, external commitments, and thus partly distancing participants from external social demands on embodiment and identity. However, it is far less time spent free of all rules, and indeed, it is based on shared rules and rigidly codified practices. As suggested, fitness gyms filter social distinctions and bring together widely diverse social groups, at the cost of officially favouring rather self-contained and polite relationships. Although opposed to work, it is organised also through elements which derive from the world of work. For many participants, exercise is experienced as being time dedicated to themselves, but this is based on what they have learned about themselves in the gym. Time spent in training is not a distraction which produces no results, it is productive time. Even fun and involvement in training has serious outcomes as it allows for sustained participation. The gym both reveals and controls individualism. Although it is the result of voluntary adherence, in order to give value to training and the bodily transformations it produces, clients do not feel they have to trust only their own freedom of choice. On the contrary, they believe that by exercising with weights, on treadmills, or by taking exercise-to-music classes, they can rediscover their own body and its naturalness.

Looking at how fitness culture is accomplished in a consumer space such as the fitness centre helps in considering this particular culture of consumption as lived culture. While buying a fitness pass is a punctual purchase decision predicated on normative visions of the body, effective use of a gym and participation in the fitness scene is an ongoing practice, based on the engagement with routine and discovery. A dialectic between routine and discovery is often organised by consumer practices: too much routine can get boring, too much discovery can get stressful. A fine balance of both helps present consumer practices as both legitimate and pleasurable, a dual concern which is the crux of contemporary consumer culture.

Notes

Introduction: Bodies, Consumers and the Ethnography of Commercial Gyms

1. Both focused on the US, these are in fact two quite different endeavors: a more polemic and general reflection on late-modern body culture the former, and a more precisely focused institutional study of the fitness industry the latter. To these I must add my own earlier ethnography of two fitness gyms in Italy (Sassatelli, 2000c) and Kari Steen-Johnsen's (2004) work on keep-fit exercise in Norway, both of which take more seriously the perspective of the fitness consumer. Linda Spielvogel's (2003) monograph on female fitness participants in Tokyo may also be mentioned as a perspective on a non-Western reality which provides interesting observations on the domestication of American-driven trends in Japan especially among fitness professionals.

2. While the commercialisation of the fitness sector has been very strong in the last decade in the USA (see Smith Maguire, 2007), in Italy and Britain the pace of commercialisation appears to be clear and yet slower (see also Crossley, 2006). Of course this needs to be further qualified in terms of other institutional variables, as Steen-Johnsen (2004) has shown for the Scandinavian context, where, given very similar levels of economic development, there is a marked difference in penetration rate between Denmark, on the one hand, and Norway and Sweden, on the other. A larger and more complex non-profit fitness sector exists in Denmark, where there is a mix of fitness centres owned by voluntary sports clubs, by municipalities and by independent non-profit institutions often belonging to the Danish Gymnastics and Sports Associations, with the result that commercial fitness clubs are less widespread than in the other two Scandinavian countries. Other important factors may be the urban configuration of a region or nation, with large metropolitan areas being those where, generally, commercial fitness penetration among the population is stronger.

3. Interaction entails a notion of "procedural order" or "operational consensus" (Goffman, 1959, 20–1). This makes it possible to take into consideration the "conditions and limits placed on the way in which aims are sought, or activities brought to a conclusion", considering them as relatively autonomous from the "choice of goals or the way in which these goals can be integrated into a single system of activity" (Goffman, 1971, x–xi, 1963a, 7–8, 1982).

4. I have not in any way wished to compare the many fitness gyms I have observed: via the use of a variety of sufficiently different, if not extreme cases – ranging from women-only informal studios, to up-market health centres, from local leisure centres to international chains – my main aim was to describe what characterises fitness gyms as a specific social environment and reach a number of analytical generalisations on mechanisms witnessed in different gyms.

5. Through fieldwork I tried not only to address clients' various social profiles in terms of gender and class, but also, their gym careers (interviewing neophytes, regular gym-goers, enthusiasts, irregulars and quitters) and training preferences (from aerobics lovers to weight-lifters). Trainers were mostly chosen from the premises

I visited or via email contacts to increase variety. The choice of informants was made according to the principles of "theoretical sampling" (Glaser and Strauss, 1967) with a rather loose interview schedule that has helped cover some key areas (Seidman, 2005). While fitness fans were easier to get hold to, quitters were difficult, and the sample is clearly skewed in favour of more regular and enthusiastic gym-goers. In order to put interviewees at ease, most clients were interviewed in their homes, while most trainers were interviewed in the gym. All the interviews were recorded, some were very long and lasted over two hours, others were much briefer taking less than one hour. Words or phrases in inverted commas, unless a specific biographical reference is made, have come directly from interviews and informal conversations, or were spoken during gym activities. In analysing the material I have used typological plans and identified relations, contrasts and similarities (Silverman, 1993).

6. This mediation is creative, but it is predicated on the interaction between production and consumption. As proposed by Paul Hirsch's (1972) well-known model of the "cultural industry system", mass-marketed cultural goods are the result of a collective process of production which entails various different actors (artists, gatekeepers, talent scouts, managers, journalists) responding to different institutional and personal interest and, what is more, involves considerable feedback from consumers (Du Gay et al., 1997, Miller 1987).

7. In particular these are: *Salve, Starbene, Vitality*, and *Siluhette* for Italy; *Ultrafit, Health & Fitness, Zest* and *Top Santè* for Britain; *Shape, Self* and *Men's Health* for the USA. Much more could have been done in terms of discourse and visual analysis of these rich and varied texts. However, also because my initial ethnography did not (regrettably) rely on directly recorded images of training bodies, I preferred to use them more to complement my understanding of expert and commercial discourse on fitness than use them in their own right.

8. Many of these texts are available both in English and Italian, thus allowing for the local-global dialectic. An interesting spin-off of such concern is the dialectic between McDonaldised fitness premises and local appropriation (O'Toole, 2009, see Chapter 7).

1 The Cultural Location of Fitness Gyms

1. On the commercialisation of physical recreational activity, see Andrieu (1987), Green (1986) and Hargreaves (1987) who maintain that this particular cultural collocation kept a check on the increasing tension between the disciplined utility of the body and disorderly hedonism. The removal of exercise from the explicitly political sphere had ambivalent outcomes. On the one hand, it had a liberating effect, encouraging the development of public or private initiatives which were not necessarily bureaucratised (Hargreaves, 1987), and giving rise to flourishing activities not related to those sanctioned by national sports federations (Perrin, 1985) and the search for new forms of exercise (Grover, 1989; Jackson Lears, 1981; Pociello, 1981). On the other hand, it weakened the political impact of physical activity, and reclassified it, so that it simply became a form of youth entertainment (Defrance, 1981).

2. Aerobic workouts were originally developed by Kenneth H. Cooper in the 1960s to improve astronauts' and pilots' level of fitness and established the basis for this specific kind of aerobic training (Cooper, 1967). "The Cooper Institute" elaborated different training methods that enhanced endurance, based on ideas of variation,

moderation and balance. This model was further developed in the 1970s to address beauty as well as health through the work of Jackie Sorensen, who created a dance programme for US cable television based on Cooper's ideas of aerobic fitness training. Rhythmic dance music was integral to this, and became a feature of the slightly more aggressive vision of aerobic exercise proposed by Jane Fonda's idea of the "workout" (see also Chapter 2).

3. In his subsequent and classic work on distinction and taste, Bourdieu (1984) more fully conceptualises taste – including attitudes towards one's own body – as an expression of *habitus*. *Habitus* is a set of dispositions which guides actors in their choices. It varies according to different capital endowments (economic, cultural and social) which it helps to reproduce as an infinitely applicable and creative classificatory instrument. Taste is therefore seen as a form of "symbolic power" through which objective and subjective classifications coincide, enabling a naturalisation and reproduction of the existing system of differences (Bourdieu, 1977 see also Leberge and Kay, 2002; Wacquant, 2003, 2005 for a broader view of Bourdieu's theory as applied to sport activities).

4. Taking seriously the formation of taste as negotiated in actual consumer practices whose structure is not co-terminous with income or occupational structure, and indeed considering the role of such practices in the consolidation of a "middle-class identity" is being recognised as important in contemporary studies of class and class *habitus*. On this basis, what has been traditionally called "middle class" can be considered as a social space where one may share, but also competitively confront, tastes, goods and lifestyles. In other terms, rather than being considered dependent variables, consumer choices are co-constitutive elements of social standing (Sassatelli et al., 2008).

2   Spatiality and Temporality

1. This is part of a larger trend, comprising the organisation of work as well as of consumption, which is well captured by Boltanski and Chiapello in their book *Le Nouvel Esprit du Capitalism* (1999). Looking at management manuals they consider how the logic of "project" – which requires a total investment on the part of the worker mixing work and leisure – is taking over many productive realities (see Chapter 7).

2. The notion of "passage ritual" only partially accounts for the changing room. A classic passage ritual is one-way, occurs between rigidly defined, mutually exclusive identities, and provides the "liminal" space in which the implementation of new attributes is strictly prescribed and symbolically sustained. For Turner liminality is a "structured anti-structural moment" where clear ceremonial rules and shared symbolic meanings allow for the collective management of meaning transformations. We may consider changing rooms as primary examples of the individualisation of the liminal, something that Turner (1977, 1982) called the "liminoid".

3. The wellness wave is probably part of a larger culture of wellbeing (Sointu, 2005) and responds, partly, to the very practical need of participants to "do something without fatigue".

4. Gym instructors, and more broadly, fitness trainers, defy the distinction between task and emotional leaders that is often made in small group research. As I shall show more fully (see Chapter 3) they are probably better understood as experts,

task and emotional leaders (on their role in the emotional structure of gym scenes, see also Chapter 5).
5. This, of course, is not true of circuit training, a type of machine-based exercise, whereby a group of clients is led jointly through a sequence of machines (see Crossley, 2004). Also, the joint use of machines is promoted in some female-only studios, such as that studied by Leeds Craig and Liberti (2007). These types of exercise, mixing machine workout, light sociability and trainer leadership are quite often characterised by some kind of gender reappraisal (see also Chapter 6).

3   Interaction and Relational Codes

1. The kind of environment which is provided by community sports centres and informal and local gyms may partly respond to similar anxieties: where such options are less available, such as in the USA, there seems a trend for the development of women-only studios (Craig and Liberti, 2007). This points to the continuous articulation between the differentiation within the fitness industry and its public.
2. Incidentally, these sentiments have been tapped into by the fitness industry broadly understood, not only with home videos, but also with manuals such as *The Kitchen Gym* by Anne Maria Millard (2005) where the whole house, with its shelves, steps, chairs and so on, and its cleaning and maintenance routines becomes a rather familiar training arena for the housewife.
3. In my experience, in most fitness gyms marginalisation compels groups who are overtly homosexual to either use the gym outside its busiest hours, or to choose a premise frequented by like-minded clients (Chapter 2). For research into physical activity and sexuality, see Aoki (1996), Klein (1993), Lowe (1998), Mansfield and McGinn (1993), Monaghan (1999) and Wacquant (1995). See also Alvarez (2008) for an insider perspective on gym gay culture.
4. On this, we may add a note concerning what associations are often considered conducive to, that is, politics. A recent study conducted on sports clubs, scouts and environmental groups has shown that while cultural or environmental associations (concerned with some form of common or public good) are conducive to political active members, membership of leisure and sports associations (concerned with more individualistic goals) tends not to command increased political participation (Quintelier, 2008).
5. This may be a rewarding aspect of the job, which has paradoxical effects. As a survey-based research of fitness instructors in Queensland, Australia, has shown, a disproportionally young, female, casual workforce may be "willing to trade-off standard condition of employment" for emotional rewards such as the "exposure of physical capital or bodily prowess" (Sappey and Maconachie, 2009).
6. Currently, the three main formats are BodyStep, Body Pump and BodyJam; they are offered in some 10,000 venues across 55 countries with an estimated 4 million participants a week (http://www.LesMills.com).
7. By and large, in contemporary consumer capitalism, McDonaldisation (the efficiency, predictability, calculability and control which increasingly characterise global commodity production and circulation) is countered by aestheticisation. The latter takes the form of local, quality oriented business and retail, of various kind of associations which promote taste refinement, tradition and

territorial awareness and, above all, of consumer practices which stress quality and uniqueness, and may pursue irregularity as a sign of charismatic elements (Sassatelli, 2007).

8. This is a rather broadly distributed magazine, reaching more than 25,000 subscribers (including owners and operators of fitness centres, health clubs and YMCAs) (http://www.athleticbusiness.com/fitnessmanagement/).

9. *Il Nuovo Club*, 2, 1999, p. 7. Although more developed in Britain and especially the USA than in Italy, publications for trainers and fitness managers are generally becoming very important. While there is research available on fitness magazines for the general public (see Markula, 2001; Smith Maguire, 2007), there is still a shortage of research on marketing and exercise discourse addressed to trainers and gym staff. This endeavour would certainly be important to capture the figure of the personal trainer as opposed to the gym instructor.

4   Framing Fitness

1. Goffman develops an idea expressed by Gregory Bateson in his famous essay on play and fantasy (see also Chapter 5). Bateson (1972) showed that play illustrates the human being's capacity to create relatively separated areas of meaning which temporarily overturn "normal" expectations. Goffman (1961, 1967) has used the concept of "frame" in his work on games, and later developed this idea in detail in *Frame Analysis* (1974) in which he analyses the experience of social actors in everyday life as an absorbing oscillation of a multiplicity of different frames (see Gonos, 1977; Tannen, 1993; Verhoven, 1984).

2. Even if the development of athleticism from the nineteenth century onwards has long been acknowledged (see Bourdieu, 1978; Gruneau, 1983; Guttman, 1978; McIntosh, 1963), other sport styles may be identified. In studying rugby, for example, Alain Garrigou (1987) maintains that athleticism gains ground against two other styles, stressing community (*fête*) or warlike-utilitarian motives (*travail*), both referring to values external to sport. The author relates the increasing dominance of athleticism to the relative autonomisation of sport, and to its professionalisation.

3. Here I have reworked the well-known Weberian distinction between modern and pre-modern forms of legitimation (Weber, 1922, vol. 1). This helps understand the rise of bourgeois techniques of the body and the birth of physical education (Chambat, 1987; Defrance, 1976, 1981; Hargreaves, 1987; Vigarello, 1978, 1988; see also Chapters 1 and 7).

4. Body building and keep-fit training appear quite different in terms of both the physical characteristics they promote and their motivational logics. Professional and semi-professional body building works on contests. Body builders will periodically enter into competitions and compete against other contestants. At a difference with sport, rather than being the public display of a highly specific task performance, these competitions are a display of highly specific physical appearances (see Courtine, 1991; Klein, 1993).

5. Bateson starts from the idea that meta-communication – that is, communication on how to interpret signals – is crucial for framed activities as play, thus creating relatively autonomous spheres of meaning. Far more than in other daily situations, in which meta-communication and communication are continually intertwined, as a framed activity keep-fit training provides relatively clear meta-communicative indications on what is right or wrong and on what is expected of the participants (see also Chapter 5 for a comparison with play).

5 Discipline and Fun

1. Goffman (1961, p. 38) defines framed activities as those in which "the world made up of the objects of our spontaneous involvement and the world carved out by the encounter's transformation rules can be congruent, one coinciding perfectly with the other. In such circumstances, what the individual is obliged to attend to, and the way in which he is obliged to perceive what is around him, will coincide with what can and what does become real to him through the natural inclination of his spontaneous attention." Similar to Arlie Russell Hochschild (1983) and drawing on Goffman, I have tried to offer a sociological perspective on emotions, observing the way in which involvement can be favoured by a particular local organisation of experience. This, incidentally, amounts to considering "frames" less as structural givens and more as toolkits for the ongoing negotiation of social reality (see Reese, 2007).
2. The characterisation of play as an intrinsically pleasurable activity, as an aim in itself, has been widely used, starting from the classic works of Johan Huizinga (1955) and Roger Caillois (1958). The de-contextualised and uncritical adoption of this definition of play has, however, inspired considerable criticism, summarised in the well-known essay by Brian Sutton-Smith and Diana Kelly-Byrne (1984). On the difficulty of drawing an immediate analogy between athleticism and play, see Booth (1993), Giulianotti (2005) and Guttmann (1978).
3. Role distance can be defined as behaviour geared towards expressing personal identity, which involves introducing a specific "margin of freedom and manoeuvrability, of pointed dis-identification between himself and the self virtually available for him in the situation" (Goffman, 1961, p. 117; see also Turner, 1968). In every situation there is always, therefore, a simultaneous multiplicity of selves, yet the situations vary according to how the moments of dis-identification can be managed, and of how much room for manoeuvre is left to the subject.
4. On the different importance of "physical capital" for the social classification of individuals into different categories, see primarily Bourdieu (1978; 1990), Bourdieu and Wacquant (1992), Shilling (1993) and Wacquant (1995).
5. Seppo Iso-Ahola's (1989) reviews of social psychology studies on free time shows that they view analogous phenomena as being the result of a trade-off between intrinsic motivation (carrying out an activity for the pleasure of doing so) and extrinsic motivation (to include external control, ultimate benefits and competition). What can be observed in the gym clearly shows that there is a strong correlation between informality – in other words, the possibility of deviating from the rigid requirements of role and interaction – and the perception of doing something which corresponds to the expression of oneself, and between these two characteristics of interaction and the definition of something as enjoyment (Samdahl, 1988). Nonetheless, this should not lead to an idealisation of the notion of free time (see Allison, 1993; Horne et al., 1987; Rojek, 1985, 2000).
6. See, for example, the work by Robert Yeung and David Hemsley (1997) which shows that the perception of being able to follow the exercises explains alone the 15 per cent variation in effective capacity to continue an aerobics programme through time.

6 The Culture of the Fit Body

1. The relationship between knowledge and discipline is crucial in Foucault's work. As we know from his work on disciplinary institutions (Foucault, 1975, 1977; see also

Rabinow and Dreyfus, 1983, pp. 168–209), disciplinary techniques have both passive and active subjectivity effects: they subject individual bodies to specific control
techniques, while simultaneously embodied subjects acquire ability and knowledge. In commercial institutions, such as fitness gyms, the active effects appear to
be accentuated: emphasis is on the sentient participant to be kept motivated, the
demanding client to be kept satisfied.

2. See http://www.together.uk.com. By and large, this may be a function of the
increase in obesity. But such trends are mediated by context-specific cultural and
social configurations as well as institutional features. The Italian fitness industry,
for example, has been much slower in jumping on the bandwagon of weight control compared to the British one, partly as a feature of its fragmented, small-scale
nature, which limits the offering of a variety of secondary services; partly as the
management of diet is far less medicalised in Italy, being still largely conceived as
a "family" matter.

3. Something of the kind has been suggested by Goffman in his *Stigma*, when dealing with how individuals deal with stigmatising attributes, essentially via direct
attempts to correct the attribute, indirect correction through the pursuit of success in other, apparently incompatible areas and through the breaking of social
reality – that is, "employ[ing] an unconventional interpretation of the character of his social identity" (Goffman, 1963b, p. 19). Feminist readings of aerobics
may be seen as one such unconventional interpretation (see Collins, 2002). More
broadly, the view of keep-fit activities as coping devices through which normative
femininity, and gendered embodiment more in general, is negotiated rather than
reproduced are corroborated by recent fieldwork research, in Canada and the USA,
among women gym-goers (Leeds Craig and Libeti, 2007; MacNevin, 1999).

4. Body ideals may be analytically placed on a matrix defined by the intersection
of the surface/depth axis and the means/measure axis (Sassatelli, 2000c, 2003; see
also Feher et al., 1989; Turner, 1984). The ensuing four analytical dimensions may
thus refer to different ways of intervening on the body: the body can be modified and ameliorated as a tool or a sign to be preserved, a tool or a sign to be
presented. Health is typically something to be preserved, beauty something to be
presented. Fitness culture appears to work at the intersection of health and beauty,
indeed contemporary commercial gyms reframe both beauty and health in terms
of fitness.

5. Numerous studies on the development of medicine in modern times have stressed
that the body has been seen as an organic, pure system, threatened on all fronts
(Crawford, 1985; Haley, 1979; O'Neill, 1985, pp. 118–47; Turner, 1984). The development of a positive idea of health (Park, 1994) and, later, of medicine centred
on genetics (Haraway, 1991) is partly contributing to the modification of this
image, and shifting attention to the use of the body and the flow of information
within it.

6. In addition, Anne Bolin (1992) stresses that other activities, in addition to body
building, can make the most of women's athletic qualities: in other words, the
female body should not be fat in order to challenge dualistic definitions of gender.

7. While body building is the clearest example of muscular work for aesthetic ends
(Courtine, 1991; Klein, 1993), in most exercise techniques there are movements
involving muscles which are rarely used in everyday life, and seem to serve more
to improve body appearance than to increase its functionality (Kagan and Morse,
1988; Maguire and Mansfield, 1998; Markula, 1995). And yet the study of Pirkko
Markula (1995, p. 443) on women and aerobics shows that those who exercise

may begin to doubt the "logic" of certain exercises "since they have no functional value" and demand "uncomfortable" or "unpleasant" positions.

7 Fit Bodies, Strong Selves

1. A number of different dimensions may be considered in looking at the use of space for fitness and sporting reasons. On the one hand, even reimmersion in nature can happen via more rationalised – fitness-like – procedures, such as evident in the current development of Nordic walking (see Shove and Pantzar, 2005). Nordic walking combines displacement and emplacement in that paths come complete with expected times, lights and even calories. On the other hand, phenomena such as Parkour – that is, the use of the urban built environment as a "gym" for spectacular moves – appear to rely on forms of non-commercial institutionalisation akin to sub-cultural formations of an "anarcho-environmental kind" (Atkinson, 2009). There seems to be a dialectic between the "immuring of physical activity" and the aspiration to "go back into the open" (Heichberg, 1998) which finds expression, among other things, in the provision of virtualised natural settings inside ever more "green", rounder, natural-looking gym environments.
2. Giddens (1990, pp. 27–9, 1991, p. 81) asserts that "as tradition loses its authority, the cumulative choices that combine to form a lifestyle define the central nucleus of a person's identity and the continual invention and re-invention of their character", even if they feel unable to rely purely on themselves and feel compelled to seek "expert" opinion that will guide them in those choices.
3. Clearly, fitness discourse participates into a current trend towards what I call *promotional reflexivity* (Sassatelli, 2009), which is evident not only in the marketing strategies of an "alternative" cosmetic company such as The Body Shop but also in initiatives taken by more traditional multinationals, such as the Dove Campaign for Real Beauty, whose consultant was feminist psychotherapist Susie Orbach.
4. In comments made by clients, the idea of the "mind" often refers to the "self" or at least to the characteristics that appear to distinguish it. It corresponds perfectly with a common practice in our culture that depicts the mind as the key dimension of the self. One talks about the mind in order to question the individuality and autonomy of the "human being" (Feher et al., 1989; Haraway, 1991; Rorty, 1980).
5. A similar interpretation has been deployed not only to understand fitness activities beyond the gym such as jogging (Gillick, 1984), but also gym activities beyond fitness such as body building (Klein, 1993).
6. Of course there is an element of ambiguity in the cross-referencing between recognition and self-recognition. Fitness fans are often quite vocal about the fact that how "other people see you" depends on how "you feel about yourself". However, how you feel about yourself may depend on how much you manage to consider yourself "adequate" – "to your age", "your body type", "your work", that is, to a set of generalised cultural ideals which, as suggested, are mediated by practices such as keep-fit bodywork. While self-recognition relies inevitably on addressivity (Perinbanayagam, 2006) fitness training is organised in non-dialogic form, emphasising another paradoxical trait of the gym.
7. For a discussion of how Protestant asceticism and hedonism have been intermeshed in the consolidation of modern consumer culture see Campbell's classic work (1987). See also Lears (1981, 1983), Green (1986) and Grover (1989) for a discussion applied to the development of the leisure industry in the USA.

8. The phenomenon is relatively small, but merits consideration. A recent, exploratory study of exercise addiction in Britain found that out of 100 self-selected gym participants (who are likely to be themselves among the most regular and enthusiastic participants) around 8 per cent could actually be classified as exercise addicts (Warner and Griffiths, 2005).

Conclusion: Embodiment, Subjectivity and Consumer Culture

1. In leisure studies and marketing, decisional models for consumer choice tend to make a clear distinction between various dimensions of action (cognitive, affective and conative) and seem to separate them into those befitting rational choice and those closer to the various theories of learning. In the first case, attitude is defined as a mechanism which, following an active search for information and sustained comparison, controls behaviour; in the second case, attitude is defined as an evaluation, a modality which gives meaning to behaviour, which follows purchase and collection of specific information. With regard to services, those who defend the more rationalistic approaches also tend to recognise the fact that consumers do not have many other possibilities of being aware of the attributes of an activity unless they try them. For a review of decisional models used in sports psychology, see Godin and Shepard (1990).
2. In studies on sports psychology, the geographical proximity of the exercise environment (to home or work) has been identified as being one of the clearest indicators of attendance at a fitness programme (Le Unes and Nation, 1996, p. 528 ff.). However, very few of the regular clients I have encountered were prepared to change their gym for one which is nearer. Indeed, they say that they left more convenient, well-known or cheaper gyms because they did not offer what they were looking for.
3. See, among others, Mannell and Zuzanek (1991) and Vanden Auweele et al. (1997). The most frequent justification given by those who say they are interested in but do not practise physical activity – "lack of time" – seems to be a way of recognising the social value of fitness and a rationalisation of the lack of any deep subjective interest.
4. Nagi Noda, who died in 2007, created this video for Panasonic's "Ten Short Movies – Capture the Motion" series for the 2004 summer Olympics. The film is a word-for-word parody of American fitness guru Susan Powter's first workout video except the video's instructor is dressed in a body suit giving her the appearance of having muscles shaped like the fur of a groomed poodle dog. Also, exercising with her in the video are six actors dressed in dog costumes, with actual live dogs' heads superimposed over their real heads. The video, circulating freely on the Internet, features Californian model Mariko Takahashi, and has become very popular and debated.

References

Abbott, A. (1988) *The System of Professions*, Chicago, IL: University of Chicago Press.

Adams, J. and R. Kirby (2002) "Excessive exercise as an addiction: a review", *Addiction Research and Theory*, 10, pp. 415–37.

Alessandri, N. (2001) *Wellness. Scegli di vivere bene. La filosofia di Mr. Technogym*, Milano: Mondadori.

Allison, L. (ed.) (1993) *The Changing Politics of Sport*, Manchester: Manchester University Press.

Alvarez, E. (2008) *Muscle Boys. Gay Gym Culture*, New York: Taylor and Francis.

Amir, G. (1987) "Au menu de Vital: Un concentre d'idéologie de rapport aux sport", in *Sport et changement social. Actes des premières journées d'études*, Bourdeaux: Maison des science de l'homme d'Aquitaine, pp. 100–18.

Andrieu, G. (1987) "La gymnastique commerciale", in P. Arnaud (ed.), *Les athlètes de la République*, Toulouse: Bibliothéque Historique Private, pp. 80–100.

Ang, I. (1985) *Watching Dallas: Soap Opera and the Melodramatic Imagination*, London: Methuen.

Aoki, D. (1996) "Sex and muscle: the female bodybuilder meets Lacan", *Body and Society*, 2 (4), pp. 59–74.

Appadurai, A. (1996) *Modernity at Large. Cultural Dimensions of Globalization*, Minneapolis, MN: University of Minnesota Press.

Archer, J. (2006) *Fitness*, London: Hodder Education.

Aron, J. P. (1987) "La tragédie de l'apparence à l'époque contemporaine", *Communication*, 46, pp. 305–14.

Arnaud, P. (ed.) (1987) *Les athlètes de la République. Gymnastique, sport et idéologie républicaine, 1870/1914*, Toulouse: Bibliothéque Historique Privat.

Arsac, L. (1992) "Le corps sportif, machine en action", in G. Genzling (ed.), *Le corps surnaturé. Les sports entre science et conscience*, Paris: Editions Autrement, pp. 79–91.

Ashton, D. (2001) *Body Business*, Victoria: Viking.

Atkinson, M. F. (2009) "Parkour, Anarcho-Environmentalism and Poiesis", *Journal of Sport and Social Issues*, 33 (2), pp. 169–94.

Avedon, E. M. and B. Sutton-Smith (1971) *The Study of Games*, New York: Wiley.

Baer, H. (2001) *Biomedicine and Alternative Healing Systems in America: Issues of Class, Race, Ethnicity, and Gender*, Madison, WI: University of Wisconsin Press.

Bamber, D., I. M. Cockerill, S. Rodgers and D. Caroll (2000) "It's exercise or nothing: a qualitative analysis of exercise dependence", *British Journal of Sport Medicine*, 34, pp. 125–32.

Baudrillard, J. (1998) *The Consumer Society*, London: Sage (1st edn, 1970).

Baumann, Z. (2007) *Consuming Life*, Cambridge: Polity Press.

Bateson, G. (1972) *Steps to an Ecology of Mind*, New York: Chandler Publishing Company.

Beck, U. and E. Gernsheim (2001) *Individualisation*, London: Sage.

Bennett, T., M. Savage, E. Silva, A. Warde, M. Gayo-Cal and D. Wright (2009) *Culture, Class, Distinction*, London: Routledge.

Berger, P. and T. Luckmann (1966) *The Social Construction of Reality. A Treatise in the Sociology of Knowledge*, London: Penguin.

Bernabè, N., G. Iacobelli and F. Moroni (eds) (2007) *A che punto è la New Economy in Italia?* Milano: Angeli.

Berryman, J. (1992) *Exercise and the Medical Tradition from Hippocrates through Antebellum America*, in J. Berryman and R. Park (eds), *Sport and Exercise Science: Essays in the History of Sport Medicine*, Urbana, IL: University of Illinois Press, pp. 1–57.

Bessy, O. (1987) "Les salles de gymnastique: un marché du corps et de la forme", *Esprit*, 4, pp. 79–94.

Bluin Le Baron, J. (1981) "Expression corporelle: le flou et la forme", in C. Pociello (ed.), *Sport et société. Approche socio-culturelle des pratiques*, Paris: Vigot, pp. 100–12.

Bolin, A. (1992) "Flex appeal, food and fat: competitive bodybuilding, gender and diet", *Play and Culture*, 5, pp. 378–400.

Bolin, A. and J. Granskog (2003) *Athletic Intruders. Ethnographic Research on Women, Culture and Exercise*, Albany, NY: SUNY Press.

Boltanski, L. (1971) "Les usages sociaux du corps", *Annales ESC*, 26 (1), pp. 205–33.

Boltanski, L. and E. Chiapello (1999) *Le nouvel esprit du capitalisme*, Paris: Gallimard.

Bonetta, G. (1990) *Corpo and nazione. L'educazione ginnastica, igienica and sessuale nell'Italia liberale*, Milan: Angeli.

Booth, D. (1993) "The consacration of sport: idealism in social science theory", *International Journal of the History of Sport*, 10 (1), pp. 1–19.

Bordo, S. (1993) *Unbearable Weight. Feminism, Western Culture and the Body*, Berkeley, CA: University of California Press.

Bordo, S. (1999) *The Male Body. A New Look at Men in Public and Private*, New York: Farrar, Strauss & Giroux.

Bourdieu, P. (1977) *Outline of a Theory of Practice*, Cambridge: Cambridge University Press (1st edn, 1972).

—— (1978) "Sport and social class", *Social Science Information*, 17 (6), pp. 819–40.

—— (1983) "Erving Goffman, discoverer of the infinitely small", *Theory, Culture and Society*, 2 (1), pp. 112–14.

—— (1984) *Distinction: A Social Critique of the Judgement of Taste*, London: Routledge (1st edn, 1979).

—— (1990) *The Logic of Practice*, Stanford, CA: Stanford University Press (1st edn, 1980).

Bourdieu, P. and Y. Delsaut (1975) "Le couturier et sa griff: contribution à une théorie de la magie", *Actes de la Recherche en Sciences Sociales*, 1 (1), pp. 7–35.

Bourdieu, P. and L. Wacquant (1992) *An Invitation to Reflexive Sociology*, Chicago, IL: University of Chicago Press.

Brace-Govan, J. (2002) "Looking at bodywork. Women and three physical activities", *Journal of Sport and Social Issues*, 26 (4), pp. 403–20.

Brehm, B. (2004) *Successful Fitness Motivation Strategies*. Champaign, IL: Human Kinetics.

Brewer, J. and F. Trentmann (2006) *Consuming Cultures, Global Perspectives. Historical Trajectories, Transnational Exchanges*, Oxford: Berg.

Brohm, J. M. (1989) *Sport: A Prison of Measured Time*, London: Pluto Press.

Brown, S. (2003) *The Energy Booster Workout*, London: Eddison Sadd Editions.

Brusati, P. (1992) *Ginnastica estetica femminile*, Padova: Muzzio.

Bryant, G. A. and D. Jary (ed.) (1991) *Giddens' Theory of Structuration. A Critical Appreciation*, London: Routledge.

Bryman, A. (1999) "Theme parks and McDonaldization", in B. Smart (ed.), *Resisting McDonaldization*, London: Sage, pp. 101–15.

Burgess, G. R.; S. Grogan, and L. Burwitz, (2007) "Effects of a 6-week aerobic dance intervention on body image and physical self-perceptions in adolescent girls", in *Body Image*, 3, 57–66.

Burke, K. (1962) *A Grammar of Motives and a Rhetoric of Motives*, Cleveland, OH: World Publishing.

Burns, T. (1992) *Erving Goffman*, London: Routledge.

Butler, J. (1990) *Gender Trouble. Feminism and the Subversion of Identity*, London: Routledge.

Caillois, R. (1958) *Les jeux et les hommes*, Paris: Gallimard.

Caldwell, L. L. (2005) "Leisure and health. Why is leisure therapeutic?", *British Journal of Councelling and Psychology*, 1, pp. 7–26.

Calhoun, C., E. LiPuma and M. Postone (eds) (1993) *Bourdieu: Critical Perspectives*, Cambridge: Polity Press.

Campbell, C. (1994) "Capitalism, consumption and the problem of motives", in J. Friedman (ed.), *Consumption and Identity*, Chur: Harwood Academic Publishers, pp. 23–46.

Canby, V. (1985) " 'Perfect', gym and jouranlism", *New York Times*, 7 June, 1985.

Caplin, C. (1992) *Il metodo holistix*, Milano: Sperling and Kupfer.

Castiglione, C. and E. Arcelli (1996) *In palestra è bello*, Milano: Sperling and Kupfer.

Cella, G. (1989) *Sentirsi in Forma*, Milano: Feltrinelli.

Chambat, P. (1987) "La gymnastique, sport de la République", *Esprit*, 4, pp. 22–35.

Chambliss, D. F. (1989) "The mundanity of eccelence. An ethnographic report on stratification and Olympic swimmers", *Sociological Theory*, 7 (1), pp. 70–86.

Cianti, G. (1994) *Sempre giovani*, Milano: Sonzogno.

Coalter, F. (1998) "Leisure studies, leisure policy and social citizenship: the failure of welfare or the limits of welfare?", *Leisure Studies*, 17, pp. 21–36.

Cole, C. L. (1993) "Resisting the canon: feminist cultural studies, sport and the technologies of the body", *Journal of Sport and Social Issues*, 17, pp. 77–97.

Collins, L. H. (2002) "Working out the contradictions. Feminism and aerobics", *Journal of Sport and Social Issues*, 26 (1), pp. 85–109.

Connell, R. (2002) *Gender*, Cambridge: Polity Press.

Council of Europe (1980) *European Sport for All Charter*, Council of Europe, Strasbourg: Institutional Publication.

Cooper, K. H. (1967) *Aerobics*, New York: Bantam.

Courtine, J. J. (1991) "Les stakhanovistes du narcissisme", *Communication*, 56, pp. 225–45.

Crawford, R. (1985) "A cultural account of health. Self-control, release and social body", in J. McKinlay (ed.), *Issues in the Political Economy of Health Care*, New York: Methuen, pp. 60–103.

Crompton, R. (1996) "Consumption and class analysis", in S. Edgell, K. Hetherington and A. Warde (eds), *Consumption Matters*, Oxford: Blackwell, pp. 113–32.

Crossley, N. (2001) *The Social Body. Habit, Identity and Desire*, London: Sage.

—— (2004) "The circuit trainer's habitus: reflexive body techniques and the sociality of the workout", *Body and Society*, 10 (1), pp. 37–69.

—— (2005) "Mapping reflexive body techniques: on body modification and maintenance", *Body and Society*, 32 (5–6), pp. 653–77.

—— (2006) "In the gym: motives, meanings and moral careers", *Body and Society*, 12 (3), pp. 23–50.

Csikszentmihalyi, M. (1982) *Beyond Boredom and Anxiety*, New York: Jossey-Bass.

—— (1997) *Finding Flow: The Psychology of Engagement within Everyday Life*, New York: Basic Books.

Cullum, R. and L. Mowbray (2005) *The English YMCA Guide to Exercise to Music*, London: Pelham.

Dallal, T. and R. Harris (2005) *Belly Dancing for Fitness*, London: Eddison Sadd Editions.

Dant, T. (1998) "Playing with things. Objects and subjects in windsurfing", *Journal of Material Culture*, 3 (1), pp. 77–95.

De Certeau, M. (1984) *The Practice of Everyday Life*, Berkeley, CA: University of California Press (1st edn, 1979).

Dechevanne, N. (1981) "La division sexuelle du travail gymnique", in C. Pociello (ed.), *Sports et société. Approche socio-culturelle des pratiques*, Paris: Vigot, pp. 83–99.

De Coverley Veale, D. M. W. (1987) "Exercise dependence", *British Journal of Addiction*, 82, pp. 735–40.

Defrance, J. (1976) "Esquisse d'une histoire sociale de la gymnastique, 1760–1870", *Actes de la recherche en sciences sociales*, 6, pp. 22–46.

—— (1981) "Se fortifier pour se soumettre?", in C. Pociello (ed.), *Sport et société. Approche socio-culturelle de pratiques*, Paris: Vigot, pp. 70–82.

Di Maggio, P. and H. Louch (1998) "Socially embedded consumer transactions", *American Sociological Review*, 63, pp. 619–37.

Dinnerstein, M. and R. Weitz (1998) "Jane Fonda, Barbara Bush and other aging bodies: femininity and the limits of resistance", in R. Weitz (ed.), *The Politics of Women's Bodies. Sexuality, Appearance and Behaviour*, Oxford: Oxford University Press, pp. 189–203.

Dishman, R. K. (1988) "Exercise adherence research: future directions", *American Journal of Health Promotion*, 3, pp. 52–6.

Dittmar, H. (2008) *Consumer Culture, Identity and Well-Being. The Search for the "Good Life" and the "Body Perfect"*, Hove: Psychology Press.

Douglas, M. (1966) *Purity and Danger. An Analysis of Concepts of Pollution and Taboo*, London: Routledge.

—— (1992) "Wants", in M. Douglas (ed.), *Risk and Blame: Essays in Cultural Theory*, London: Routledge, pp. 149–54.

Douglas, M. and B. Isherwood (1979) *The World of Goods. Towards an Anthropology of Consumption*, New York: Basic Books.

Du Gay, P., S. Hall, L. Janes, H. Mckay and K. Negus (1997) *Doing Cultural Studies. The Story of the Sony Walkman*, Milton Keynes: Open University Press.

Dworkin, S. L. (2003) "A woman's place is in the cardiovascular room? Gender relations, the body and the gym", in A. Bolin and J. Granskog (eds), *Athletic Intruders: Ethnographic Research on Women, Culture and Exercise*, Albany, NY: SUNY Press, pp. 131–58.

Eccles, S. (2002) "The lived experiences of additive consumers", *Journal of Research for Consumer Issues*, 4, pp. 1–17.

Elias, N. (1978/1982) *The Civilizing Process*, 2 vols, Oxford: Basil Blackwell (1st edn, 1936/1939).

Elias, N. and E. Dunning (1986) *The Quest for Excitement: Sport and Leisure in the Civilizing Process*, Oxford: Basil Blackwell.

Elster, J. (1979) *Ulysses and the Sirens. Studies in Rationality and Irrationality*, Cambridge: Cambridge University Press.

Eskes, T. B., M. C. Duncan and E. M. Miller (1998) "The discourse of empowerment. Foucault, Marcuse and women's fitness texts", *Journal of Sport Issues*, 22 (3), pp. 317–44.

Ewen, S. (1988) *All Consuming Images. The Politics of Style in Contemporary Culture*, New York: Basic Books.

Faure, S. (2000) *Apprendre par le corps. Socio-anthropologie de techniques de danse*, Paris: La Dispute.

Featherstone, M. (1982) "The body in consumer culture", *Theory, Culture and Society*, 1 (2), pp. 18–33.

—— (1991) *Consumer Culture and Postmodernism*, London: Sage.

Featherstone, M. and M. Hepworth (1982) "Ageing and inequality: consumer culture and the new middle age", in D. Robbins Caldwell, L., G. Day, K. Jones and H. Ras (eds), *Rethinking Social Inequality*, Aldershot: Gower, pp. 97–126.

Feher, M., R. Naddaff and N. Tazi (eds) (1989) *Fragments for a History of the Human Body*, 3 vols, New York: Zone.

Felstead, A., A. Fuller, N. Jewson, K. Kakavelakis and L. Unwin (2007) "Grooving to the same tune? Learning, training and productive systems in the aerobic studio", *Work, Employment and Society*, 21 (2), pp. 189–208.

Ferrara, P. (1992) *L'Italia in Palestra. Storia, documenti and immagini della ginnastica dal 1833 al 1973*, Rome: La Meridiana Editori.

Fine, G. A. (1983) *Shared Fantasy: Role Playing Games As Social Worlds*, Chicago, IL: University of Chicago Press.

—— (1998) *Morel Tales: The Culture of Mushrooming*, Cambridge, MA: Harvard University Press.

—— (2003) "Towards a peopled ethnography. Developing theory from group life", *Ethnography*, 4 (1), pp. 41–60.

Fishwick, L. (2001) "Be what you wanna be. A sense of identity down at the local gym", in N. Watson and S. Cunningham-Burley (eds), *Reframing the Body*, Basingstoke: Palgrave Macmillan, pp. 195–209.

Fonda, J. (1981) *Jane Fonda's Workout Book*, New York: Simon and Schuster.

Foster, R. J. (2008) *Coca-Globalization. Following Soft Drinks from New York to New Guinea*, Basingstoke: Palgrave Macmillan.

Foucault, M. (1978) *History of Sexuality. Vol. 1*, Harmondsworth: Penguin (original edn, 1976).

—— (1983) "The subject and power", in H. Dreyfus and P. Rabinow (eds), *Michel Foucault: Beyond Structuralism and Hermeneutics*, Chicago, IL: University of Chicago Press, pp. 208–26.

—— (1984a) *L'usage des plaisirs*, Paris: Gallimard.

—— (1984b) *Le souci de soi*, Paris: Gallimard.

—— (1984c) "What is enlightenment?", in P. Rabinow (ed.), *The Foucault Reader*, London: Penguin, pp. 32–50.

—— (1988) "On power", in L. D. Kritzman (ed.), *Michel Foucault. Politics, Philosophy, Culture*, London: Routledge, pp. 96–109.

—— (1991) *Discipline and Punish*, London: Penguin (1st edn, 1975).

—— (1993) "About the beginning of the hermeneutics of the self", *Political Theory*, 21 (2), pp. 198–227.

Frankel, R. M. (1984) "From sentence to 'sequence'. Understanding the medical encounter through microinteractional analysis", *Discourse Processes*, 7, pp. 135–70.

Frankfurt, H. G. (1988) *The Importance of What We Care About*, Cambridge: Cambridge University Press.

Freidson, E. (1985) *Professional Powers. A Study of the Institutionalization of Formal Knowledge*, Chicago, IL: University of Chicago Press.

Frew, M. and D. McGillivray (2005) "Health clubs and body politics. Aesthetics and the quest for physical capital", *Leisure Studies*, 24 (2), pp. 161–75.

Garcia Canclini, N. (2001) *Consumers and Citizens. Globalization and Multicultural Conflicts*, Minneapolis, MN: University of Minnesota Press.

Garcia, A. W. and A. C. King (1991) "Predicting long-term adherence to aerobic exercise: a comparison of two models", *Journal of Sport and Exercise Psychology*, 13, pp. 394–410.

Garfinkel, H. (1956) "Conditions of successful degradation ceremonies", *American Journal of Sociology*, LXI, pp. 420–4.

—— (1984) *Studies in Ethnomethodology*, Cambridge: Polity Press (1st edn, 1967).

Garrigou, A. (1987) "Le travail, la fête et l'athlétisme: les enjeux des styles de jeu", *Sport et changement social*, Bourdeaux: Maison des science de l'homme d'Aquitaine, pp. 81–99.

Geertz, C. (1973) *Interpretation of Cultures*, New York: Basic Books.

Giddens, A. (1984a) "Corpo, riflessività, riproduzione sociale: Erving Goffman e la teoria sociale", *Rassegna Italiana di Sociologia*, 25 (3), pp. 369–400.

—— (1984b) *The Constitution of Society. Outline of the Theory of Structuration*, Cambridge: Polity Press.

—— (1990) *The Consequences of Modernity*, Cambridge: Polity Press.

—— (1991) *Modernity and Self-Identity*, Cambridge: Polity Press.

Gillett, J. and P. White (1992) "Male bodybuilding and the reassertion of hegemonic masculinity", *Play and Culture*, 5, pp. 358–69.

Gillick, M. (1984) "Health promotion, jogging and the pursuit of the moral life", *Journal of Health Politics, Policy and the Law*, 9 (3), pp. 369–87.

Gilroy, S. (1989) "The embodiment of power. Gender and physical activity", *Leisure Studies*, 8, pp. 163–71.

Gimlin, D. (2002) *Bodywork. Beauty and Self-Image in American Culture*, Berkeley, CA: University of California Press.

Ginsberg, L. (2000) "The hard work of working out. Defining leisure, health and beauty in a Japanese fitness club", *Journal of Sport and Social Issues*, 24 (3), pp. 260–81.

Giulianotti, R. (2005) *Sport. A Critical Sociology*, Cambridge: Polity Press.

Glaser, B. G. and A. L. Strauss (1978) *The Discovery of Grounded Theory: Strategies of Qualitative Research*, London: Weidenfeld and Nicolson.

Glassner, B. (1990) "Fit for postmodern selfhood", in H. S. Becker and M.McCall (eds), *Symbolic Interaction and Cultural Studies*, Chicago, IL: University of Chicago Press.

—— (1992) *Bodies. Overcoming the Tyranny of Perfection*, Chicago, IL: Contemporary Books.

Godbey, G. (1985) "Non-use of public leisure services: a model", *Journal of Park and Recreation Administration*, 3 (2), pp. 1–12.

Godin, G. and R. J. Shephard (1990) "Use of attitude behaviour models in exercise promotion", *Sports Medicine*, 10 (2), pp. 103–21.

Goffman, E. (1959) *The Presentation of the Self in Everyday Life*, New York: Doubleday Anchor.

—— (1961) *Encounters: Two Studies in the Sociology of Interaction*, London: Penguin.

—— (1963a) *Behaviour in Public Places. Notes on the Social Organization of Gatherings*, New York: The Free Press.

—— (1963b) *Stigma. Notes on the Management of Spoiled Identities*, Englewood Cliffs, NJ: Prentice-Hall.

—— (1967) *Interaction Rituals. Essays on Face-to-Face Behavior*, New York: Pantheon Books.

—— (1971) *Relations in Public. Microstudies of the Public Order*, New York: Basic Books.

—— (1974) *Frame Analysis: An Essay on the Organization of Experience*, New York: Harper and Row.

—— (1979) *Gender Advertisements*, Cambridge, MA: Harvard University Press.

—— (1981) *Forms of Talk*, Oxford: Basil Blackwell.

—— (1982) "The interaction order", *American Sociological Review*, 47, pp. 1–17.

Goldstein, M. S. (1992) *The Health Movement. Promoting Fitness in America*, New York: Twayne Press.

Gonos, G. (1977) "Situation vs. frame: the interactionist and the structuralist analysis of everyday life", *American Sociological Review*, 42, pp. 854–67.

Goodman, N. (1983) *Fact, Fiction and Forecast*, Cambridge, MA: Harvard University Press.

Goodsell, A. (1995) *Obiettivo forma*, Milan: IdeaLibri.

Gori, G. (1996) *L'atleta e la nazione*, Rimini: Panozzo.

Gottdiener, M. (1997) *The Theming of America: Dreams, Visions and Commercial Spaces*, Boulder, CO: Westview Press.

Green, H. (1986) *Fit for America: Health, Fitness, Sport and American Society*, Baltimore, MD: Johns Hopkins University Press.

Griffiths, M. D. (1999) "Exercise addiction. A case study", *Addiction Research*, 5, pp. 161–8.

Grogan, S. (1999) *Body Image. Understanding Body Dissatisfaction in Men, Women and Children*, London: Routledge.

Grover, K. (ed.) (1989) *Fitness in American Culture. Images of the Health, Sport, and the Body 1830–1940*, Amherst, MA: University of Massachusetts Press.

Gruneau, R. (1983) *Class, Sport and Social Development*, Amherst, MA: University of Massachusetts Press.

Guerrier, Y. and A. Adib (2003) "Working at leisure and leisure at work: a study of emotional labour in tour reps", *Human Relations*, 56 (11), pp. 1399–417.

Guthrie, S. R. and S. Castelnuovo (1992) "Elite women bodybuilders: models of resistance or compliance?", *Play and Culture*, 5, pp. 401–8.

Guttmann, A. (1978) *From Ritual to Record: The Nature of Modern Sports*, New York: Columbia University Press.

Haley, B. (1979) *The Healthy Body and Victorian Culture*, Cambridge, MA: Harvard University Press.

Hallett, T. (2007) "Between deference and distinction: interaction ritual through symbolic power in an educational institution", *Social Psychology Quarterly*, 70 (2), pp. 148–71.

Halliwell, E., H. Dittmar and A. Osborn (2007) "The effects of exposure to muscular male models amongst men who use the gym and non-exercisers", *Body Image*, 4 (3), pp. 278–87.

Hammersley, M. and P. Atkinson (1983) *Ethnography*, London: Tavistock.

Haraway, D. (1991) *Simians, Cyborgs and Women*, London: Free Association.

Hargreves, J. (1986) *Sport, Power and Culture. A Social and Historical Analysis of Popular Sports in Britain*, London: Polity Press.

—— (1987) "The body, sport and power relations", in J. Horne, D. Jary and A. Tomlinson (eds), *Sport Leisure and Social Relations*, London: Routledge, pp. 139–59.

Heichberg, H. (1998) *Body Cultures. Essays on Sport, Space and Identity*, London: Routledge.

Heikkala, J. (1993) "Discipline and excel: techniques of the self and body and the logic of competing", *Sociology of Sport Journal*, 10, pp. 397–412.

Hirsch, P. (1972) "Processing fads and fashions: an organization-set analysis of cultural industry systems", *American Journal of Sociology*, 77, pp. 639–59.

Hirschman, A. O. (1979) *Exit, Voice and Loyalty*, Cambridge, MA: Harvard University Press.

Hochschild, A. R. (1983) *The Managed Heart: Commercialization of Human Feeling*, Berkeley, CA: University of California Press.

Horne, J., D. Jary and A. Tomlinson (eds) (1987) *Sport Leisure and Social Relations*, London: Routledge.

Hughes, E. C. (1963) "Professions", *Daedalus*, 92, pp. 655–68.

Huizinga, J. (1955) *Homo Ludens. A Study of the Play Element in Culture*, Boston, MA: Beacon Press.

IHRSA (2006) *European Market Report*, 2006, IHRSA.

Iso-Ahola, S. (1989) "Motivation for leisure", in E. L. Jackson and T. L. Burton (eds), *Understanding Leisure and Recreation*, State College, PA: Venture Publishing, pp. 113–34.

Jackson, G. (1992) *Forma fisica e benessere*, Milan: Vallardi.

Jakowski, E. J. (2001) *Escape Your Shape. How to Work Out Smarter, Not Harder*, New York: Fireside.

Kagan, E. and M. Morse (1988) "The body electronic: aerobic exercise video", *The Drama Review*, 32, pp. 164–80.

Kelly, J. (1983) *Leisure Identities and Interactions*, London: Allen and Unwin.

Kenen, R. L. (1987) "Double messages, double images: physical fitness, self-concepts and women's exercise classes", *Journal of Physical Education, Recreation and Dance*, 56 (6), pp. 76–9.

Kern, S. (1975) *Anatomy and Destiny: A Cultural History of the Human Body*, New York: Bobbs-Merrill.

Klein, A. M. (1993) *Little Big Men. Bodybuilding Subculture and Gender Construction*, New York: SUNY Press.

Laberge, S. and J. Kay (2002) "Pierre Bourdieu's Sociocutural theory and sport practice", in J. Maguire and K. Young (eds), *Theory, Sport and Society*, Oxford: Elsevier, pp. 239–66.

Lahire, B. (2004) *La culture des individus. Dissonances culturelles et distinction de soi*, Paris: La Découverte.

Lamont, M. and V. Molnàr (2002) "The study of boudaries in the social sciences", *Annual Review of Sociology*, 28, pp. 167–95.

Lasch, C. (1979) *The Culture of Narcissism*, New York: Norton.

Lash, S. and J. Urry (1987) *The End of Organized Capitalism*, Cambridge: Polity Press.

Lears, T. J. J. (1981) *No Place of Grace: Antimodernism and the Transformation of American Culture 1880–1920*, New York: Norton.

Lears, T. J. J. (1983) "From salvation to self-realization: advertising and the therapeutic roots of the consumer culture, 1880–1930", in R. W. Fox and T. J. Lears (eds), *The Culture of Consumption: Critical Essays in American History, 1880–1980*, New York: Pantheon Books, pp. 3–38.

Le Breton, D. (1990) *Anthropologie du corps et Modernité*, Paris: PUF.

Leeds Craig, M. and R. Liberti (2007) " 'Cause that's what girls do'. The making of a feminized gym", *Gender and Society*, 21 (5), pp. 676–99.

Lenskyi, H. (1994) "Sexuality and femininity in sport contexts: issues and alternatives", *Journal of Sport and Social Issues*, 18, pp. 356–76.

Le Unes, A. and J. A. Nation (1996) *Sport Psychology. An Introduction*, Chicago, IL: Nelson-Hall.

Lewis, J. (1991) *The Ideological Octopus*, London: Routledge.

Liuti, M. (1998) "Il mercato del fitness in Italia. Attualità and tendenze del settore fitness italiano", *Il Nuovo Club*, 43, pp. 35–42.

Lloyd, M. (1996) "Feminism, aerobics and the politics of the body", *Body and Society*, 2 (2), pp. 79–98.

Loland, N. W. (2000) "The art of concealment in a culture of display: aerobicizing women's and men's experience and use of their own bodies", *Sociology of Sport Journal*, 17, pp. 111–29.

Louveau, C. (1981) " 'La forme, pas les formes!' Simulacres et équivoques dans les pratiques physiques féminines", in C. Pociello (ed.), *Sports et société. Approche socio-culturelle des pratiques*, Paris: Vigot, pp. 113–28.

Lowe, M. (1998) *Women of Steel. Female Body Builders and the Struggle for Self-Definition*, New York: New York University Press.

Lupton, D. (1994) "Consumerism, commodity culture and health promotion", *Health Promotion International*, 9 (2), pp. 111–8.

MacNeill, M. (1998) "Sex, lies and videotapes: the political and cultural economy of celebrity fitness videos", in G. Rail (ed.), *Sport in Postmodern Times*, New York: SUNY Press, pp. 163–84.

MacNevin, A. (1999) "Every body has a dream: a social inquiry into the relationship between the pursuit of physical fitness and conceptions of the self", Unpublished PhD Dissertation, Memorial University of Newfoundland, Canada.

Maguire, J. and L. Mansfield (1998) " 'No-body's perfect'. Women, aerobics and the body beautiful", *Sociology of Sport Journal*, 15 (2), pp. 109–37.

Malaby, T. M. (2007) "Beyond play. A new approach to games", *Games and Culture*, 2 (2), pp. 95–113.

Mandell, R. D. (1984) *A Cultural History of Sport*, New York: Columbia University Press.

Mangan, J. A. (2000) *Superman Supreme. Fascist Body as a Political Icon*, London: Routledge.

Mangano, M. (1995) *Esercizi per cosce, glutei e fianchi*, Rome: Edizioni Mediterraneo.

Mannell, R. C. and J. Zuzanek (1991) "The nature and variability of leisure constraints in daily life: the case of the physically active leisure of older adults", *Leisure Sciences*, 13, pp. 337–51.

Mansfield, A. and B. McGinn (1993) "Pumping irony: the muscular and the feminine", in S. Scott and D. Morgan (eds), *Body Matters. Essays on the Sociology of the Body*, London: Falmer Press, pp. 49–68.

March, K. (2000) "Who do I look like? Gaining a sense of self-authenticity through the physical reflections of others", *Symbolic Interaction*, 23 (4), pp. 359–73.

Markland, D. and L. Hardy (1993) "The exercise motivations inventory. Preliminary development and validity of a measure of individuals' reasons for participation in regular physical exercise", *Personality and Individual Differences*, 15 (3), pp. 289–96.

Markula, P. (1995) "Firm but shapely, fit but sexy, strong but thin: the postmodern aerobicizing female bodies", *Sociology of Sport Journal*, 12 (4), pp. 424–53.

—— (2001) "Women's body image distortion in fitness magazine discourse", *Journal of Sport and Social Issues*, 25 (2), pp. 158–79.

Marshall, D. (2004) *Bodydoctor*, London: Harper-Collins.

Massey, D. (1994) *Space, Place and Gender*, Minneapolis, MN: University of Minnesota Press.

McCracken, G. (1988) *Culture and Consumption: New Approaches to the Symbolic Character of Consumer Goods and Activities*, Bloomington, IN: Indiana University Press.

McDermott, L. (2000) "A qualitative assessment of the significance of body perception to women's physical activity experiences", *Sociology of Sport Journal*, 17, pp. 331–63.

McIntosh, P. C. (1963) *Sport in Society*, London: Watts and Co.

Mehan, H. (1979) *Learning Lessons*, Cambridge, MA: Harvard University Press.

Metoudi, M. (1987a) "Sportivité et apparence", in *Sport et changement social*, Bourdeaux: Maison des science de l'homme d'Aquitaine, pp. 119–31.

—— (1987b) "De nouveaux usages pour les sports d'hier", *Esprit*, 4, pp. 42–52.

Millard, A.-M. (2005) *The Kitchen Gym. Get Lean While You Clean*, London: Hamlyn.

Miller, D. (1987) *Material Culture and Mass Consumption*, Oxford: Basil Blackwell.

Mills, M. (2006) *Mind & Body Metamorphosis*, Chichester: Summersdale Publishers.

Monaghan, L. F. (1999) "Creating 'the perfect body'", *Body and Society*, 2–3, pp. 267–90.

—— (2001) "Looking good, feeling good: the embodied pleasures of vibrant physicality", *Sociology of Health and Illness*, 23 (3), pp. 330–56.

Morse, M. (1987) "Artemis aging: exercise and the female body on video", *Discourse*, 10, pp. 19–53.

Nixon, S. and B. Crewe (2004) "Pleasure at work? Gender, consumption and work-based identities in the creative industries", *Consumption, Markets and Culture*, 7 (2), pp. 129–47.

Oja, P. and B. Tuxworth (1995) *Eurofit for Adults. Assessment of Health-Realted Fitness*, Tampere: Council of Europe.

O'Neill, J. (1985) *Five Bodies: The Human Shape of Modern Society*, Ithaca, NY: Cornell University Press.

O'Toole, J. (2009) "McDonald's at the gym? A tale of two curves@", *Qualitative Sociology*, 32 (1), pp. 75–91.

Park. R. J. (1994) "A decade of the body: researching and writing about the history of health, fitness, exercise and sport, 1983–1993", *Journal of Sport History*, 21 (1), pp. 59–82.

Park, S. H. (1996) "Relationship between involvement and attitudinal loyalty constructs in adult fitness programs", *Journal of Leisure Research*, 28 (4), pp. 233–50.

Perinbanayagam, R. (2006) *Games and Sport in Everyday Life. Dialogues and Narratives of the Self*, Boulder, CO: Paradigm.

Perrin, E. (1985) *Les cultes du corps. Enquête sur les nouvelles pratiques corporelles*, Lausanne: Favre.

Perrot, Ph. (1987) "Pour un généalogie de l'austerité des apparences", *Communication*, 46, pp. 157–80.

Peterson, R. (1992) "Understanding audience segmentation: from elite and mass to omnivore and univore", *Poetics*, 21, pp. 243–58.

Peterson, R. and R. Kern (1996) "Changing highbrow taste: from snob to omnivore", *American Sociological Review*, 61, pp. 900–7.

Phillips, J. and M. Drummond (2001) "An investigation into body image perception, body satisfaction and exercise expectation of male fitness leaders: implication for professional practice", *Leisure Studies*, 20 (1), pp. 95–105.

Pinckney, C. (1992) *Callanetics*, London: Vermilion Press.

Pine, B. J. and J. H. Gilmore (1998) "Welcome to the experience economy", *Harvard Business Review*, 73 (2), pp. 103–13.

Pociello, C. (ed.) (1981) *Sports et société. Approche socio-culturelle des pratiques*, Paris: Vigot.

Podilchak, W. (1991) "Establishing the fun in leisure", *Leisure Sciences*, 13, pp. 123–36.

Price, J. (2003) *The Anytime, Anywhere Exercise Book*, Avon, MA: Adams Media Corporation.

Pronger, B. (2002) *Body Fascism. Salvation in the Technology of Physical Fitness*, Toronto: University of Toronto Press.

Punzo, M. (1992) *La ginnastica energetica*, Milan: De Vecchi.

Quintelier, E. (2008) "Who is politically active: the athlete, the scout member or the environmental activist?", *Acta Sociologica*, 51 (4), pp. 355–70.

Rabinbach, A. (1990) *The Human Motor. Energy, Fatigue, and the Origins of Modernity*, New York: Basic Books.

Rabinow, P. and H. P. Dreyfus (1983) *Michel Foucault: Beyond Structuralism and Hermeneutics*, Chicago, IL: University of Chicago Press.

Rader, B. J. (1991) "The quest for self-sufficiency and the new strenousity", *Journal of Sport History*, 18 (2), pp. 255–66.

Reese, S. D. (2007) "The framing project. A bridging model for media research revisited", *Journal of Communication*, 57 (1), pp. 148–54.

Reid, I. S. and J. L. Crompton (1993) "A taxonomy of leisure purchase decision paradigms based on level of involvement", *Journal of Leisure Research*, 25 (2), pp. 182–202.

Ricci, G. (2005) *Innova Marketing, Il nuovo approccio al marketing per le aziende di fitness e wellness*, Bologna: Il Campo.

Ritzer, G. (1993) *The McDonaldization of Society*, Newbury Park, CA: Pine Forge Press.

Rizzi, A. (1992) *Corso pratico di stretching per tutti*, Milan: Mariotti.

Robinson, J. I. and M. A. Rogers (1994) "Adherence to exercise programs", *Sport Medicine*, 17, pp. 39–52.

Rojek, C. (1985) *Capitalism and Leisure Theory*, London: Routledge.

—— (2000) *Leisure and Culture*, Basingstoke: Palgrave Macmillan.

Rorty, R. (1980) *Philosophy and the Mirror of Nature*, Oxford: Basil Blackwell.

Roskies, E.; P. Seraganian; R. Oseasohn; J.A. Hanley; R. Collu; N. Martin; and C. Smilga (1986) "The Montreal Type A Intervention Project", *Health Psychology*, 5, pp. 45–69.

Ruffier, J. E. (1991) *La ginnastica per la nostra salute*, Aosta: Musumeci.

Samdahl, D. M. (1988) "A symbolic interactionist model of leisure. Theory and empirical support", *Leisure Sciences*, 10, pp. 27–39.

Sappey, J. and G. J. Maconachie (2009) "The new world of work and employment: fitness workers and what they want from the employment relationship", *in Proceedings of the 15th World Congress of the International Industrial Relations Association*, Sydney, Australia, available at http://www.iceaustralia.com/IIRA2009/, accessed October 2009.

Sassatelli, R. (1999a) "Interaction order and beyond. A field analysis of body culture within fitness gyms", *Body and Society*, 5 (2–3), pp. 227–48.

—— (1999b) "Fitness gyms and the local organization of experience", *Sociological Research Online*, 4 (3), http://www.socresonline.org.uk/.

—— (2000a) "Tamed hedonism: choice, desires and deviant pleasures", in A. Warde and J. Gronow (eds), *Ordinary Consumption*, London: Harwood, pp. 93–106.

—— (2000b) "The commercialization of discipline. Fitness and its values", *Journal of Italian Studies, Special Issue on Sport*, 9 (4), pp. 332–49.

—— (2000c) *Anatomia della Palestra*, Bologna: Il mulino.

—— (2001) "Trust, choice and routine: putting the consumer on trial", *Critical Review of International Social and Political Philosophy*, 4 (4), pp. 84–105.

—— (2003) "Bridging health and beauty. A critical perspective on keep-fit culture", in G. Boswell and F. Poland (eds), *Women's Bodies*, London: Macmillan, pp. 77–88.

—— (2007) *Consumer Culture. History, Theory and Politics*, London: Sage.

—— (2009) "Promotional reflexivity. Irony, de-fetishization and moralization in the body shop promotional rhetoric", in G. Benvenuti (ed.), *Cultural Studies*, Bologna: Odoya, pp. 65–89.

—— (2010) "Indigo bodies. Fashion, mirror work and sexual identity in Milan", in D. Miller and S. Woodward (eds), *Global Denim*, Oxford: Berg, pp. 101–22.

Sassatelli, R., M. Santoro and G. Semi (2008) "Quello che i consumi rivelano. Spazi, pratiche and confini del ceto medio", in A. Bagnasco (ed.), *Ceto medio. Perché e come occuparsene*, Bologna: Il Mulino, pp. 165–210.

Savage, M. (2000) *Class Analysis and Social Transformation*, Milton Keynes: Open University Press.

Sheper-Hughes, N. and L. Wacquant (eds) (2001) "Commodifying bodies", special issue *Body and Society*, 7, pp. 2–3.

Searle, M. S., J. B. Mactavish and R. E. Brayley (1993) "Integrating ceasing participation with other aspects of leisure behavior: a replication and extension", *Journal of Leisure Research*, 25 (4), pp. 389–404.

Segal, L. (2007) *Slow Motion. Changing Masculinities, Changing Men*, 3rd edn, Basingstoke: Palagrave Macmillan.

Seidman, I. (2005) *Interviewing as Qualitative Research*, 3rd edn, New York: Teachers College Press.

Selby, J. (1994) *Come eliminare la pancia senza fatica*, Milan: Tea Pratica.

Sennett, R. (1998) *The Corrosion of Character*, New York: Norton.

Shepard, R. J. (1995) "Physical activity, fitness and health. The current consensus", *Quest*, 47, pp. 3: 288–303.

Shilling, C. (1993) *The Body and Social Theory*, London: Sage.

Shove, E. and M. Pantzar (2005) "Consumers, producers and practices: understanding the invention and reinvention of Nordic walking", *Journal of Consumer Culture*, 5, pp. 43–64.

Silverman, D. (1993) *Interpreting Qualitative Data. Methods for Analysing Talk, Text and Interaction*, London: Sage.

Simmel, G. (1917) *Grundfragen der Soziologie. Individuum und Gesellschaft*, Berlin: Goschen.

—— (1950) *The Sociology of Georg Simmel*, New York: Free Press (1st edn, 1908).

—— (1971) "The metropolis and mental life", in G. Simmel (ed.), *On Individuality and Social Forms*, Chicago, IL: Chicago University Press, pp. 324–39 (1st edn, 1903).

—— (1990) *Philosophy of Money*, 2nd edn, London: Routledge (2nd edn, 1907).

Slater, D. (2009) "The ethics of routine. Consciousness, tedium and value," in E. Shove, F. Trentmann and R. Wilk. (eds), *Time, Consumpiton and Everyday Life*, Oxford: Berg, pp. 217–30.

Smith Maguire, J. (2002) "Body lessons. Fitness publishing and the cultural production of the fitness consumer", *International Review for the Sociology of Sport*, 37, pp. 449–64.

—— (2007) *Fit For Consumption. Sociology and the Business of Fitness*, London: Routledge.

Snow, D. A., E. B. Rochford, S. K. Worden and R. D. Benford (1986) "Frame alignment processes, micromobilization, and movement participation", *American Sociological Review*, 51 (4), pp. 464–81.

Sointu, E. (2005) "The rise of an ideal. Tracing changing discourses of wellbeing", *Sociological Review*, 52 (2), pp. 255–74.

Solomon, H. A. (1984) *The Exercise Myth*, New York: Harcourt.

Spielvogel, L. (2003) *Working Out in Japan. Shaping the Female Body in Tokyo Fitness Clubs*, Durham, NC: Duke University Press.

Spitzack, C. (1990) *Confessing Excess: Women and the Politics of Body Reduction*, Albany, NY: University of New York Press.

St Martin, L. and N. Gavey (1996) "Women's bodybuilding: feminist resistance and/or femininity's recuperation", *Body and Society*, 2 (4), pp. 45–58.

Stebbins, R. A. (2009) "Serious leisure and work", *Sociology Compass*, 3, July, pp. 764–74.

Steen-Johnsen, K. (2004) "Individualised communities. Keep-fit exercise organisations and the creation of social bonds", PhD Dissertation, Norwegian University of Sport and Physical Education.

Strauss, A. (2002) "Adapt, adjust, accommodate: The production of yoga in a transnational world", *History and Anthropology*, 13 (3), pp. 231–51.

Stockdale, J. E. (1989) "Concepts and measures in leisure participation and preference", in E. L. Jackson and T. L. Burton (eds), *Understanding Leisure and Recreation*, State College, PA: Venture Publishing, pp. 421–49.

Sutton-Smith, B. and D. Kelly-Byrne (1984) "The idealization of play", in P. K. Smith (ed.), *Play in Animals and Humans*, Oxford: Basil Blackwell, pp. 305–21.

Swartz, D. (1997) *Culture and Power. The Sociology of Pierre Bourdieu*, Chicago, IL: University of Chicago Press.

Tannen, D. (ed.) (1993) *Framing in Discourse*, Oxford: Oxford University Press.

Theberge, N. (1991) "Reflections on the body in the sociology of sport", *Quest*, 43, pp. 123–34.

Thirion, J. F. (1987) "Les nouvelles pratiques et la notion de développement personnel", in *Sport et changement social*, Bourdeaux: Maison des science de l'homme d'Aquitaine, pp. 131–49.

Time Out London (2006) *Health and Fitness 2006*, London: Universal House.

—— (2007) *Health and Fintess 2007*, London: Universal House.

Trentmann, F. (ed.) (2006) *The Making of the Consumer: Knowledge, Power and Identity in the Modern World*, Oxford: Berg.

Turner, B. S. (1984) *The Body and Society*, Oxford: Blackwell.

—— (1987) "The rationalization of the body: reflections on modernity and discipline", in S. Whimster and S. Lash (eds), *Max Weber*, London: Allen and Unwin, pp. 222–41.

Turner, R. H. (1968) "The self-conception in social interaction", in C. Gordon and K. J. Gergen (eds), *The Self in Social Interaction*, New York: Wiley, pp. 93–106.

Turner, V. (1967) *The Forest of Symbols: Aspects of Ndembu Ritual*, Ithaca, NY: Cornell University Press.

—— (1969) *The Ritual Process: Structure and Anti-Structure*, London: Routledge.

—— (1977) "Variations on the theme of liminality", in S. Moore and B. Meyerhoff (eds), *Secular Rituals*, Assen: Van Gorcum, pp. 43–65.

—— (1982) *From Ritual to Theatre. The Human Seriousness of Play*, New York: Performing Arts Journal Publications.

Ulmann, J. (1971) *De la gynastique aux sports modernes. Histoire des doctrine de l'éducation physique*, Paris: Librairie Philosophique.

Unger, J. B. and C. A. Johnson (1995) "Social relationships and physical activity in health club members", *American Journal of Health Promotion*, 9 (5), pp. 340–51.

Urry, J. (1995) *Consuming Places*, London: Routledge.

Vanden Auweele, Y., R. Rzewnick and V. Van Mele (1997) "Reasons for not exercising and exercise intentions", *Journal of Sports Sciences*, 15 (2), pp. 151–65.

Verhoeven, J. C. (1985) "Goffman's frame analysis and modern micro-sociological paradigms", in S. N. Eisenstadt and J. Helle (eds), *Micro-Sociological Theory*, London: Sage, pp. 71–100.

Vigarello, G. (1978) *Le corps redressé: Histoire d'un pouvoir pédagogique*, Paris: Delarge.

—— (1988) *Un histoire culturelle du sport: techniques d'hier et d'aujourd'hui*, Paris: Revue EPS.

—— (1992) "Mécanique, corps, incorporel", in L. Giard (ed.), *Michel Foucault: lire l'oeuvre*, Paris: Jerome Millon, pp. 193–200.

Vigarello, G. and O. Mongin (eds) (1987) *Le nouvel age du sport*, special issue of *"Esprit"*, 4 April.

Volkvein, K. (ed.) (1998) *Fitness as a Cultural Phenomenon*, New York: Waxmann Münster.

Vugt, M. V., C. Howard and S. Moss (1998) "Being better than some, but not better than average", *British Journal of Social Psychology*, 37 (2), pp. 185–201.

Wacquant, L. (1995) "Why men desire muscles", *Body and Society*, 1 (1), pp. 163–81.

—— (2003) *Body and Soul*, Chicago, IL: Chicago University Press.

—— (2005) "Carnal connections: on embodiment, apprenticeship and membership", *Qualitative Sociology*, 28 (4), pp. 445–74.

Wagemaker, H. and L. Goldstein (1980) "The runner's high", *Journal of Sports, Medicine and Physical Fitness*, 20, pp. 227–9.

Ward, J. (2004) " 'Not all differences are created equal': multiple jeopardy in a gendered organization", *Gender and Society*, 18, pp. 82–102.

Warde, A. (2006) "Cultural capital and the place of sport", *Cultural Trends*, 15 (2–3), pp. 107–22.

Warner, R. and M. Griffiths (2005) "A qualitative thematic analysis of exercise addiction. An exploratory study", *International Journal of Mental Health Addiction*, 4, pp. 13–26.

Weber, M. (1930) *The Protestant Ethic and the Spirit of Capitalism*, London: Allen and Unwin (1st edn, 1905).

—— (1968) *Economy and Society*, edited by Guenther Roth and Claus Wittich, New York: Bedminister Press, vol. 1 (1st edn 1922).

Weitz, R. (ed.) (1998) *The Politics of Women's Bodies. Sexuality, Appearance and Behaviour*, Oxford: Oxford University Press.

Wernick, A. (1991) *Promotional Culture. Advertising, Ideology and Symbolic Expression*, London: Sage.

White, P., K. Young and J. Gillett (1995) "Bodywork as a moral imperative. Some critical notes on health and fitness", *Loisir et Société*, 18 (1), pp. 159–81.

Whorton, J. C. (1982) *Crusaders for Fitness. The History of American Health Reformers*, Princeton, NJ: Princeton University Press.

Wilk, R. (2004) "Morals and metaphors. The meaning of consumption", in K. M. Ekström and H. Brembeck (eds), *Elusive Consumption*, Oxford: Berg, pp. 11–26.

Willis, P. (1979) *Profane Culture*, London: Routledge.

Wright Mills, C. (1940) "Situated actions and vocabularies of motives", *American Sociological Review*, 5, pp. 904–13.

Wynne, D. (1998) *Leisure, Lifestyle and the New Middle Class: A Case Study*, London: Routledge.

Yates, A. (1991) *Compulsive Exercise and Eating Disorders. Toward an Integrated Theory of Activity*, New York: Brunner/Mazel.

Yeung, R. R. and D. R. Hemsley (1997) "Exercise behaviour in an aerobic class", *Personality and Individual Differences*, 23 (3), pp. 425–31.

Young, I. R. (1990) *Throwing Like a Girl and Other Essays in Feminist Philosophy and Social Theory*, Bloomington, IN: United Press.

Zelizer, V. (2004) *The Purchase of Intimacy*, Princeton, NJ: Princeton University Press.

Index